HIV and Liver Disease

Kenneth E. Sherman
Editor

HIV and Liver Disease

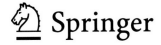
Springer

Editor
Kenneth E. Sherman, MD, PhD
Gould Professor Medicine
Director, Division of Digestive Diseases
University of Cincinnati College of Medicine
Cincinnati, OH, USA
Kenneth.sherman@uc.edu

ISBN 978-1-4419-1711-9   e-ISBN 978-1-4419-1712-6
DOI 10.1007/978-1-4419-1712-6
Springer New York Dordrecht Heidelberg London

Library of Congress Control Number: 2011936393

© Springer Science+Business Media, LLC 2012
All rights reserved. This work may not be translated or copied in whole or in part without the written permission of the publisher (Springer Science+Business Media, LLC, 233 Spring Street, New York, NY 10013, USA), except for brief excerpts in connection with reviews or scholarly analysis. Use in connection with any form of information storage and retrieval, electronic adaptation, computer software, or by similar or dissimilar methodology now known or hereafter developed is forbidden.
The use in this publication of trade names, trademarks, service marks, and similar terms, even if they are not identified as such, is not to be taken as an expression of opinion as to whether or not they are subject to proprietary rights.
While the advice and information in this book are believed to be true and accurate at the date of going to press, neither the authors nor the editors nor the publisher can accept any legal responsibility for any errors or omissions that may be made. The publisher makes no warranty, express or implied, with respect to the material contained herein.

Printed on acid-free paper

Springer is part of Springer Science+Business Media (www.springer.com)

Preface

The 1980s saw the emergence of HIV as a devastating disease whose social, political, and scientific ramifications have globally impacted humankind. During the late 1980s and early 1990s, the role and significance of liver disease in the setting of HIV merited little more than a footnote as huge numbers of people died of AIDS-related complications. My own nascent research in the area of hepatitis virus infections in the liver was discouraged by some senior mentors, who considered research effort to study liver disease in patients who faced certain death from AIDS to be both useless and futile. Despite these admonitions, a small cadre of physician-scientists in the USA and Europe were drawn to the scientific window afforded by this experiment of nature that permitted study of liver disease in the setting of a rapidly declining immunologic milieu. The urgency of our investigations was driven by the tragic plight of the patients afflicted with this terrible disease. During this same time period, the hepatitis C virus was "unlocked" and characterized using newly developed molecular tools, which opened the door to study this virus in the setting of HIV infection. New methods also permitted a fresh look at hepatitis B, which had been described early in the AIDS epidemic as a nonissue. By 1991, the era of treating HCV and HBV with nonspecific antiviral agents such as interferon alfa had begun, and most investigators focused on one viral disease and not the mix of two or even three in one individual.

The early 1990s witnessed the emergence of targeted treatments for HIV culminating in the development of multidrug "cocktails" that provided effective suppression of HIV replication. This suppression was accompanied by reemergence of T-helper cells resulting in immune reconstitution among those whose declining CD4 levels had led to development of overt AIDS complications. This miracle of medicine changed the lives of hundreds of thousands of people whose prior death sentence was converted to life with a chronic disease. Suddenly, people with HIV infection had a future, but by the late 1990s it became apparent that their future was somewhat clouded by the recognition that other comorbid conditions could affect survival. As rates of *Mycobacterium avium*, cryptococcal meningitis, and Kaposi's sarcoma declined, liver disease, coronary artery disease, and other metabolic disorders emerged and took on greater importance. Multiple epidemiologic studies suggested that liver disease was the leading or second most important cause of morbidity and mortality among those with HIV in countries and cohorts where antiretroviral therapy was available. The etiologies were multifactorial; hepatitis C and hepatitis B are now considered the most important etiologic entities, but direct hepatotoxicity from antiretroviral drugs is an important cofactor, as is alcohol-associated liver injury.

The genesis of a book on HIV and Liver Disease is derived from a series of NIH-supported conferences which were designed to bring together a cross-disciplinary mix of experts to address issues of liver disease in this population of patients. The experts, which included hepatologists, infectious disease physicians, epidemiologists, toxicologists, government regulatory experts, and drug-developers from industry and academia discussed, debated, and synthesized the information and defined the course of future research efforts. Meetings were held in 2006,

2008 and 2010. Many of those experts contributed to this book, which attempts to comprehensively describe the state of the field, identify the gaps in knowledge and provide insights into how these deficiencies might be addressed.

The book begins by defining the current state of the HIV epidemic and the importance of liver disease in 2011. It summarizes the treatment and management of HIV and then focuses on the assessment of liver injury, including a detailed description of liver pathologies in those with HIV. Next is a series of chapters that examine mechanisms of liver injury focusing on those with the greatest impact in the HIV-infected patient. The role of hepatotrophic viruses and the host genetics are discussed. The material includes interesting new information regarding HIV's direct effects on the liver. There is an excellent chapter that summarizes recommendations regarding practical management and prevention of hepatitis viral infections in those with HIV and a chapter that focuses on the recognition and management of the patient with advanced liver disease. Treatment is also given to drug hepatotoxicity. The last chapters of the book move to social, psychological, and behavioral issues including management of drug and alcohol abuse, an examination of racial disparities in HIV and liver disease and a discussion of quality-of-life issues that impact our patient's well-being, even when the effects are difficult to measure.

"HIV and Liver Disease" is designed to be a useful reference for all health-care providers who manage patients with HIV. For those less familiar with issues related to liver disease, it will serve as a guide to evaluation and management. For the cognoscenti, those physician-scientists who have contributed to this field, the text will provide an up-to-date source for describing where we are, and in what direction the field is moving. For the student, it will hopefully provide a roadmap to discover the excitement of this rapidly evolving field.

Cincinnati, OH   Kenneth E. Sherman

Acknowledgments

First and foremost, I would like to thank the many patients with HIV and liver disease whose stories have inspired my focus and interest in this field. When I first proposed this book, I received an enthusiastic response from Springer, and I am grateful for the support and efforts of Elektra McDermott who served as my primary contact with the publisher throughout the long process of synthesizing the publication plan and bringing together all the chapters from our distinguished authors. The contributing authors are spectacular…all experts in their areas of assignment and committed to bringing forth a book that would be both understandable and useful for a wide audience of potential readers. Finally, I would like to thank my wife, and sometimes research collaborator, Susan Nacht Sherman, who has been a source of continuous and unwavering support in my career as an academic physician-scientist.

Contents

1. The HIV Epidemic in the USA: Current Trends, 2010 1
   John T. Brooks and Mi Chen

2. Epidemiology of Liver Disease in Human Immunodeficiency
   Virus-Infected Persons 9
   Adeel A. Butt

3. Current and Future Treatment Guidelines for HIV 15
   Judith Feinberg

4. Pathology of HIV-Associated Liver Disease 23
   Amy E. Noffsinger and Jiang Wang

5. Noninvasive Markers of Liver Injury and Fibrosis 33
   Jenny O. Smith and Richard K. Sterling

6. Mechanisms of Alcoholic Steatosis/Steatohepatitis 45
   Zhanxiang Zhou, Ross E. Jones, and Craig J. McClain

7. Immunopathogenesis of Liver Injury 55
   Mohamed Tarek M. Shata

8. Host Gene Polymorphisms and Disease/Treatment Outcomes
   in HIV and Viral Coinfections 67
   Jacob K. Nattermann and Jürgen K. Rockstroh

9. Effects of HIV on Liver Cell Populations 81
   Meena B. Bansal and Jason T. Blackard

10. HIV Replication 91
    Vladimir A. Novitsky and Max Essex

11. Hepatitis C: Natural History 101
    Mark S. Sulkowski

12. Natural History of Hepatitis B Virus in HIV-Infected Patients 107
    Chloe L. Thio

13. Other Hepatitis Viruses and HIV Infection 113
    José V. Fernández-Montero and Vincent Soriano

14. Hepatitis B Virus: Replication, Mutation, and Evolution 125
    Amy C. Sherman and Shyam Kottilil

15. Hepatitis C Virus Treatment in HIV 133
    Raymond Chung and Gyanprakash Avinash Ketwaroo

16	**Treatment of Hepatitis B in HIV-Infected Persons**	141
	Ellen Kitchell and Mamta K. Jain	
17	**Prevention of Hepatitis Infection in HIV-Infected Patients**	151
	Edgar Turner Overton and Judith A. Aberg	
18	**Antiretroviral Therapy and Hepatotoxicity**	163
	Norah J. Shire	
19	**Management of End-Stage Liver Disease and the Role of Liver Transplantation in HIV-Infected Patients**	171
	Marion G. Peters and Peter G. Stock	
20	**Assessment and Treatment of Alcohol- and Substance-Use Disorders in Patients with HIV Infection**	181
	Ashley D. Bone and Andrew F. Angelino	
21	**Racial Disparities in HIV and Liver Disease**	189
	Nyingi M. Kemmer	
22	**Quality of Life in Patients with HIV Infection and Liver Disease**	195
	Cindy L. Bryce and Joel Tsevat	

Index 205

Contributors

Judith A. Aberg, MD Department of Medicine, Bellevue Hospital Center, New York University School of Medicine, New York, NY, USA

Andrew F. Angelino, MD Department of Psychiatry and Behavioral Sciences, Johns Hopkins University School of Medicine, Baltimore, MD, USA

Meena B. Bansal, MD Department of Medicine, Mount Sinai School of Medicine, New York, NY, USA

Jason T. Blackard, PhD Division of Digestive Diseases, University of Cincinnati College of Medicine, Cincinnati, OH, USA

Ashley D. Bone, MD Department of Psychiatry and Behavioral Sciences, Johns Hopkins University School of Medicine, Baltimore, MD, USA

John T. Brooks, MD Division of HIV/AIDS Prevention, US Centers for Disease Control and Prevention, Atlanta, GA, USA

Cindy L. Bryce, PhD School of Medicine, University of Pittsburgh, Pittsburgh, PA, USA

Adeel A. Butt, MD, MS School of Medicine/Division of Infectious Diseases, University of Pittsburgh, Pittsburgh, PA, USA

Mi Chen, MS Division of HIV/AIDS Prevention, National Center for HIV/AIDS, Viral Hepatitis, and TB Prevention, Centers for Disease Control and Prevention, Atlanta, GA, USA

Raymond Chung, MD Department of Gastroenterology, Massachusetts General Hospital, Boston, MA, USA

Max Essex, DVM, PhD Department of Immunology and Infectious Diseases, Harvard School of Public Health, Boston, MA, USA

Judith Feinberg, MD Department of Medicine/Division of Infectious Diseases, University of Cincinnati College of Medicine, Cincinnati, OH, USA

José V. Fernández-Montero, MD Department of Infectious Diseases, Carlos III Hospital, Madrid, Spain

Mamta K. Jain, MD, MPH Department of Internal Medicine, UT Southwestern Medical Center, Dallas, TX, USA

Ross E. Jones, MD Department of Medicine, University of Louisville, Louisville, KY, USA

Nyingi M. Kemmer, MD, MPH Division of Digestive Diseases, Department of Internal Medicine, University of Cincinnati, Cincinnati, OH, USA

Gynaprakash Avinash Ketarwoo, MD, MSc Department of Gastroenterology, Beth Israel Deaconess Medical Center, Boston, MA, USA

Ellen Kitchell, MD Department of Internal Medicine, University of Texas, Southwestern Medical Center, Dallas, TX, USA

Shyam Kottilil, MD, PhD Department of Laboratory Immunoregulation, National Institute of Allergy and Infectious Diseases, Bethesda, MD, USA

Craig J. McClain, MD Department of Medicine, University of Louisville, Louisville, KY, USA

Jacob K. Nattermann, MD Department of Internal Medicine I, University of Bonn, Bonn, Germany

Amy E. Noffsinger, MD Caris Life Center, Camp Dennison, OH, USA

Vladimir A. Novitsky, MD, PhD Department of Immunology and Infectious Diseases, Harvard School of Public Health, Boston, MA, USA

Edgar Turner Overton, MD Department of Internal Medicine/Infectious Diseases Division, Washington University School of Medicine, St. Louis, MO, USA

Marion G. Peters, MD, BS Department of Medicine, University of California, San Francisco, CA, USA

Jürgen K. Rockstroh, MD Department of Internal Medicine I, University of Bonn, Bonn, Germany

Mohamed Tarek M. Shata, MD, MSc, PhD Department Viral Immunology Lab/Division of Digestive Diseases, University of Cincinnati, Cincinnati, OH, USA

Amy C. Sherman, BA Department of Laboratory Immunoregulation, National Institute of Allergy and Infectious Diseases, Bethesda, MD, USA

Kenneth E. Sherman, MD, PhD Division of Digestive Diseases, University of Cincinnati College of Medicine, Cincinnati, OH, USA

Norah J. Shire, PhD, MPH Experimental Medicine, Infections Diseases, Merck, Sharp, and Dohme Corp., North Wales, PA, USA

Jenny O. Smith, MD Department of Gastroenterology, Hepatology, and Nutrition, Virginia Commonwealth University Medical Center/Medical College of Virginia, Richmond, VA, USA

Vincent Soriano, MD, PhD Department of Infectious Diseases, Carlos III Hospital, Madrid, Spain

Richard K. Sterling, MD, MSc Virginia Commonwealth University Medical Center/Medical College of Virginia, Richmond, VA, USA

Peter G. Stock, MD, PhD Department of Surgery, University of California - San Francisco, San Francisco, CA, USA

Mark S. Sulkowski, MD Division of Infectious Diseases and Gastroenterology/Hepatology Department of Medicine, Johns Hopkins University School of Medicine, Baltimore, MD, USA

Chloe L. Thio, MD Department of Medicine, Johns Hopkins University School of Medicine, Baltimore, MD, USA

Joel Tsevat, MD, MPH University of Cincinnati and Cincinnati VA Medical Center, Cincinnati, OH, USA

Jiang Wang, MD, PhD Pathology and Laboratory Medicine, University of Cincinnati College of Medicine, Cincinnati, OH, USA

Zhanxiang Zhou, PhD Department of Nutrition, University of North Carolina Greensboro, Kannapolis, NC, USA

The HIV Epidemic in the USA: Current Trends, 2010

John T. Brooks and Mi Chen

Disclaimers

The findings and conclusions in this report are those of the authors and do not necessarily represent the official position of the Centers for Disease Control and Prevention.

Background

The Centers for Disease Control (CDC) estimates that 1.1 million persons in the USA are living with HIV infection [1], of whom 21% are unaware of that they are HIV infected [2]. The incidence of new infections in 2006 was approximately 56,000 [3] and had remained unchanged between 50,000 and 60,000 annual new infections during the preceding decade. As a result, the estimated annual rate of HIV transmission, calculated as the number of new infections each year (numerator, a value that has remained steady at about 55,000) resulting from the population of persons with prevalent infection (denominator, a value that has increased each year by about 55,000) has been declining slowly from 6.8 to 5.0 transmissions per 100 persons living with HIV between 1999 and 2006 [4].

Prevalence Rates and Trends

Data on prevalent HIV diagnoses has been collected by CDC from 37 states with mature confidential name-based HIV infection reporting systems that report diagnosis of both chronic asymptomatic HIV infections and of AIDS; this subset of states does not include some jurisdictions with concentrated urban HIV epidemics [1]. The estimated prevalence rate of diagnoses of HIV infection in 2007 was 275.4 per 100,000 population and has increased steadily from 2005 (259.0) to 2006 (267.1). Of the estimated 580,371 persons who by the end of 2007 were living with HIV infection in these 37 states, the largest percentages were aged 40–44 years (20%) and 45–49 years (19%). The highest HIV prevalence rates continued to be observed among men and members of racial and ethnic minority groups [1–3]: 492.8 per 100,000 among men, and 967.5 among blacks, 133.3 among whites, and 364.0 among Hispanics. Among the 417,797 men, 64% had been exposed through male-to-male sexual contact, 16% through injection drug use (IDU), 7% through both male-to-male sexual contact and IDU, and 12% through heterosexual contact; among 153,814 women, 73% had been exposed through heterosexual contact and 26% had been exposed through IDU. During 2005–2007, the estimated number of persons living with a diagnosis of HIV infection increased by 13 and 11% among MSM persons exposed through heterosexual contact, respectively, but remained essentially stable among persons exposed through IDU.

Differences by Race and Gender

As indicated earlier, blacks, both males and females, experienced the highest prevalence rates of HIV infection compared with other racial/ethnic groups [1]. In 2007, the prevalence rate of HIV infection (per 100,000 persons) was 2.7 times the corresponding rate for Hispanics, and 7.3 times the corresponding rate for whites. Among other subgroups, the corresponding rates were 126.7 for American Indians/Alaska Natives, 55.4 for Asians, 173.6 for Native Hawaiians/Other Pacific Islanders, and 187.2 for persons of multiple races.

Among persons of color, women are at considerably higher risk of HIV infection compared with white women than are men of color compared with white men. Figure 1.1 depicts rates of new diagnoses of HIV infections in 2008. Whereas the rates of new diagnosis of HIV among black men

J.T. Brooks (✉)
Division of HIV/AIDS Prevention,
US Centers for Disease Control and Prevention,
1600 Clifton Rd NW, Atlanta, GA 30333, USA
e-mail: zud4@cdc.gov

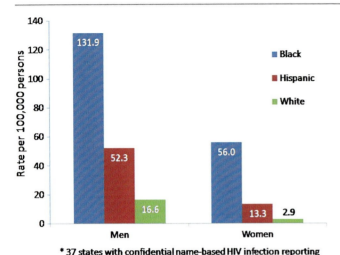

Fig. 1.1 Estimated rates of diagnoses of HIV infection among adults and adolescents, by sex and race/ethnicity, 2008 – 37 states with confidential name-based HIV infection reporting. Centers for Disease Control and Prevention. HIV Surveillance Report 2008, Volume 20. http://www.cdc.gov/hiv/topics/surveillance/resources/reports. Published June 2010

and Hispanic/Latino men were 7.9 and 3.2 times higher than for white men, respectively, the same rates among black women and Hispanic/Latino women were 19.3 and 4.6 times higher than their white counterparts, respectively.

Although white men, especially MSM, were most affected in the early years of the US epidemic, currently the majority of new diagnoses of HIV infection occur among racial and ethnic minority males, particularly young men many of whom are MSM [1, 5]. Between 2005 and 2008, the estimated number of new diagnoses of HIV infection among all young (aged 13–24 years) black and young Hispanic/Latino MSM were essentially double the same number for white young MSM: among blacks, from 1,841 to 3,188 new diagnoses with an estimated annual percentage change (EAPC) of 20.0; for Hispanics/Latinos 520–820 infections, EAPC 18.1; among whites 663–917 cases, EAPC 10.7 [6].

Geography

Four states (California, Florida, New York and Texas) carried the greatest burden of HIV disease in the USA as of the end 2008: 51% of cumulative adult and adolescent diagnoses of AIDS, and 46 and 43% of all new diagnoses of AIDS and of HIV infection, respectively, in 2008 [1]. The burden of HIV disease is approximately three times greater among residents of metropolitan areas (populations ≥ 500,000) compared with residents of nonmetropolitan or rural areas (populations < 50,000), whether considering the rates of new HIV or of AIDS diagnosis during 2008, or the rates of persons living with HIV or with AIDS at the end of 2007. In a CDC survey conducted between 2005 and 2007 [7], HIV prevalence among high-risk heterosexuals within impoverished areas of major urban centers was 2.1%, a rate that exceeded the cutoff of 1% that defines a generalized epidemic and that was similar to rates in several low-income sub-Saharan African nations where the HIV epidemic is driven by heterosexual transmission [8]. In contrast to overall HIV prevalence in the USA, HIV prevalence rates in urban poverty areas did not differ significantly by race or ethnicity. Lastly, both the prevalence rates of persons living with HIV infection in the 34 states with mature reporting systems as of 2007, and the rates of new HIV diagnoses nationwide were notably elevated across the southeastern USA [9] Indeed, in 2008, nine of the top ten metropolitan statistical areas with the highest rates of new HIV diagnoses were in the southeast (the exception was New York NY): Atlanta GA, Baton Rouge LA, Charlotte NC, Jackson MS, Jacksonville FL, Memphis TN, Miami FL, New Orleans LA, and Orlando FL [1].

Incidence Rates and Trends

Using new testing technology and statistical extrapolation methods, CDC has recently estimated that 56,300 new HIV infections occurred in the USA in 2006 for an overall incidence rate of 22.8 per 100,000 population [3]. Forty five percent of the infections were among black, 53% were among MSM, and 27% were among women. The majority of new infections in 2006 occurred among persons age 13–39 years. However, 25% of new infections occurred among persons aged 40–49 years, and 10% of new infections occurred among persons age 50 years and older.

Similar to prevalence data, the HIV incidence for blacks was 7.3 times as high as incidence among whites (83.7 per 100,000 vs. 11.5 per 100,000) and almost 2.9 times as high as incidence among Hispanics (29.3 per 100,000) [3]. An independent historical trend analysis (back-calculation of HIV incidence from HIV surveillance data) corroborated these findings, yielding an estimate of approximately 55,400 new HIV infections per year during 2003–2006. The study also documented that despite early progress in the epidemic, since 1999 HIV incidence (and corresponding prevalence) has been steadily increasing among MSM, whereas reductions in new HIV infections occurred among both injecting drug users and heterosexuals.

Persons Living with a Diagnosis of Aids

With advent of highly active combination antiretroviral therapy in 1996, the number of persons living with HIV infection who have been diagnosed with AIDS and the annual estimated number of deaths dropped precipitously from their

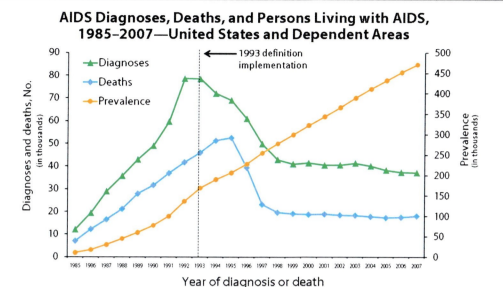

Fig. 1.2 Estimated numbers of AIDS cases, deaths, and persons living with AIDS, 1985–2007 – the USA and dependent areas

peak years: 52 and 72%, respectively (Fig. 1.2) [1]. Both values have remained stable since 2005 and 82% percent of persons diagnosed with AIDS in 2000–2004 were alive at the end of 2007. As a result, there has been a steady increase in the prevalence of persons living with AIDS, which includes persons who have ever experienced an AIDS-defining opportunistic illness or had a CD4 cell count <200 cells/mm^3 even if they have subsequently experienced immune reconstitution and achieved a CD4 cell count ≥200 cells/mm^3.

Continued improvements in the potency and tolerability of antiretroviral agents together with increased emphasis on treatment adherence have paralleled a threefold decline in the incidence rate of multiple regimen treatment failure: 56 to 16 events per 100 person-years from 1996–1997 to 2005 [10]. Maintaining antiretroviral therapy even in patients who cannot achieve an undetectable HIV RNA viral load significantly reduces their risk of experiencing an AIDS-defining event [11]; however, following exhaustion of effective treatment options, changes in survival have been modest at best, declining only from 6.5 to 5.0 deaths per 100 person-years from 1996–1997 to 2003 with a cumulative mortality of 26% at 5 years after failure [10].

Late HIV Diagnoses

Although early identification of HIV infection and prompt linkage to care and treatment improve survival and prolong the period of disease free survival on effective therapy, late diagnosis of HIV infection remains a major US public health dilemma. Two CDC studies have estimated that the fraction of persons who received a diagnosis of AIDS at or within the subsequent 12 months after diagnosis of their HIV infection ranged between 38% (based on nationally reported surveillance data from 1996 to 2005) [12] and 45% (based on an a supplemental surveillance project that conducted interviews with recently diagnosed patients in 16 states between 2000 and 2003) [13]. Another national surveillance report found that from 2001 through 2003, the median first CD4 cell count within 12 months of HIV diagnosis ranged 167–175 cells/mm^3 [14]. A South Carolina study conducted during 2004–2005 of 759 persons with newly diagnosed HIV infection found that 34% had CD4 cell counts ≤200 cells/mm^3 and 56% had CD4 cell counts ≤350 cells/mm^3 around the time of their HIV diagnosis [15] and in the Johns Hopkins HIV Clinical Cohort in Baltimore, the median CD4 cell count at presentation among antiretroviral-naïve HIV-infected patients decreased significantly from 371 cells/mm^3 in 1990–1994 to 276 cells/mm^3 in 2003–2006 [16].

Two recent reports suggest improvements may be occurring. The first study reported findings using data from a large multicenter North American cohort that included observations from 44,491 persons of whom 95% received care in the USA The investigators found that the median CD4 count at first presentation for care after HIV diagnosis increased from 256 cells/mm^3 (interquartile range [IQR], 96–455 cells/mm^3) to 317 cells/mm^3 (IQR, 135–517 cells/mm^3) from 1997 to 2007 ($P<0.01$) with an estimated adjusted mean CD4 count increase of 6 cells/mm^3 per year (95% confidence interval, 5–7 cells/mm^3 per year) [17]. A second report from the District of Columbia, found that with increased effort to expand HIV testing from 16,748 tests in 2004 to 72,684 tests in 2008 [18], the median CD4 cell count at HIV diagnosis increased from 216 to 340 cells/mm^3 ($p<0.01$) [19]. Although encouraging, in both reports more than 50% of persons had CD4 cell counts below currently recommended threshold of 500 cells/mm^3 for initiating antiretroviral therapy [20] at the time of their initial HIV diagnosis.

Need for Routine HIV Testing

The Washington DC experience highlights the value of expanded HIV testing. Approximately 21% of persons living with HIV in the U.S. are unaware of their HIV-positive status [2]. Persons who do not know that they are HIV infected are more likely to engage in high-risk sexual behavior capable of transmitting HIV infection than persons who have learned their status and had the opportunity to modify their behaviors [21]. To increase the number of persons who know their HIV status and, if positive, who are linked to clinical and preventive services early, the CDC has recommended since 2006 universal routine (i.e., opt-out) voluntary HIV screening for all persons age 13–64 years in public and private care settings, and repeat annual testing for persons at high risk for HIV (i.e., injection-drug users and their sex partners, persons who exchange sex for money or drugs, sex partners of HIV-infected persons, and MSM or heterosexual persons who themselves or whose sex partners have had more than one sex partner since their most recent HIV test [22]. Recent advances in HIV screening diagnostics, such as the use of rapid HIV-antibody tests and of HIV RNA tests to detect acute HIV infections, offer opportunities to diagnose HIV earlier among persons unaware of their status.

A 2008 CDC report indicates there is room for improvement. Using the National Health Interview Survey, the investigators reported that between 1987 and 2006 the number of persons reporting having ever been tested for HIV infection rose from 6 to 38%, while the number reporting having been tested in the preceding 12 months remained essentially stable at 10% between 2001 and 2006 [23]. When asked of persons at risk for HIV infection as defined in the preceding paragraph, 23.0% of respondents reported having been tested in the preceding 12 months. Continued national efforts to improve HIV testing methods, to reduce legal barriers that require informed signed consent, and to further integrate HIV testing into the routine care of all patients and also make testing available in other venues enriched in high-risk patients (e.g., needle exchange facilities, gay and lesbian community centers) are critical to reach the 2015 target in the President's July 2010 National HIV/AIDS Strategy that 90% of persons living with HIV infection know their status [24].

Despite long-standing recognition that MSM and African-Americans are at substantially increased risk of HIV infection, self-awareness of risk in these groups appears poor, emphasizing the importance of routine testing. Two studies have focused on MSM. A survey conducted during 1994–2000 among 5,649 younger urban MSM ages 15–29 years found that 77% were unaware of their infection prior to testing [25]. A subsequent survey in 2005 of 1,767 urban MSM with a median age of 32 years (range: 18–81) found that among the 450 men who tested HIV positive, 48% reported they were unaware of their infection prior to the test, of whom over half had never been tested for HIV infection or had been tested >1 year earlier [26].

Three studies have focused specifically on African-Americans. A sub-study of the 1994–2000 survey conducted among 909 young urban black MSM ages 15–22 years during 1994–1998 reported that 93% of the 139 men diagnosed with HIV infection were unaware of their status prior to the test and 71% believe they were at low risk of HIV infection [27]. A subsequent survey of young black MSM college students in North Carolina diagnosed with HIV infections during 2001–2003 indicated little change in the intervening years: 70% reported that at the time of their positive HIV test that they believed they were unlikely to be infected [28]. A similar survey of black women diagnosed with HIV infection in North Carolina during 2003–2004 (median age 29 years, range 18–42) found that 58% believed they were unlikely or very unlikely to have HIV infection at the time of their positive test [29].

Trends in All-Cause Morbidity and Mortality

Studies continue to demonstrate that widespread use of highly active antiretroviral therapy (HAART) since 1996 has led to sustained and continually improving reductions in morbidity and mortality among HIV-infected adults and children in the USA [30–32] and other industrialized countries [33–36]. In the USA, life expectancy after HIV infection has increased from 10.5 to 22.5 years from 1996 to 2005, respectively [37]. Similar findings have been reported among Canadians patients: from 9.1 to 23.6 years for a person 20 years of age initiating antiretrovirals at CD4 cell counts <200 cells/mm^3 diagnosed with HIV during 1993–1994 and 2002–2004, respectively [33]. Analyses of data from over 16,000 Europeans found that the excess mortality rate among HIV-seroconverters compared with mortality in the general population was 94% lower during 2002–2006 than the period prior to 1996 [36]. In that study, mortality rates in the first 5 years following infection for persons infected sexually with HIV were comparable to mortality rates of the general population; however, HIV-infected persons experienced excess mortality over the longer term.

Much of the morbidity and mortality benefit associated with widespread use of HAART has been derived from the associated profound reductions in AIDS-defining opportunistic illnesses (Fig. 1.3) [38, 39]. As a result, among treated patients, chronic diseases and conditions not typically associated with HIV have increasingly predominated both as causes for hospitalization [40, 41] and as causes of death [31, 42, 43].

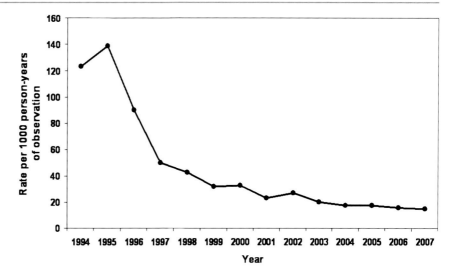

Fig. 1.3 Annual incidence of first AIDS-defining opportunistic infection in the HIV Outpatient Study, 1994–2007. Reprinted with permission from Brooks JT, Kaplan JE, Holmes KK, Benson C, Pau A, Masur H. HIV-associated opportunistic infections-going, going, but not gone: the continued need for prevention and treatment guidelines. Clin Infect Dis. 2009;48(5):609–11

The introduction of simplified formulations of more tolerable and durable antiretrovirals and the recent development of multiple new antiretroviral treatment options (e.g., integrase inhibitors, CCR5 inhibitors) have allayed some of the concerns that earlier treatment (i.e., at higher CD4 cell counts) exposes patients to unnecessary pill burden, expense, and antiretroviral-related toxicities, and might limit future treatment options due to the emergence of antiretroviral drug resistance.

The timing of antiretroviral therapy initiation ("when to start") has been an area of considerable interest and controversy. There is now broad agreement based on the Strategies for Management of Antiretroviral Therapy that structured treatment interruptions are harmful and should be avoided. Increasing evidence from this seminal clinical trial [44] and multiple large observational cohort studies [45–47] suggests that patients initiating antiretroviral therapy to suppress HIV viremia at higher CD4 cell counts experience improved survival but also reduces their risk for non-AIDS defining illnesses, including chronic diseases as well as complications and toxicities of antiretroviral treatment [44, 48–51]. Reassuringly, initiation of antiretroviral therapy at higher CD4 cell counts does not appear to increase the risk of developing antiretroviral resistance [52] or of exhausting available treatment options and failing therapy [53]. Current US guidelines [20] recommend initiating antiretroviral therapy at CD4 cell counts <500 cells/mm^3 with the option of initiating at higher CD4 cell counts especially under certain circumstances (e.g., when initiating therapy against hepatitis B infection, to prevent HIV transmission between serodiscordant sexual partners or injection-drug-using partners).

Non-AIDS Morbidity and Mortality

As noted above, with improved survival on HAART and aging of the cohorts, HIV-infected patients are increasingly affected by chronic illnesses. These conditions include cardiovascular disease, hepatic and renal disorders, osteopenia, endocrine and metabolic abnormalities (including insulin resistance with consequent hyperglycemia, hyperlipidemia, diabetes, and lipodystrophy) and non-AIDS-defining cancers, particularly anal cancer, Hodgkin's lymphoma, lung cancer, oropharyngeal cancers, and hepatocellular carcinoma [54–58]. Three factors can contribute to risk for these conditions: (1) HIV and the effects of chronic viral infection and attendant inflammation, (2) antiretroviral treatment and its associated toxicities and adverse events, and (3) the host, most notably the population and psychosocial context in which the HIV disease occurs. For example, rates of hepatitis B and C infection, obesity, and tobacco use, all of which raise a patient's risk for a variety of chronic illnesses, are highly prevalent among HIV-infected patients, often at rates that substantially exceed comparable rates in the general population [59–63]. Most US HIV-infected patients in care are able to achieve complete virologic suppression with increasingly less toxic and more durable antiretroviral therapy; however, further reductions in mortality and morbidity will likely depend on effective prevention and treatment of the frequent chronic comorbidities these HIV-infected patients experience [64].

Summary

The US HIV epidemic is increasing among men who have sex with men and disproportionately affects black and Hispanic persons. In urban poverty areas, prevalence of HIV infection among heterosexuals now equals that of some sub-Saharan Africa nations. Early diagnosis of HIV infection and entry into care, prompt initiation of HAART when indicated, and continued high adherence to treatment can substantially reduce HIV-related morbidity and mortality. In the current era, HIV-infected persons in care have, on average, a much improved survival prognosis. However, as patients live longer they are increasingly affected not by the direct consequences of HIV infection but by chronic diseases. HIV infection in the USA has evolved into a chronic disease for persons in care, for which providers increasingly need to focus attention on the prevention of comorbid conditions and early identification and treatment of long-term complications.

References

1. CDC. HIV surveillance report, 2008. Vol 20. In: Division of HIV/AIDS Prevention NCfHA, Viral Hepatitis, STD, and TB Prevention, Centers for Disease Control and Prevention (CDC), U.S. Department of Health and Human Services, Atlanta, Georgia, editor; 2010.
2. Campsmith ML, Rhodes PH, Hall HI, Green TA. Undiagnosed HIV prevalence among adults and adolescents in the United States at the end of 2006. J Acquir Immune Defic Syndr. 2010;53(5):619–24.
3. Hall HI, Song R, Rhodes P, et al. Estimation of HIV incidence in the United States. JAMA. 2008;300(5):520–9.
4. Holtgrave DR, Hall HI, Rhodes PH, Wolitski RJ. Updated annual HIV transmission rates in the United States, 1977–2006. J Acquir Immune Defic Syndr. 2009;50(2):236–8.
5. Trends in HIV/AIDS diagnoses among men who have sex with men – 33 States, 2001–2006. MMWR Morb Mortal Wkly Rep. 2008;57(25):681–6.
6. Hall I, Helms D, Walker F, Belle E. Trends in HIV diagnoses and testing among U.S. adolescent and young adult males XVIII International AIDS Conference; 2010; Vienna, Austria; 2010.
7. Denning P, DiNenno E. Communities in crisis: is there a generalized HIV epidemic in impoverished urban areas of the United States? XVIII International AIDS Conference; 2010; Vienna, Austria; 2010.
8. UNAIDS. 2008 report on the global AIDS epidemic; 2008.
9. CDC. 2010 [cited; Available from: http://www.cdc.gov/hiv/topics/surveillance/resources/slides/general/index.htm. Last accessed August 19, 2010. Slides #14 ands #22.
10. Deeks SG, Gange SJ, Kitahata MM, et al. Trends in multidrug treatment failure and subsequent mortality among antiretroviral therapy-experienced patients with HIV infection in North America. Clin Infect Dis. 2009;49(10):1582–90.
11. Kousignian I, Abgrall S, Grabar S, et al. Maintaining antiretroviral therapy reduces the risk of AIDS-defining events in patients with uncontrolled viral replication and profound immunodeficiency. Clin Infect Dis. 2008;46(2):296–304.
12. CDC. Late HIV testing – 34 states, 1996–2005. MMWR Morb Mortal Wkly Rep. 2009;58(24):661–5.
13. CDC. Late versus early testing of HIV – 16 Sites, United States, 2000–2003. MMWR Morb Mortal Wkly Rep. 2003;52(25):581–6.
14. CDC. Reported CD4+ T-lymphocyte results for adults and adolescents with HIV/AIDS-33 states, 2005. HIV/AIDS Surveill Suppl Rep. 2005;11(2).
15. Ogbuanu IU, Torres ME, Kettinger L, Albrecht H, Duffus WA. Epidemiological characterization of individuals with newly reported HIV infection: South Carolina, 2004–2005. Am J Public Health. 2007;99 Suppl 1:S111–7.
16. Keruly JC, Moore RD. Immune status at presentation to care did not improve among antiretroviral-naive persons from 1990 to 2006. Clin Infect Dis. 2007;45:1369–74.
17. Althoff KN, Gange SJ, Klein MB, et al. Late presentation for human immunodeficiency virus care in the United States and Canada. Clin Infect Dis. 2010;50(11):1512–20.
18. Expanded HIV testing and trends in diagnoses of HIV infection – District of Columbia, 2004–2008. MMWR Morb Mortal Wkly Rep. 59(24):737–41
19. Castel A, Samala R, Griffin A, et al. Monitoring the impact of expanded HIV testing in the District of Columbia using population-based HIV/AIDS surveillance data. 17th Conference on Retroviruses and Opportunistic Infections; 2010; San Francisco, CA, 2010.
20. Panel on Antiretroviral Guidelines for Adults and Adolescents. Guidelines for the use of antiretroviral agents in HIV-1-infected adults and adolescents. December 1, 2009: Department of Health and Human Services.
21. Marks G, Crepaz N, Janssen RS. Estimating sexual transmission of HIV from persons aware and unaware that they are infected with the virus in the USA. AIDS. 2006;20(10):1447–50.
22. Branson BM, Handsfield HH, Lampe MA, et al. Revised recommendations for HIV testing of adults, adolescents, and pregnant women in health-care settings. MMWR Recomm Rep. 2006;55(RR-14):1–17.
23. CDC. Persons tested for HIV – United States, 2006. MMWR Morb Mortal Wkly Rep. 2008;57(31):845–9.
24. The national HIV/AIDS strategy for the United States and the national HIV/AIDS strategy: federal implementation plan. In: House W, editor. Washington, DC; 2010.
25. MacKellar DA, Valleroy LA, Secura GM, et al. Unrecognized HIV infection, risk behaviors, and perceptions of risk among young men who have sex with men - Opportunities for advancing HIV prevention in the third decade of HIV/AIDS. J Acquir Immune Defic Syndr. 2005;38(5):603–14.
26. CDC. HIV prevalence, unrecognized infection, and HIV testing among men who have sex with men – five U.S. cities, June 2004–April 2005. MMWR Morb Mortal Wkly Rep. 2005;54(24):597–601.
27. CDC. Unrecognized HIV infection, risk behaviors, and perceptions of risk among young black men who have sex with men – six U.S. cities, 1994–1998. MMWR Morb Mortal Wkly Rep. 2002;51(33):733–6.
28. CDC. HIV transmission among black college student and non-student men who have sex with men – North Carolina, 2003. MMWR Morb Mortal Wkly Rep. 2004;53(32):731–4.
29. CDC. HIV transmission among black women – North Carolina, 2004. MMWR Morb Mortal Wkly Rep. 2005;54(4):89–94.
30. Palella FJ, Delaney KM, Moorman AC, et al. Declining morbidity and mortality among patients with advanced human immunodeficiency virus infection. N Engl J Med. 1998;338(13):853–60.
31. Palella Jr FJ, Baker RK, Moorman AC, et al. Mortality in the highly active antiretroviral therapy era: changing causes of death and disease in the HIV outpatient study. J Acquir Immune Defic Syndr. 2006;43(1):27–34.
32. Patel K, Hernan MA, Williams PL, et al. Long-term effectiveness of highly active antiretroviral therapy on the survival of children and adolescents with HIV infection: a 10-year follow-up study. Clin Infect Dis. 2008;46(4):507–15.
33. Lima VD, Hogg RS, Harrigan PR, et al. Continued improvement in survival among HIV-infected individuals with newer forms of highly active antiretroviral therapy. AIDS. 2007;21(6):685–92.
34. Ewings FM, Bhaskaran K, McLean K, et al. Survival following HIV infection of a cohort followed up from seroconversion in the UK. AIDS. 2008;22(1):89–95.
35. May M, Sterne JA, Sabin C, et al. Prognosis of HIV-1-infected patients up to 5 years after initiation of HAART: collaborative analysis of prospective studies. AIDS. 2007;21(9):1185–97.
36. Bhaskaran K, Hamouda O, Sannes M, et al. Changes in the risk of death after HIV seroconversion compared with mortality in the general population. JAMA. 2008;300(1):51–9.
37. Harrison KM, Song RG, Zhang XJ. Life expectancy after HIV diagnosis based on national HIV surveillance data from 25 states, United States. J Acquir Immune Defic Syndr. 2010;53(1):124–30.
38. Buchacz K, Baker RK, Palella FJ, et al. AIDS-defining opportunistic illnesses in US patients, 1994–2007: a cohort study. AIDS. 2010;24(10):1549–59.

39. Brooks JT, Kaplan JE, Holmes KK, Benson C, Pau A, Masur H. HIV-associated opportunistic infections-going, going, but not gone: the continued need for prevention and treatment guidelines. Clin Infect Dis. 2009;48(5):609–11.
40. Kourtis AP, Bansil P, Posner SF, Johnson C, Jamieson DJ. Trends in hospitalizations of HIV-infected children and adolescents in the United States: analysis of data from the 1994–2003 Nationwide Inpatient Sample. Pediatrics. 2007;120(2):e236–e43.
41. Buchacz K, Baker RK, Moorman AC, et al. Rates of hospitalizations and associated diagnoses in a large multisite cohort of HIV patients in the United States, 1994–2005. AIDS. 2008;22(11): 1345–54.
42. Lau B, Gange SJ, Moore RD. Risk of non-AIDS-related mortality may exceed risk of AIDS-related mortality among individuals enrolling into care with CD4(+) counts greater than 200 cells/mm(3). J Acquir Immune Defic Syndr. 2007;44(2):179–87.
43. Hooshyar D, Hanson DL, Wolfe M, Selik RM, Buskin SE, McNaghten AD. Trends in perimortal conditions and mortality rates among HIV-infected patients. AIDS. 2007;21:2093–100.
44. El-Sadr WM, Lundgren JD, Neaton JD, et al. CD4+count-guided interruption of antiretroviral treatment. N Engl J Med. 2006;355(22):2283–96.
45. Kitahata MM, Gange SJ, Abraham AG, et al. Effect of early versus deferred antiretroviral therapy for HIV on survival. N Engl J Med. 2009;360(18):1815–26.
46. Sterne JAC, May M, Costagliola D, et al. Timing of initiation of antiretroviral therapy in AIDS-free HIV-1-infected patients: a collaborative analysis of 18 HIV cohort studies. Lancet. 2009;373(9672):1352–63.
47. Funk MJ, Fusco JS, Cole SR, et al. HAART initiation and clinical outcomes: insights from the CASCADE cohort of HIV-1 seroconverters on "When to Start." XVIII International AIDS Conference; 2010; Vienna, Austria; 2010.
48. Baker JV, Peng G, Rapkin J, et al. CD4+ count and risk of non-AIDS diseases following initial treatment for HIV infection. AIDS. 2008;22(7):841–8.
49. Emery S, Neuhaus JA, Phillips AN, et al. Major clinical outcomes in antiretroviral therapy (ART)-naive participants and in those not receiving ART at baseline in the SMART study. J Infect Dis. 2008;197(8):1133–44.
50. Lichtenstein KA, Armon C, Buchacz K, et al. Initiation of antiretroviral therapy at CD4 cell counts >/=350 cells/mm³ does not increase incidence or risk of peripheral neuropathy, anemia, or renal insufficiency. J Acquir Immune Defic Syndr. 2008;47(1):27–35.
51. Reekie J, Kosa C, Engsig F, et al. Relationship between current level of immunodeficiency and non-acquired immunodeficiency syndrome-defining malignancies. Cancer. 2010;published ahead of print July 26 2010 [DOI: 10.1002/cncr.25311].
52. Uy J, Armon C, Buchacz K, Brooks JT, The HOPS Investigators. Initiation of HAART at higher CD4 cell counts is associated with a lower frequency of antiretroviral drug resistance mutations at virologic failure. J Acquir Immune Defic Syndr. 2009;51(4):450–3.
53. Phillips AN, Leen C, Wilson A, et al. Risk of extensive virological failure to the three original antiretroviral drug classes over long-term follow-up from the start of therapy in patients with HIV infection: an observational cohort study. Lancet. 2007; 370(9603):1923–8.
54. Patel P, Hanson DL, Sullivan PS, et al. Incidence of types of cancer among HIV-Infected persons compared with the general population in the United States, 1992–2003. Ann Intern Med. 2008;148(10): 728–U29.
55. Bedimo R. Non-AIDS-defining malignancies among HIV-infected patients in the highly active antiretroviral therapy era. Curr HIV/AIDS Rep. 2008;5(3):140–9.
56. Simard EP, Pfeiffer RM, Engels EA. Spectrum of cancer risk late after AIDS onset in the United States. Arch Intern Med. 2010;170(15):1337–45.
57. Polesel J, Franceschi S, Suligoi B, et al. Cancer incidence in people with AIDS in Italy. Int J Cancer. 2010;127(6):1437–45.
58. Franceschi S, Lise M, Clifford GM, et al. Changing patterns of cancer incidence in the early- and late-HAART periods: the Swiss HIV Cohort Study. Br J Cancer. 2010;103(3):416–22.
59. Spradling PR, Richardson, Buchacz K, Moorman AC, Brooks JT, and the HIV Outpatient Study (HOPS) Investigators. Prevalence of chronic hepatitis B virus infection among patients in the HIV Outpatient Study, 1996–2007. J Viral Hepatitis. 2010;(published ahead of print doi:10.1111/j.1365-2893.2009.01249.x).
60. Spradling PR, Richardson JT, Buchacz K, et al. Trends in hepatitis C virus infection among patients in the HIV Outpatient Study, 1996–2007. J Acquir Immune Defic Syndr. 2010;53(3):388–96.
61. Crum-Cianflone N, Roediger MP, Eberly L, et al. Increasing rates of obesity among HIV-infected persons during the HIV epidemic. PLoS One. 2010;5(4):e10106.
62. Tedaldi EM, Brooks JT, Weidle PJ, et al. Increased body mass index does not alter response to initial highly active antiretroviral therapy in HIV-1-infected patients. J Acquir Immune Defic Syndr. 2006; 43(1):35–41.
63. Vidrine DJ. Cigarette smoking and HIV/AIDS: health implications, smoker characteristics and cessation strategies. AIDS Educ Prev. 2009;21(3 Suppl):3–13.
64. Justice AC. Prioritizing primary care in HIV: comorbidity, toxicity, and demography. TopHIV Med. 2006;14(5):159–63.

Epidemiology of Liver Disease in Human Immunodeficiency Virus-Infected Persons

Adeel A. Butt

Introduction

In the era of combination antiretroviral therapy (CART) and improved survival [1], liver disease has become a leading cause of morbidity and mortality among HIV-infected persons [2–4]. The term "liver disease" encompasses a wide spectrum, ranging from asymptomatic mild elevations of liver enzymes (aspartate aminotransferase, AST; alanine aminotransferase, ALT; alkaline phosphatase, ALP) to cirrhosis and end stage liver disease with all its complications (e.g., ascites, esophageal varices, hepatic encephalopathy). Liver disease in HIV-infected persons may be due to the virus itself, combination antiretroviral therapy (CART) used to treat HIV, infectious and noninfectious complications of HIV, or a combination of the above. Since several potential factors may be at play in any given HIV-infected person with liver disease, at times it is very difficult to clearly ascribe etiology. In addition to opportunistic infections and cancers, several conditions that are common in the general population may be seen with increasing frequency in HIV-infected persons. In this chapter, we discuss the epidemiology of liver disease in HIV-infected patients by etiology. Pathogenesis, natural history, and treatment for these conditions are discussed separately in other chapters.

While the majority of liver related morbidity and mortality is due to coinfection with hepatitis C virus (HCV) and excess alcohol use [5–7], the list of causes is extensive. Liver disease is implicated as the cause of death in 15–17% of the deaths in HIV-infected persons of which two thirds to three quarter are attributed to HCV coinfection [7, 8]. The proportion of liver related deaths among HIV-infected persons increased from <2% in 1995 to 17% in 2005 [8]. Excessive alcohol was reported in 48% of those patients, and 62% had undetectable HIV RNA levels [8]. The prevalence of liver enzyme elevation in HIV-infected persons in the absence of HCV or HBV coinfection is approximately 16%, with an incidence of 3.9 per 100 person years [9, 10]. Such elevations are associated with higher HIV RNA levels higher body mass index, and excess alcohol use. However, mild to moderate elevations do not seem to have a significant effect upon disease progression or mortality [9, 11]. Liver cirrhosis is a more serious consequence in HIV-infected persons, with an estimate overall prevalence of 8.3% (95% CI 7.2–9.5). The presence of liver cirrhosis in HIV-infected persons in the absence of viral hepatitis or alcohol use is 1.1% (95% CI 0.5–1.8) [12].

Combination Antiretroviral Therapy

Therapy with combination antiretroviral therapy is associated with liver enzyme elevation in 6–30% of patients [13]. Severe CART-related hepatotoxicity is reported in approximately 10% of patients, and life-threatening events are reported at a rate of 2.6 per 100 person years [14]. Most antiretroviral drugs used to treat HIV infection can lead to liver injury, but is particularly true for nonnucleoside reverse transcriptase inhibitors and protease inhibitors. Even within a class, there may be differences in the degree of liver injury potential. In a prospective study of 568 subjects, nevirapine-containing regimen was associated with twice as many grade 3 or 4 liver enzyme elevations compared with efavirenz-containing regimens [13]. Concomitant alcohol use and HCV coinfection may increase risk of liver injury in these people. However, the overall risk is small and is usually reversible when recognized in time. In one study, 88% of HIV–HCV coinfected persons on combination antiretroviral therapy remained free of any liver toxicity [15]. Risk of liver toxicity was higher among those who were on a ritonavir-based regimen. The risk of liver enzyme abnormalities in most studies was substantially higher in patients with HCV or HBV coinfection.

While most protease inhibitor-based regimen may cause liver enzyme elevation, other effects may be seen and differ by drug. For example, the typical pattern of liver abnormality associated with the protease inhibitors indinavir and atazanavir is an asymptomatic elevation of unconjugated bilirubin in the absence of AST/ALT elevation, seen in 6–40% of patients treated with these agents [16]. Progression to overt clinical jaundice is uncommon (7–8%), and the usual course of action is to observe such patients unless clinical jaundice or other liver abnormalities are found.

HIV and HCV–HBV Coinfection

Due to shared routes of transmission and similarities in behavioral patterns, there is a high risk of HCV and HBV coinfection among HIV-infected persons. In large national cohorts, the prevalence of HCV coinfection among HIV-infected persons is 18% [17–19]. In comparison, the prevalence of HCV infection in the general population in the USA is 1.6% [20].

HIV–HCV coinfected persons are more likely to have advanced liver disease and an accelerated progression of liver disease [21, 22]. But the effect of liver disease upon HIV progression is less well established. Some studies have demonstrated that HIV–HCV coinfected persons have more AIDS at baseline, more rapid progression to AIDS and decreased rate of CD4+ lymphocyte recovery [23, 24], while others have not found any such association [25, 26].

The prevalence of chronic HBV coinfection among HIV-infected persons is reported to be 7–11% [27, 28]. HIV-infected persons with negative serologic markers still have a substantial risk of occult chronic HBV infection defined as the presence of HBV DNA. In a study by Lo Re et al., 10% of HIV-infected subjects with negative HBsAg/anti-HBc had detectable HBV DNA [29].

Approximately 25–30% of HCV monoinfected persons have persistently normal liver enzymes. Some studies have found no significant difference in liver enzyme abnormalities between HCV monoinfected and HIV–HCV coinfected persons, while other have reported higher levels in the coinfected persons. Nearly 30% of HIV–HCV coinfected persons with persistently normal liver enzymes have stage F2 fibrosis on liver biopsy [30]. A recent clinical trial in HIV–HCV coinfected persons failed to show a significant benefit of long term pegylated interferon maintenance therapy in slowing progression of liver fibrosis. The trial was halted due to very slow rates of liver fibrosis progression in patients on CART [31].

Other Infectious Diseases

Viruses from the herpesviridae family (HSV, CMV), parasites (*Toxoplasma gondii*), mycobacteria (*M. tuberculosis, M. avium* complex), and fungi (*Cryptococcus, Histoplasma*) can all affect liver and manifest mostly as elevated liver enzymes. Many of these infections are classified as "opportunistic infections" and most are more common in HIV-infected persons compared to HIV-uninfected controls. In HIV-infected patients with elevated liver enzymes and appropriate clinical setting and epidemiologic exposure, these should be considered in the differential diagnosis.

Noninfectious Comorbidities

Alcohol Use

The prevalence of alcohol abuse or dependence is much higher in HIV-infected persons compared to the general population [32]. In an urban cohort of HIV-infected persons in the USA, 10.4% of the patients reported hazardous alcohol drinking. The overall prevalence of liver fibrosis as determined by an AST to platelet ratio (APRI) of >1.5 was 11.6% [33]. Among those without HCV coinfection, 5.3% had APRI >1.5 with hazardous alcohol drinking associated with an adjusted relative risk ratio of 3.72. Among the HCV coinfected persons, 18.3% had APRI >1.5, and in this population hazardous alcohol use was not independently associated with APRI.

Nonalcoholic Fatty Liver Disease (NAFLD)

NAFLD is defined as accumulation of fat in the hepatocytes exceeding 5% of the liver weight [34, 35]. NAFLD is not a static disease and may progress over a period of time. At one end of the spectrum is the relatively benign mild fatty infiltration of the liver, while the more severe forms, or nonalcoholic steatohepatitis (NASH) are characterized by significant steatosis with increasing degree of lobular and/or portal inflammation as the disease progresses [34].

NAFLD is a common liver condition. It is estimated that 20–30% of the US adults have some degree of hepatic steatosis or NAFLD, with 2–3% having the more severe form, NASH [34–37]. NAFLD is a common cause of elevations in serum alanine aminotransferase (ALT) levels accounting for 60–90% of ALT elevations in afflicted patients [38–40]. NAFLD is associated with accelerated liver fibrosis progression [41], as well as increased all-cause and liver-related mortality [41, 42].

There are scant data about the prevalence of NAFLD in patients with HIV alone. Using magnetic resonance spectroscopy, Hadigan and colleagues identified hepatic steatosis in 42% of HIV-infected subjects [43]. Another recent study

Table 2.1 Studies showing the relationship between antiretroviral use and steatosis

Author	Year	N	% With steatosis	None (minimal)	Grade 1 (mild)	Grade 2 (moderate)	Grade 3 (severe)	F3/F4 fibrosis
Castera et al. [47]	2007	137	67	33	35	20	12	32
Neau et al. [48]	2007	148	67	33	36	19	12	32
McGovern et al. [49]	2006	183	69	31	27	18	1	NR
Gaslightwala and Bini [50]	2006	154	72	NR	24	37	11	43
Bani-Sadr et al. [53]	2006	241	61	NR	38	16	7	NR
Marks et al. [51]	2005	106	56	44	47	7	2	25
Monto et al. [54]	2005	92	NR	52	45	2	0	21

NR not reported

using liver–spleen attenuation of CT scan found steatosis in 37% of HIV-infected persons [44]. In this study, factors associated with NAFLD included a higher serum ALT–AST ratio, male sex, greater waist circumference, and longer NRTI use [44]. HIV-infected subjects with NAFLD have a lower BMI and a lower percentage of fat mass when compared with HIV-uninfected subjects with NAFLD [45]. Hepatic steatosis can progress rapidly to cirrhosis in HIV-infected persons, even in the absence of HCV coinfection, and despite effective control of HIV replication [46].

Hepatic steatosis/NAFLD is even more common among HCV–HIV coinfected patients, being reported in 67–69% of patients [47–49]. While HCV genotype 3 and BMI are associated with NAFLD/steatosis in this population, this association persists even after adjusting for BMI and HCV genotype [47, 48]. Hepatic steatosis in HCV–HIV coinfected subjects has been associated with more advanced fibrosis in multiple studies [49–52], and fibrosis progression correlates with the degree of steatosis [50]. The relationship between antiretroviral use and steatosis is less clear, with some studies reporting an increased risk [49, 52], while others did not find such an association (Table 2.1) [53, 54]. There was no association between steatosis and HIV RNA or CD4 counts [47, 48, 53, 54].

Hepatocellular Carcinoma

Globally, HCV, HBV, and alcoholic cirrhosis are the leading causes of hepatocellular carcinoma (HCC) [55]. An association between HIV and HCC has been reported by some recent studies. Since HCV, HBV, and excessive alcohol use are all more prevalent in HIV-infected persons, careful study of the role of each of these factors is important. In an analysis of HIV-infected veterans in the USA, McGinnis et al. found that while HIV-infected veterans were at a greater risk for HCC compared to uninfected veterans, this was largely explained by the higher prevalence of HCV and alcohol abuse or dependence [56]. However, among HIV-infected population with liver related death, HCC accounts for an increasing proportion of deaths, increasing from 15% in 2000 to 25% in 2005 [57]. Screening for HCC is important among HIV-infected persons, especially those with HCV or HBV coinfection or excessive alcohol use.

Other Conditions

A newer entity called "nodular regenerative hyperplasia" has been recently reported [58]. The prevalence of nodular regenerative hyperplasia in the general population has been estimated between 0.7 and 2.6% based on autopsy series, but may be as high as 8% in the HIV-infected persons [58, 59]. While some studies have suggested an association with CART, the number of reported patients in literature is too small to make any definitive conclusions.

Summary

Liver injury and liver disease are common among HIV-infected persons, and liver disease is now a leading cause of morbidity and mortality in this group. While nearly all antiretrovirals have been associated with liver injury, the overall risk from such therapy is relatively small and reversible. NAFLD is another common condition that needs to be considered. Excessive alcohol use is more prevalent among HIV-infected persons and has significant consequences, both in terms of liver disease as well as nonadherence to HIV medication and progression of HIV disease. Opportunistic infections are another important cause of liver injury. Finally, the incidence of HCC is on the rise among HIV-infected persons. For almost all conditions listed above, coinfection with HCV substantially increases the risk.

References

1. Palella Jr FJ, Delaney KM, Moorman AC, et al. Declining morbidity and mortality among patients with advanced human immunodeficiency virus infection. HIV Outpatient Study Investigators. N Engl J Med. 1998;338(13):853–60.
2. Palella Jr FJ, Baker RK, Moorman AC, et al. Mortality in the highly active antiretroviral therapy era: changing causes of death and

disease in the HIV outpatient study. J Acquir Immune Defic Syndr. 2006;43(1):27–34.
3. Bonnet F, Morlat P, Chene G, et al. Causes of death among HIV-infected patients in the era of highly active antiretroviral therapy, Bordeaux, France, 1998–1999. HIV Med. 2002;3(3):195–9.
4. Krentz HB, Kliewer G, Gill MJ. Changing mortality rates and causes of death for HIV-infected individuals living in Southern Alberta, Canada from 1984 to 2003. HIV Med. 2005;6(2):99–106.
5. Darby SC, Ewart DW, Giangrande PL, et al. Mortality from liver cancer and liver disease in haemophilic men and boys in UK given blood products contaminated with hepatitis C. UK Haemophilia Centre Directors' Organisation. Lancet. 1997;350(9089):1425–31.
6. Bica I, McGovern B, Dhar R, et al. Increasing mortality due to end-stage liver disease in patients with human immunodeficiency virus infection. Clin Infect Dis. 2001;32:492–7.
7. Weber R, Sabin CA, Friis-Moller N, et al. Liver-related deaths in persons infected with the human immunodeficiency virus: the D:A:D study. Arch Intern Med. 2006;166(15):1632–41.
8. Rosenthal E, Salmon-Ceron D, Lewden C, et al. Liver-related deaths in HIV-infected patients between 1995 and 2005 in the French GERMIVIC Joint Study Group Network (Mortavic 2005 study in collaboration with the Mortalite 2005 survey, ANRS EN19). HIV Med. 2009;10(5):282–9.
9. Kovari H, Ledergerber B, Battegay M, et al. Incidence and risk factors for chronic elevation of alanine aminotransferase levels in HIV-infected persons without hepatitis b or c virus co-infection. Clin Infect Dis. 2010;50(4):502–11.
10. Sterling RK, Chiu S, Snider K, Nixon D. The prevalence and risk factors for abnormal liver enzymes in HIV-positive patients without hepatitis B or C coinfections. Dig Dis Sci. 2008;53(5):1375–82.
11. Vergara S, Macias J, Mira JA, et al. Low-level liver enzyme elevations during HAART are not associated with liver fibrosis progression among HIV/HCV-coinfected patients. J Antimicrob Chemother. 2007;59(1):87–91.
12. Castellares C, Barreiro P, Martin-Carbonero L, et al. Liver cirrhosis in HIV-infected patients: prevalence, aetiology and clinical outcome. J Viral Hepat. 2008;15(3):165–72.
13. Sulkowski MS, Thomas DL, Mehta SH, Chaisson RE, Moore RD. Hepatotoxicity associated with nevirapine or efavirenz-containing antiretroviral therapy: role of hepatitis C and B infections. Hepatology. 2002;35(1):182–9.
14. Puoti M, Nasta P, Gatti F, et al. HIV-related liver disease: ARV drugs, coinfection, and other risk factors. J Int Assoc Physicians AIDS Care (Chic Ill). 2009;8(1):30–42.
15. Sulkowski MS, Thomas DL, Chaisson RE, Moore RD. Hepatotoxicity associated with antiretroviral therapy in adults infected with human immunodeficiency virus and the role of hepatitis C or B virus infection. JAMA. 2000;283(1):74–80.
16. Sulkowski MS. Drug-induced liver injury associated with antiretroviral therapy that includes HIV-1 protease inhibitors. Clin Infect Dis. 2004;38 Suppl 2:S90–7.
17. Sherman KE, Rouster SD, Chung RT, Rajicic N. Hepatitis C Virus prevalence among patients infected with Human Immunodeficiency Virus: a cross-sectional analysis of the US adult AIDS Clinical Trials Group. Clin Infect Dis. 2002;34(6):831–7.
18. Goulet JL, Fultz SL, McGinnis KA, Justice AC. Relative prevalence of comorbidities and treatment contraindications in HIV-mono-infected and HIV/HCV-co-infected veterans. AIDS. 2005;19 Suppl 3:S99–S105.
19. Spradling PR, Richardson JT, Buchacz K, et al. Trends in hepatitis C virus infection among patients in the HIV Outpatient Study, 1996–2007. J Acquir Immune Defic Syndr. 2010;53(3):388–96.
20. Armstrong GL, Wasley A, Simard EP, McQuillan GM, Kuhnert WL, Alter MJ. The prevalence of hepatitis C virus infection in the United States, 1999 through 2002. Ann Intern Med. 2006;144(10):705–14.
21. Vogel M, Rockstroh JK. Liver disease: the effects of HIV and antiretroviral therapy and the implications for early antiretroviral therapy initiation. Curr Opin HIV AIDS. 2009;4(3):171–5.
22. Benhamou Y, Bochet M, Martino VD, et al. Liver fibrosis progression in human immunnodeficiency virus and Hepatitis C virus coinfected patients. Hepatology. 1999;30:1054–8.
23. Greub G, Ledergerber B, Battegay M, et al. Clinical progression, survival, and immune recovery during antiretroviral therapy in patients with HIV-1 and hepatitis C virus coinfection: the Swiss HIV cohort study. Lancet. 2000;356:1800–5.
24. De Luca A, Bugarini R, Lepri AC, et al. Coinfection with hepatitis viruses and outcome of initial antiretroviral regimens in previously naive HIV-infected subjects. Arch Intern Med. 2002;162(18):2125–32.
25. Dorrucci M, Pezzotti P, Phillips AN, Lepri AC, Rezza G. Coinfection of hepatitis C virus with Human Immunodeficiency virus and progression to AIDS. J Infect Dis. 1995;172:1503–8.
26. Sulkowski MS, Moore RD, Mehta SH, Chaisson RE, Thomas DL. Hepatitis C and progression of HIV disease. JAMA. 2002;288(2):199–206.
27. Kellerman SE, Hanson DL, McNaghten AD, Fleming PL. Prevalence of chronic hepatitis B and incidence of acute hepatitis B infection in human immunodeficiency virus-infected subjects. J Infect Dis. 2003;188(4):571–7.
28. Chun HM, Fieberg AM, Hullsiek KH, et al. Epidemiology of Hepatitis B virus infection in a US cohort of HIV-infected individuals during the past 20 years. Clin Infect Dis. 2010;50(3):426–36.
29. Lo Re III V Frank I, Gross R, et al. Prevalence, risk factors, and outcomes for occult hepatitis B virus infection among HIV-infected patients. J Acquir Immune Defic Syndr. 2007;44(3):315–20.
30. Sanchez-Conde M, Berenguer J, Miralles P, et al. Liver biopsy findings for HIV-infected patients with chronic hepatitis C and persistently normal levels of alanine aminotransferase. Clin Infect Dis. 2006;43(5):640–4.
31. Sherman KE, Andersen J, Butt AA, Umbleja T, Alston B, Koziel MJ, Peters MG, Sulkowski M, Goodman ZD, Chung RT; for the Aids Clinical Trials Group A5178 Study Team. Sustained Long-term Antiviral Maintenance Therapy in HCV/HIV Coinfected Patients (SLAM-C). J Acquir Immune Defic Syndr 2010; October 1, Epub ahead of publication.
32. Kraemer KL, McGinnis KA, Skanderson M, et al. Alcohol problems and health care services use in human immunodeficiency virus (HIV)-infected and HIV-uninfected veterans. Med Care. 2006;44(8 Suppl 2):S44–51.
33. Chaudhry AA, Sulkowski MS, Chander G, Moore RD. Hazardous drinking is associated with an elevated aspartate aminotransferase to platelet ratio index in an urban HIV-infected clinical cohort. HIV Med. 2009;10(3):133–42.
34. Neuschwander-Tetri BA, Caldwell SH. Nonalcoholic steatohepatitis: summary of an AASLD Single Topic Conference. Hepatology. 2003;37(5):1202–19.
35. Angulo P. GI epidemiology: nonalcoholic fatty liver disease. Aliment Pharmacol Ther. 2007;25(8):883–9.
36. Williams R. Global challenges in liver disease. Hepatology. 2006;44(3):521–6.
37. Browning JD, Szczepaniak LS, Dobbins R, et al. Prevalence of hepatic steatosis in an urban population in the United States: impact of ethnicity. Hepatology. 2004;40(6):1387–95.
38. Angulo P. Nonalcoholic fatty liver disease. N Engl J Med. 2002;346(16):1221–31.
39. Ioannou GN, Boyko EJ, Lee SP. The prevalence and predictors of elevated serum aminotransferase activity in the United States in 1999–2002. Am J Gastroenterol. 2006;101(1):76–82.
40. Clark JM, Brancati FL, Diehl AM. The prevalence and etiology of elevated aminotransferase levels in the United States. Am J Gastroenterol. 2003;98(5):960–7.

41. McCullough AJ. Pathophysiology of nonalcoholic steatohepatitis. J Clin Gastroenterol. 2006;40(3 Suppl 1):S17–29.
42. Adams LA, Lymp JF, St SJ, et al. The natural history of nonalcoholic fatty liver disease: a population-based cohort study. Gastroenterology. 2005;129(1):113–21.
43. Hadigan C, Liebau J, Andersen R, Holalkere NS, Sahani DV. Magnetic resonance spectroscopy of hepatic lipid content and associated risk factors in HIV infection. J Acquir Immune Defic Syndr. 2007;46(3):312–7.
44. Guaraldi G, Squillace N, Stentarelli C, et al. Nonalcoholic fatty liver disease in HIV-infected patients referred to a metabolic clinic: prevalence, characteristics, and predictors. Clin Infect Dis. 2008;47(2):250–7.
45. Mohammed SS, Aghdassi E, Salit IE, et al. HIV-positive patients with nonalcoholic fatty liver disease have a lower body mass index and are more physically active than HIV-negative patients. J Acquir Immune Defic Syndr. 2007;45(4):432–8.
46. Loulergue P, Callard P, Bonnard P, Pialoux G. Hepatic steatosis as an emerging cause of cirrhosis in HIV-infected patients. J Acquir Immune Defic Syndr. 2007;45(3):365.
47. Castera L, Loko MA, Le BB, et al. Hepatic steatosis in HIV-HCV coinfected patients in France: comparison with HCV monoinfected patients matched for body mass index and HCV genotype. Aliment Pharmacol Ther. 2007;26(11–12):1489–98.
48. Neau D, Winnock M, Castera L, et al. Prevalence of and factors associated with hepatic steatosis in patients coinfected with hepatitis C virus and HIV: Agence Nationale pour la Recherche contre le SIDA et les hepatites virales CO3 Aquitaine Cohort. J Acquir Immune Defic Syndr. 2007;45(2):168–73.
49. McGovern BH, Ditelberg JS, Taylor LE, et al. Hepatic steatosis is associated with fibrosis, nucleoside analogue use, and hepatitis C virus genotype 3 infection in HIV-seropositive patients. Clin Infect Dis. 2006;43(3):365–72.
50. Gaslightwala I, Bini EJ. Impact of human immunodeficiency virus infection on the prevalence and severity of steatosis in patients with chronic hepatitis C virus infection. J Hepatol. 2006;44(6):1026–32.
51. Marks KM, Petrovic LM, Talal AH, Murray MP, Gulick RM, Glesby MJ. Histological findings and clinical characteristics associated with hepatic steatosis in patients coinfected with HIV and hepatitis C virus. J Infect Dis. 2005;192(11):1943–9.
52. Sulkowski MS, Mehta SH, Torbenson M, et al. Hepatic steatosis and antiretroviral drug use among adults coinfected with HIV and hepatitis C virus. AIDS. 2005;19(6):585–92.
53. Bani-sadr F, Carrat F, Bedossa P, et al. Hepatic steatosis in HIV-HCV coinfected patients: analysis of risk factors. AIDS. 2006;20(4):525–31.
54. Monto A, Dove LM, Bostrom A, Kakar S, Tien PC, Wright TL. Hepatic steatosis in HIV/hepatitis C coinfection: prevalence and significance compared with hepatitis C monoinfection. Hepatology. 2005;42(2):310–6.
55. El Serag HB. Hepatocellular carcinoma: an epidemiologic view. J Clin Gastroenterol. 2002;35(5 Suppl 2):S72–8.
56. McGinnis KA, Fultz SL, Skanderson M, Conigliaro J, Bryant K, Justice AC. Hepatocellular carcinoma and non-Hodgkin's lymphoma: the roles of HIV, hepatitis C infection, and alcohol abuse. J Clin Oncol. 2006;24(31):5005–9.
57. Salmon-Ceron D, Rosenthal E, Lewden C, et al. Emerging role of hepatocellular carcinoma among liver-related causes of deaths in HIV-infected patients: The French national Mortalite 2005 study. J Hepatol. 2009;50(4):736–45.
58. Dinh MH, Stosor V, Rao SM, Miller FH, Green RM. Cryptogenic liver disease in HIV-seropositive men. HIV Med. 2009;10(7):447–53.
59. Mallet V, Blanchard P, Verkarre V, et al. Nodular regenerative hyperplasia is a new cause of chronic liver disease in HIV-infected patients. AIDS. 2007;21(2):187–92.

Current and Future Treatment Guidelines for HIV

Judith Feinberg

Introduction

Combination antiretroviral therapy (CART), consisting of 3 drugs with at least two different viral targets, has changed HIV/AIDS from an invariably lethal disease to a manageable one [1]. As potent antiretroviral combination therapy has improved the disease-free survival of HIV-infected individuals, adding millions of years of additional life to those receiving these drugs [2]. Large European and North American cohort studies have demonstrated that even patients who are diagnosed and begin treatment late in the disease process no longer die of AIDS or an AIDS-associated opportunistic disease – rather, mortality is increasingly due to end-stage liver and kidney disease, cardiovascular disorders, and non-AIDS-defining malignancies [3–11]. A recent study from Haiti shows similar results that patients starting combination antiretroviral therapy with a CD4 count between 200 and 350 cells/mm^3 had decreased rates of death and incident tuberculosis so the advances in HIV therapy hold true in resource-poor settings as well as in the industrialized world [12]. Consequently, preventing and treating these newer causes of morbidity and mortality has been a dominant theme in the research efforts of the last few years.

In the late 1990s, as the number of drugs approved for the treatment of HIV increased, the US Public Health Service developed a set of guidelines to assist those caring for HIV-infected patients. The pace of drug development and new knowledge in the management of HIV infection has been brisk, leading to near-annual revisions of the Department of Health and Human Services (DHHS) Guidelines for the Treatment of Adults and Adolescents. In fact, since management options can change swiftly, midyear updates to the guidelines are regularly posted on the federal AIDSinfo Web site (http://aidsinfo.nih.gov). Initially, the guidelines were presented as columns of drugs with the recommendation to chose two from the nucleoside reverse transcriptase inhibitor (NRTI) column and one from either the protease inhibitor (PI) or the nonnucleoside reverse transcriptase inhibitor (NNRTI) columns. Since then, the guidelines have evolved to recommend specific regimens as "preferred," "alternative" or "not recommended." This represents a significant change driven by clear evidence from randomized (and, in some cases, double-blinded, placebo-controlled) clinical trials that have demonstrated the improved efficacy, safety, and tolerability of newer regimens. With the rapid development of a number of drugs to which multidrug resistant HIV is sensitive, as well as the introduction of three new classes of antiretroviral agents, the goal of avoiding morbidity and mortality by complete viral suppression has become a reality for both the highly antiretroviral-experienced and the previously untreated patient alike.

The DHHS Guidelines [13] address all of the key issues in managing persons with HIV infection. Baseline evaluation, including laboratory testing; the goals of therapy; individualizing therapy; therapeutic options; when to initiate and when to change therapy; the importance of patient adherence to achieve optimal outcomes and prevent the emergence of resistance; antiretroviral therapy-associated adverse effects; management of acute HIV infection; special considerations in adolescents, pregnant women, injection drug users, and those coinfected with hepatitis B, hepatitis C, and tuberculosis are all discussed in detail. The guidelines also include recommendations for counseling HIV-infected patients on preventing transmission.

Currently recommended initial therapy HIV infection consists of two NRTIs, the oldest class of antiretroviral drugs, combined with either an NNRTI a ritonavir-boosted PI, or most recently, an integrase inhibitor (INI) [13]. These preferred regimens represent a departure from previously "preferred" initial regimens, with only an efavirenz (NNRTI)-based

J. Feinberg (✉)
Department of Medicine/Division of Infectious Diseases,
University of Cincinnati College of Medicine,
University Hospital Eden Ave/Albert Sabin Way, Holmes Hospital,
Room 3112, Cincinnati, OH 45267, USA
e-mail: FEINBEJ@UCMAIL.UC.EDU

regimen persisting in this category. Changes in the "preferred" initial therapy are based on research in two directions: (1) clinical trials indicating that newer ritonavir-boosted PIs (atazanavir and darunavir) are not inferior to lopinavir/ritonavir and offer better tolerability and safety profiles [14, 15] and (2) the development of the first integrase inhibitor, raltegravir [16], which has been shown to be highly potent, well tolerated, and safe.

At the same time that HIV drug development has been driving changes in the "preferred" category, data have been evolving to support earlier initiation of treatment based on immunologic status (CD4 cell counts) while recognition of longer-term toxicities have influenced the guidelines in a more conservative direction. In 1998, the DHHS guidelines recommended offering combination antiretroviral therapy to asymptomatic patients with CD4 counts <500 cells/mm^3, acknowledging that while many experts would delay therapy and observe asymptomatic patients with CD4+ T-cell counts >500, other experts would treat at that level [17]. By 2004, as a result of mounting concerns about short- and long-term toxicities, CART was recommended for symptomatic or asymptomatic patients with CD4+ T-cell counts <200. Treatment "should be offered to asymptomatic patients with CD4+ T-cell counts from 201 to 350," although this was not mandated [18]. In 2008, the guidelines had evolved to recommending initiation of antiretroviral therapy in patients with a history of an AIDS-defining illness or with a CD4+ T-cell count <350 [19].

By 2009, recommendations for even earlier initiation of treatment were based on data from several observational cohorts, suggesting that therapy may be considered in some patients with CD4+ T-cell counts >350 [13]. Although evidence from randomized controlled trials showing benefit for patients with higher CD4 cell counts is not yet available, cumulative observational cohort data clearly demonstrate benefit for earlier initiation of treatment. Arguments for beginning treatment at CD4 counts >350 are based on the fact that potent CART may improve and preserve immune function in most patients with virologic suppression, regardless of their baseline CD4 count, and that maintaining a higher CD4 count will prevent irreversible immune system damage. In addition, data have demonstrated a decreased risk of HIV-associated complications, such as tuberculosis, HIV-associated malignancies such as non-Hodgkin lymphoma and Kaposi sarcoma, human papillomavirus (HPV)-associated malignancies such as cervical and anal carcinomas, peripheral neuropathy, and HIV-associated cognitive impairment, as well as decreased risk of nonopportunistic conditions and non-AIDS-associated malignancies. The bulk of this evidence for earlier treatment is derived from large cohort studies, suggesting that initiating treatment earlier results in increased immunologic response, [20] lower mortality rates, [21] lower risk of developing some long-term treatment-related complications, [22] and lower rates of extensive triple class virologic failure [23]. Importantly, recommendations for earlier initiation of ART were also based on the growing awareness that untreated HIV infection may be associated with development of many non-AIDS-defining diseases, including cardiovascular disease, kidney disease, liver disease, and non-AIDS-defining malignancies [24, 25]. Lastly, treatment of HIV decreases the risk of HIV transmission, whether vertical (maternal–fetal) or horizontal (between sexual partners) [26, 27]. However, the split among the panel members regarding their level of enthusiasm for treatment at CD4 cell counts above 500 cells/mm^3 indicates how heated the current discussions around initiating treatment have become in the absence of prospective, randomized trial data [13].

There are, of course, limitations to cohort data that evaluate the timing of treatment initiation. Cohort studies are not designed to demonstrate statistical significance between CD4+ cell count endpoints, although they can indicate trends in outcomes. A large, randomized, controlled trial demonstrated that continuous CART therapy was more beneficial than treatment interrupted by achievement of a CD4 cell count >350 [28], and a post hoc subanalysis has shown that initiating treatment earlier results not only in the reduced risk of AIDS-related OIs or death but also in the reduced risk of non-AIDS-related complications [24].

There is as yet no randomized trial that definitively addresses the optimal time to initiate antiretroviral therapy in patients with CD4+ cell counts >200 cells/mm^3. Currently, there are two randomized controlled trials that are evaluating early versus deferred antiretroviral therapy, and should provide crucial data in the future. One study, aptly named The Strategic Timing of ART (START), is evaluating immediate (CD4 >500 cells/mm^3) versus deferred initiation (CD4 <350 cells/mm^3) in an estimated 4,000 individuals with a CD4 count >500 cells/mm^3 [29]. A second randomized trial, HPTN 052, is designed to determine the effectiveness of immediate versus deferred therapy to prevent the sexual transmission of HIV among an estimated 1,750 HIV-serodiscordant couples where one partner has a CD4 count of 350–550 cells/mm^3 at study entry. This trial is also under way, with participants being randomized to immediate versus deferred treatment until their CD4 count falls to the ≤200–250 cells/mm^3 range or they develop an AIDS-defining illness [30].

Based on the evidence described above, the most recent version of DHHS guidelines (Dec. 1, 2009), [13] now recommends that CART should be initiated in all patients with a history of an AIDS-defining illness or with a CD4 count <350 cells/mm^3, is recommended for patients with CD4 counts between 350 and 500 cells/mm^3 (with 55% of the panel "strongly supportive" and 45% "moderately supportive"), and is an option in patients with CD4 counts >500 cells/mm^3

(panel split evenly in favor of treating with the other half considering this optional). Also, in specific clinical situations, antiretroviral therapy is indicated regardless of CD4 cell count: pregnancy (to prevent maternal morbidity and mother-to-child-transmission), HIV-associated nephropathy (which responds to HIV treatment and may delay or obviate the need for dialysis), and hepatitis B virus coinfection when treatment of hepatitis B virus is indicated (because of the anti-HBV activity of several HIV drugs).

A key limitation to starting CART earlier in the disease process is the failure to diagnosis HIV Infection early enough for patients to derive benefit. Studies have shown that the majority of patients today are not diagnosed until later stages of disease [31–33]. In the Swiss HIV Cohort Study, 31% and 10% of patients had CD4 counts <200 and <50 cells/mm^3, respectively, when they were diagnosed with HIV infection [31]. In the USA, despite CDC recommendations for routine, opt-out HIV screening published as long ago as September 2006 [34], the median CD4 count for newly diagnosed patients is in the 200 cells/mm^3 range, with the exception of pregnant women diagnosed as a routine part of prenatal care. The delay in HIV diagnosis occurs unevenly, occurring more frequently in nonwhites, injection drug users, and older patients. In fact, 38.3% of all patients [33] and 42% of injection drug users [32] have been shown to receive a diagnosis of AIDS within 1 year of testing HIV-positive.

New HIV drugs in active development include other second-generation NNRTIs, new INIs and an INI that could be termed "second generation" in that its antiviral activity includes HIV that is resistant to the first FDA-approved INI, raltegravir. Two randomized, controlled, multinational phase III trials comparing once daily TMC278 (rilpivirine) to efavirenz have just concluded, indicating that rilpivirine is non-inferior to efavirenz [35]. These data, however, were submitted for FDA review in 2010. Elvitegravir, a new InI that must be coadministered once daily with the pharmacokinetic booster cobicistat, is in the final phase of testing; [36] its resistance pattern overlaps significantly with raltegravir's. S/GSK1349572 is a promising INI that can also be administered once daily and has activity against raltegravir-resistant virus; [37, 38] phase III studies are poised to start in late 2010. Still other agents with novel targets are in earlier stages of development.

Individualizing antretroviral therapy is essential to maximizing the patient's chance of success; in HIV disease management there is no 'one size fits all'. An "alternative" regimen may be preferred for some patients, and a "preferred" regimen may not be appropriate for all patients. The activity, intrinsic genetic barrier to resistance and the possibility of cross-resistance of a regimen are topics crucial to the physician. Of equal importance to the patient is the tolerability of a given regimen (requiring specific discussion of the adverse effect profile), ease of administration, patient's lifestyle and preferences – no bus driver wants to be on medication that is likely to cause diarrhea. Other comorbid conditions and risks, such as diabetes, hyperlipidemia, heart disease, and chronic hepatitis B and/or C should also be taken into consideration. Adherence is crucial to a successful outcome, and some regimens are more forgiving in this regard than others [39]. It goes without saying that patients initiating CART should be willing and able to commit to life-long treatment and should understand both the benefits and risks of therapy and the importance of adherence. Patients may choose to postpone therapy without prejudice to their future care, and similarly, providers may elect to defer therapy based on clinical and/or psychosocial factors on a case-by-case basis.

Treating HIV in the Context of Liver Disease

As the majority of deaths in the "HAART era" in several studies are no longer AIDS-associated, end-stage liver disease (ESLD) has emerged as a common cause of mortality. Coinfection with chronic viral hepatitis B (HBV) and/or hepatitis C (HCV) play significant roles in morbidity and mortality [9, 40, 41]. Moreover, there is a bilateral interaction of chronic viral hepatitis and HIV on disease progression. Other etiologies of chronic liver disease include alcohol abuse and steatosis, and many antiretroviral drugs used have been associated with varying degrees of hepatic toxicity, including some linked to acute liver failure and death, such as nevirapine.

The presence of chronic hepatitis B coinfection has a profound effect on the choice of medications, as some of the preferred drugs for HIV have an overlapping spectrum of activity against chronic HBV. When HIV drugs with HBV activity are interrupted or stopped, patients will frequently experience a flare of their chronic HBV. Conversely, entecavir, an effective and well-tolerated nucleoside analog that was used as monotherapy for HBV in coinfected individuals who had not yet begun therapy for HIV has been shown to induce resistance to the HIV drugs lamivudine and emtricitabine [42]. There have been contradictory reports about the anti-HIV activity of telbivudine. A case report that suggests an antiretroviral effect [43] and an in vitro study that fails to demonstrate inhibition of HIV-1 [44]. Adefovir was tested in the late 1990s as an anti-HIV drug at doses of 60 and 120 mg daily, but was both nephrotoxic and ineffective at these doses. Thus far, there are no data to indicate that the hepatitis B dose, 10 mg daily, has an antiviral effect on HIV or that it induces resistance to drugs for HIV. Although there are some agents available for treating HBV that appear to have no HIV activity (e.g., adefovir, interferon), thus making treatment of HBV alone in the coinfected person plausible, these are typically not the agents of choice for HBV. There are as yet no data from randomized, controlled trials to indicate that 2 agents for chronic HBV coinfection are required. A retrospective study suggests that tenofovir plus lamivudine was associated with improved viral suppression compared with either drug alone, [45] and other studies suggest that combination therapy can decrease the development of resistance [46]. Therefore, experts recommend combination therapy with two agents active against HBV in the context of HIV infection [47].

Complicating life for the clinician is the existence of several guidelines that address the treatment of chronic hepatitis B coinfection, and while agreeing on the broad strokes, these guidelines differ in the details. The DHHS Panel on Antiretroviral Guidelines for Adults and Adolescents specifically recommends tenofovir and either lamivudine or emtricitabline for the NRTI backbone as part of a combination regimen for HIV, thus treating both infections simultaneously [13]. Patients with chronic HBV requiring treatment should nevertheless receive adequate therapy for HIV as well, as 2 NRTIs with activity against both viruses will undertreat the HIV and lead to NRTI resistance. The DHHS Opportunistic Infections Guidelines also recommend that patients initiating antiretroviral therapy should be treated for HBV, regardless of HBV DNA level, "...either with antiviral agents active against both HIV and HBV or with antiviral agents with independent activity against each virus." Anti-HBV therapy should be continued in all patients receiving antiretroviral therapy, as such treatment may reduce risk of HBV-associated immune reconstitution syndrome. However, if therapy for HIV is not yet required, coinfected patients can be managed as recommended for HBV monoinfection: treat if the patient has abnormal ALT level and HBV DNA >20,000 IU/mL (>10^5 c/mL) for HBeAg+s, and abnormal ALT and HBV DNA >2,000 IU/mL for HBeAg-s [47]. Some experts recommend treatment for patients with (1) any level of detectable HBV DNA, especially in patients with elevated ALT levels, because of the increased rate of liver disease progression, (2) substantial histologic inflammatory activity or fibrosis on liver biopsy, even if HBV DNA levels are low, and even (3) advanced fibrosis or cirrhosis on liver biopsy with any detectable HBV DNA level, if other causes for chronic liver disease have been excluded.

The DHHS Perinatal Guidelines Panel has also addressed the management of HBV/HIV coinfection [49]. Coinfected pregnant women who require HIV therapy for their own health and who will continue drugs postpartum and/or who require treatment for HBV infection should receive a 3-drug combination antiretroviral regimen that includes two agents with anti-HBV activity (e.g., tenofovir plus either lamivudine or emtricitabine) in the antepartum period that should be continued postpartum. For coinfected women who receive antiretroviral drugs during pregnancy solely as prophylaxis for prevention of mother-to-child transmission of HIV, who are expected to discontinue such prophylaxis after delivery, and who do not require treatment for HBV infection, the choice is more complex and can include the following: (1) a regimen similar to that described above for women who will continue treatment postpartum, with monitoring for HBV flare, (2) a 3-drug combination antepartum antiretroviral regimen that includes only NRTIs without anti-HBV activity (e.g., abacavir, didanosine, stavudine, or zidovudine), or (3) a 3-drug combination antepartum antiretroviral regimen including lamivudine as the sole anti-HBV agent could be considered for women presenting late in pregnancy (e.g., after 28 weeks gestation) with monitoring for HBV flare.

Chronic hepatitis C (HCV) coinfection presents a different kind of challenge. FDA-approved therapy for chronic HCV is currently limited to parenteral pegylated interferon (IFN) alfa (2a or 2b) plus oral ribavirin. This combination approach to HCV management is least successful in genotype 1, the most common genotype in the USA, and is fairly toxic. At this time, a decision whether to treat HCV or HIV first is complex and must be based on a number of factors, including the disease stage of each, liver histology and patient preference. The one exception is pregnancy, as interferon is not recommended and ribavirin is contraindicated, [48] a situation where treatment of maternal HIV and prophylaxis against neonatal HIV acquisition takes precedence.

According to the DHHS guidelines for antiretroviral therapy, all HCV-coinfected patients should be evaluated for HCV therapy, and HCV treatment is recommended "... according to standard guidelines with strong preference for treating patients with higher CD4 counts. For patients with lower CD4 counts (<200 cell/mm^3), it may be preferable to initiate antiretroviral therapy and delay HCV therapy until CD4 counts increase as a result of HIV treatment."[49] While both HIV and HCV can be treated concurrently, this approach may be complicated by pill burden, drug toxicities, and drug interactions.

Studies are being conducted that will hopefully provide further guidance on the best approach to managing the HCV-coinfected patient. In addition, the active development of over 20 small molecules with anti-HCV activity may vitiate the issue of which chronic viral infection to treat first. If they are better tolerated than IFN/ribavirin, concurrent treatment for both HIV and HCV may ultimately be possible. Telaprevir and boceprevir are two such agents that are likely to be approved by the FDA in the near future. The FDA has just published a draft guidance document, entitled "Chronic Hepatitis C Virus Infection: Developing Direct-Acting Antiviral Agents for Treatment," which is currently available for public comment at: http://www.fda.gov/downloads/Drugs/GuidanceComplianceRegulatoryInformation/Guidances/UCM225333.pdf. In contrast to IFN/ribavirin, "direct-acting antiviral agents" (DAAs) are defined as agents that interfere with specific steps in the HCV replication cycle.

As more recently developed agents for HIV have demonstrated better adverse effect profiles, it has become easier to choose less toxic combination therapy for HIV for patients also suffering from chronic liver disease. For example, we have learned that use of the newer nucleotide analog tenofovir is less likely to contribute to severe anemia in patients also undergoing IFN/ribavirin treatment than older drugs such as the nucleoside analog AZT (zidovudine). Nevirapine hepatotoxicity is more severe in women than in men, and its use should be limited to women with CD4 cell counts <250. The PI atazanavir – whether or not ritonavir-boosted – causes indirect hyperbilirubinemia in some individuals as a consequence of its hepatic metabolism by UGT1A1 (uranyl glucose transferase). While this is itself is not harmful, the frank jaundice that can sometimes occur as a result may be clinically problematic in a patient with underlying liver disease, as well as socially problematic. In general, drug-induced liver injury (DILI) following antiretroviral therapy is more common in coinfected individuals, and the risk may be greatest in advanced liver disease (cirrhosis or end-stage liver disease). It is very difficult to compare DILI incidence rates for individual drugs as they are always used in multidrug combinations and comparisons across heterogeneous clinical trial populations complicates such analyses. However, stavudine with/without didanosine, nevirapine, full-dose ritonavir, and some ritonavir-boosted PIs, such as tipranavir/ritonavir, are more hepatotoxic than other drugs [50, 51].

Therefore, it is important to monitor alanine and aspartate aminotransferase levels at 1 month after initiating or changing antiretroviral therapy, and then to repeat levels every 3–4 months. Mild to moderate fluctuations in liver enzyme levels are typical in persons with chronic HCV and should not drive changes in therapy, especially in the absence of signs and/or symptoms of worsening liver disease. However, increases in liver enzymes to >5 times the upper limit of the normal range should, "…prompt careful evaluation for signs and symptoms of liver insufficiency and for alternative causes of liver injury (e.g., acute viral hepatitis A or B infection, hepatobiliary disease, or alcoholic hepatitis)." In the HCV-coinfected patient, short-term antiretroviral interruption may be required to fully evaluate the situation. This is a more complex problem in the HBV-coinfected patient where interruption of therapy for DILI may precipitate a full-fledged HBV flare with worsening transaminase levels.

Summary

Advances in drug development with new drug targets and better-tolerated agents, evolving information about short and long-term antiretroviral drug toxicities, and emerging data about when to start antiretroviral therapy have all had a significant impact on guidelines for HIV management. Implementation of guidelines is complicated by the presence of chronic liver disease, especially chronic viral hepatitis where overlapping spectrums of antiviral susceptibility/resistance development and overlapping toxicities coincide. Nevertheless, it is important to remember that guidelines are recommendations, not absolutes. Above all, HIV therapy must be individualized.

References

1. Palella Jr FJ, Delaney KM, Moorman AC, et al. Declining morbidity and mortality among patients with advanced human immunodeficiency virus infection. HIV Outpatient Study Investigators. N Engl J Med. 1998;338(13):853–60.
2. Walensky RP, Paltiel AD, Losina E, Mercincavage LM, Schackman BR, Sax PE, et al. The survival benefits of AIDS treatment in the United States. J Infect Dis. 2006;194(1):11–9.
3. Centers for Disease Control and Prevention. HIV Mortality (through 2006) at www.cdc.gov/hiv/topics/surveillance/resources/slides/mortality/slides/mortality.pdf
4. Lewden C, Chene G, Morlat P, Raffi F, Dupon M, et al. HIV-infected adults with a CD4 cell count greater than 500 cells/mm^3 on long-term combination antiretroviral therapy reach same mortality rates as the general population. J Acquir Immune Defic Syndr. 2007;46:72–7.
5. The Data Collection on Adverse Events of Anti-HIV drugs (DAD) Study Group. Factors associated with specific causes of death amongst HIV-positive individuals in the DAD study. AIDS. 2010;24:1537–48.
6. Marin B, Thiebaut R, Bucher HC, Rondeau V, Costagliola D, et al. Non-AIDS defining deaths and immunodeficiency in the era of combination antiretroviral therapy. CASCADE, 1996–2006. AIDS. 2009;23:1743–53.
7. Study Group on Death Rates at High CD4 Count in Antiretroviral Naive Patients. Death rates in HIV-positive antiretroviral-naive patients with CD4 count greater than 350 cells per mL in Europe and North America: a pooled cohort observational study. Lancet. 2010;376:340–5.
8. Antiretroviral Therapy Cohort Collaboration. Causes of death in HIV-1-infected patients treated with antiretroviral therapy, 1996–2006: collaborative analysis of 13 HIV cohort studies. Clin Infect Dis. 2010;50(10):1387–96.
9. Palella Jr FJ, Baker RK, Moorman AC, Chmiel JS, Wood KC, Brooks JT, et al. HIV Outpatient Study Investigators. Mortality in the highly active antiretroviral therapy era: changing causes of death and disease in the HIV outpatient study. J Acquir Immune Defic Syndr. 2006;43:27–34.
10. Lau B, Gange SJ, Moore RD. Risk of non-AIDS-related mortality may exceed risk of AIDS-related mortality among individuals enrolling into care with CD4+ counts greater than 200 cells/mm^3. J Acquir Immune Defic Syndr. 2007;44:179–87.
11. Egger M, May M, Chene G, et al. Prognosis of HIV-1 infected patients starting highly active antiretroviral therapy: a collaborative analysis of prospective studies. Lancet. 2002;360(9327):119–29.
12. Severe P, Juste MAJ, Ambroise A, Eliacin L, Marchand C, et al. Early versus standard antiretroviral therapy for HIV-infected adults in Haiti. N Engl J Med. 2010;363:257–65.
13. Panel on Antiretroviral Guidelines for Adults and Adolescents. Guidelines for the use of antiretroviral agents in HIV-1-infected adults and adolescents. Department of Health and Human Services. December 1, 2009; 1–161. Available at http://www.aidsinfo.nih.gov/ContentFiles/AdultandAdolescentGL.pdf. Accessed August 30, 2010.
14. Molina JM, Andrade-Villanueva J, Echevarria J, et al. Efficacy and safety of once-daily atazanavir/ritonavir compared to twice-daily

lopinavir/ritonavir, each in combination with tenofovir and emtricitabine in ARV-naive HIV-1-infected subjects: the CASTLE study, 48-week results. CROI 2008. Boston, MA. February 3–6, 2008. Abstract 37.
15. DeJesus E, Ortiz R, Khanlou H, et al. Efficacy and safety of darunavir/ritonavir versus lopinavir/ritonavir in ARV treatment-naive HIV-1-infected patients at week 48: ARTEMIS (TMC114-C211). 47th Interscience Conference on Antimicrobial Agents and Chemotherapy. September 17–20, 2007. Chicago. Abstract H-718b.
16. Lennox JL, DeJesus E, Lazzarin A, For the STARTMRK Investigators. Safety and efficacy of raltegravir-based versus efavirenz-based combination therapy in treatment-naive patients with HIV-1 infection: a multicentre, double-blind randomised controlled trial. Lancet. 2009;374(9692):796–806.
17. CDC. MMWR. 1998; 47(No. RR-5):43,47,48.
18. Panel on Antiretroviral Guidelines for Adults and Adolescents. Guidelines for the use of antiretroviral agents in HIV-1-infected adults and adolescents. March 23, 2004;1–97.
19. Panel on Antiretroviral Guidelines for Adults and Adolescents. Guidelines for the use of antiretroviral agents in HIV-1-infected adults and adolescents. Department of Health and Human Services. November 3, 2008; 1–139.
20. Moore RD, Keruly JC. $CD4^+$ cell count 6 years after commencement of highly active antiretroviral therapy in persons with sustained virologic suppression. Clin Infect Dis. 2007;44:441–6.
21. Palella Jr FJ, Deloria-Knoll M, Chmiel JS, Moorman AC, Wood KC, et al. Survival benefit of initiating antiretroviral therapy in HIV-infected persons in different CD4 cell strata. Ann Intern Med. 2003;138:620–6.
22. Lichtenstein KA, Armon C, Buchacz K, et al. Initiation of antiretroviral therapy at CD4 cell counts ≥ 350 cells/mm^3 does not increase incidence of risk of peripheral neuropathy, anemia, or renal insufficiency. JAcquir Immune Defic Syndr. 2008;47:27–35.
23. Phillips AN, Leen C, Wilson A, For the UK Collaborative HIV Cohort (CHIC) Study. Risk of extensive virological failure to the three original antiretroviral drug classes over long-term follow-up from the start of therapy in patients with HIV infection: an observational cohort study. Lancet. 2007;370:1923–8.
24. The Strategies for Management of Antiretroviral Therapy (SMART) Study Group. Major clinical outcomes in antiretroviral therapy (ART)-naïve participants and in those not receiving ART at baseline in the SMART Study. J Infect Dis. 2008;197:1133–44.
25. M Jonsson, JS Fusco, SR Cole, and others. HAART initiation and clinical outcomes: insights from the CASCADE cohort of HIV-1 seroconverters on "When to Start." XVIII International AIDS Conference (AIDS 2010). Vienna, July 18–23, 2010. Abstract THLBB201.
26. Thea DM, Steketee RW, Pliner V, et al. The effect of maternal viral load on the risk of perinatal transmission of HIV-1. AIDS. 1997; 11(4):437–44.
27. Castilla J, Del Romero J, Hernando V, Marincovich B, García S, Rodríguez C. Effectiveness of highly active antiretroviral therapy in reducing heterosexual transmission of HIV effectiveness of highly active antiretroviral therapy in reducing heterosexual transmission of HIV. J Acquir Immune Defic Syndr. 2005;40:96–101.
28. The Strategies for Management of Antiretroviral Therapy (SMART) Study Group. CD4+ count-guided interruption of antiretroviral treatment. N Engl J Med. 2006;355:2283–96.
29. START clinical trial. Available at: http://www.clinicaltrials.gov/ct2/show/NCT00867048. Accessed on August 30, 2010.
30. HPTN 052. DAIDS Document ID: 10068. Version 3.0, 20 November 2006. http://www.hptn.org/web%20documents/HPTN_Protocols/HPTN052/HPTN052v3(A4).pdf. Accessed on August 30, 2010.
31. Wolbers M, Bucher HC, Furrer H, Rickenbach M, Cavassini M, et al. Delayed diagnosis of HIV infection and late initiation of antiretroviral therapy in the Swiss HIV Cohort Study. HIV Med. 2008;9:397–405.
32. Grigoryan A, Hall HI, Durant T, Wei X. Late HIV diagnosis and determinants of progression to AIDS or death after HIV diagnosis among injection drug users, 33 US States, 1996–2004. PLoS One. 2009;4:e4445.
33. Centers for Disease Control and Prevention. Late HIV testing – 34 states, 1996–2005. MMWR. 2009;58:661–5.
34. Branson BM, Handsfield HH, Lampe MA, Janssen RS, Taylor AW, Lyss SB, et al. Centers for Disease Control and Prevention. Revised recommendations for HIV testing of adults, adolescents, and pregnant women in health-care settings. MMWR Recomm Rep. 2006;55:1–17.
35. Cohen C, Molina JM, Cahn P, Clotet B, Fourie J, et al. Pooled week 48 efficacy and safety results from ECHO and THRIVE, two double-blind, randomised, phase III trials comparing TMC278 versus efavirenz in treatment-naïve, HIV-1-infected patients. International AIDS Conference, Vienna, Austria, July 19–23, 2010. Abstract THLBB206.
36. Elion R, Gathe J, Rashbaum B, et al. The single tablet regimen of elvitegravir/cobicistat/emtricitabine/tenofovir disoproxil fumarate (QUAD) maintains a high rate of virologic suppression, and cobicistat is an effective pharmacoenhancer through 48 weeks. 50th Interscience Conference on Antimicrobial Agents and Chemotherapy (ICAAC). September 12–15, 2010. Boston. Abstract H-938b.
37. Arribas J, Lazzarin A, Raffi F, Rakhmanova A, Richmond G, et al. Once-daily S/GSK1349572 as part of combination therapy in antiretroviral naïve adults: rapid and potent antiviral responses in the interim 16-week analysis from SPRING-1 (ING112276). International AIDS Conference, Vienna, Austria, July 19–23, 2010. Abstract THLBB205.
38. Eron J, Durant J, Poizot-Martin I, Reynes J, Soriano V, et al. Activity of a next generation integrase inhibitor (INI), S/GSK1349572, in subjects with HIV exhibiting raltegravir resistance: initial results of VIKING study (ING112961). International AIDS Conference, Vienna, Austria, July 19–23, 2010. Abstract MOAB010.
39. Bangsberg DR, Weiser S, Guzman D, Riley E. 95% adherence is not necessary for viral suppression to less than 400 copies/mL in the majority of individuals on NNRTI regimens. Conference on Retroviruses and Opportunistic Infections, Boston, MA, February 22–25, 2005. Abstract 616.
40. Weber R, Sabin CA, Friis-Møller N, et al. Liver-related deaths in persons infected with the human immunodeficiency virus: the D:A:D study. Arch Intern Med. 2006;166:1632–41.
41. Crum NF, Riffenburgh RH, Wegner S, Agan BK, Tasker SA, et al. Comparisons of causes of death and mortality rates among HIV-infected persons: analysis of the pre-, early, and late HAART (Highly Active Antiretroviral Therapy) eras. JAIDS. 2006;41:194–200.
42. http://www.fda.gov/medwatch/safety/2007/Baraclude_DHCP_02-2007.pdf. Accessed August 30, 2010.
43. Low E, Cox A, Atkins M, Nelson M. Telbivudine has activity against HIV. 16th Conference on Retroviruses and Opportunistic Infections. Montreal, Canada. February 8–11, 2009. Abstract 813a.
44. Avila C, Karwowska S, Lai C, Evans T. Telbivudine has no in vitro activity against laboratory and clinical HIV-1, including 5 clades and drug-resistant clinical isolates. 16th Conference on Retroviruses and Opportunistic Infections. Montreal, Canada. February 8–11, 2009. Abstract 813b.
45. Jain MK, Comanor L, White C, et al. Treatment of hepatitis B with lamivudine and tenofovir in HIV/HBV-coinfected patients: factors associated with response. J Viral Hepat. 2007;14:176–82.
46. Lampertico P, Vigano M, Manenti E, et al. Low resistance to adefovir combined with lamivudine: a 3-year study of 145 lamivudine-resistant hepatitis B patients. Gastroenterology. 2007;133:1445–51.
47. Centers for Disease Control and Prevention. Guidelines for Prevention and Treatment of Opportunistic Infections in HIV-

Infected Adults and Adolescents. Recommendations from CDC, the National Institutes of Health, and the HIV Medicine Association of the Infectious Diseases Society of America. MMWR 2009; 58 (No. RR-4):80–83.

48. Panel on Treatment of HIV-Infected Pregnant Women and Prevention of Perinatal Transmission. Recommendations for use of antiretroviral drugs in pregnant HIV-1-infected women for maternal health and interventions to reduce perinatal HIV transmission in the United States. May 24, 2010; pp. 1–117. Available at http://aidsinfo.nih.gov/ContentFiles/PerinatalGL.pdf. Accessed Sept. 12, 2010, 49–52.

49. Opravil M, Sasadeusz J, Cooper DA, Rockstroh JK, Clumeck N, et al. Effect of baseline CD4 cell count on the efficacy and safety of peginterferon Alfa-2a (40KD) plus ribavirin in patients with HIV/hepatitis C virus coinfection. J Acquir Immune Defic Syndr. 2008;47(1):36–49.

50. Sulkowski M. Drug-induced liver injury associated with antiretroviral therapy that includes HIV-1 protease inhibitors. Clin Infect Dis. 2004;38 Suppl 2:590–7.

51. Dieterich DT, Robinson PA, Love J, Stern JO. Drug-induced liver injury associated with the use of nonnucleoside reverse transcriptase inhibitors. Clin Infect Dis. 2004;38 Suppl 2:580–9.

Pathology of HIV-Associated Liver Disease

Amy E. Noffsinger and Jiang Wang

Introduction

Human immunodeficiency virus (HIV), commonly affects the liver and biliary tract, although the types of HIV-associated liver disorders have changed with the recent availability of highly active antiretroviral therapy (HAART) [1, 2]. Before the introduction HAART, mycobacterial infection of the liver was the most commonly diagnosed opportunistic infection. In one study that examined liver biopsies from 501 HIV-positive individuals in the USA, granulomatous hepatitis – usually due to mycobacteria – was the most common finding [3]. Mycobacterium avium complex (MAC) and *Mycobacterium tuberculosis* are most commonly isolated in patients with CD4 cell counts less than 50 cells/μl. Other opportunistic hepatobiliary infections commonly diagnosed prior to the advent of HAART, include *Cytomegalovirus*, *Toxoplasma gondii*, Leishmaniasis, and *Cryptococcus neoformans*. Since the introduction of HAART, a dramatic reduction has been observed in disseminated infections caused by Mycobacterial species, *Cytomegalovirus*, and *Cryptococcus*.

Currently, most liver disease in HIV-infected patients is the result of chronic viral hepatitis. Approximately 25% of HIV-positive individuals in the USA, Europe, and Australia also have chronic Hepatitis C [4]. Therefore, coinfection with HIV and the various hepatotropic viruses has become a critical clinical issue. Several studies have shown that HIV-1 affects outcome in patients with chronic hepatitis B (HBV) and hepatitis C viral (HCV) infections [5, 6]. HAART has improved survival rates among patients infected with HIV but may be associated with increased mortality related to progression of chronic hepatitis C viral infection and liver failure [6, 7]. In addition, HIV-positive patients consume many prescription drugs for prophylaxis and therapy some of which may be hepatotoxic. As a result, drug-induced liver disease is relatively common among HIV-infected persons. It is important to note, however, that the opportunistic infections commonly seen prior to the era of HAART are still seen commonly among HIV-positive patients in areas of the world where highly active antiretroviral drugs are not readily available.

General Features of HIV-Associated Liver Disease

Hepatomegaly is common among HIV-infected patients in industrialized countries (60–75% of cases) [8]. The frequency of this finding, however, may differ depending on the geographical location since autopsy studies from Africa show no differences in the liver size among HIV-positive versus HIV-negative patients [9]. Mild-to-moderate macrovesicular steatosis is also common in liver biopsies and autopsy material from HIV-positive patients. This is particularly true in patients affected by AIDS. Other HIV-associated biopsy findings include moderate nonspecific lymphocytic inflammation of portal tracts and hemosiderin deposition in Kupffer cells, (usually secondary to blood transfusion). Granulomas are identified in liver biopsies in up to one third of HIV-positive patients [10–12] (Fig. 4.1). The main causes of granulomas are MAC infection, tuberculosis, and fungal infections (see below). Other findings include venoocclusive disease (likely drug induced) [13] and nodular regenerative hyperplasia [14].

Liver biopsies in patients with HIV infection also commonly demonstrate evidence of bile duct injury. This injury leads to HIV-associated cholangiopathy in some patients [15, 16]. Cholestasis may also be present and under some circumstances may mimic large bile duct obstruction.

A.E. Noffsinger (✉)
Caris Life Center, 9978 Washington Street,
Camp Dennison, OH 45111, USA
e-mail: anoffsinger@carisls.com

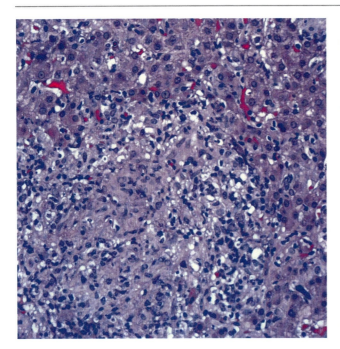

Fig. 4.1 Portal granuloma. A nonnecrotizing granuloma is present in a portal tract. It is composed of epithelioid cells and surrounding lymphocytes

HIV-Associated Liver Infection

Viral Hepatitis

HIV coinfection with hepatitis C virus (HCV), hepatitis B virus (HBV) is not uncommon given the similar risk factors for these infections. There is no evidence of an association between HIV and hepatitis A virus infection.

Hepatitis B

In the USA and Europe, approximately 8% of HIV-infected individuals are coinfected with HBV [17, 18]. In other regions of the world where the incidence of HBV infection is higher, a larger proportion of HIV-positive persons are coinfected [19]. HIV-positive men infected with hepatitis B virus are at increased risk for becoming chronic HBV carriers as CD4 lymphocyte counts decrease [20]. Additionally, HIV infection appears to facilitate reactivation of HBV in patients who had earlier become hepatitis B surface antigen negative [21]. Clinically, HIV-positive HBV patients are less likely to develop chronic hepatitis following infection than are HIV-negative individuals [22]. Overall, liver-related mortality is 17-fold higher in HIV-positive individuals with HBV than in HIV-negative HBV-infected patients [17]. Similarly, liver disease-associated mortality is higher in HIV-positive patients with HBV than those who are HBV surface antigen negative [18].

Liver biopsy studies demonstrate that HIV-positive patients have less active chronic hepatitis, less scarring and a lower incidence of cirrhosis than non-HIV-infected patients. In addition, expression of hepatitis BeAg and hepatitis B viral DNA polymerase is greater in HIV-positive patients, suggesting that HBV DNA replication is more active in these individuals [22]. HIV may also be associated with development of fibrosing cholestatic hepatitis in HBV e-antigen-positive persons [15, 23, 24].

Hepatitis C

HCV and HIV coinfection are common given the common risk factors for contracting these infections. The likelihood of HIV and HCV coinfection, however, depends on the mode of transmission of the viruses. Over 60% of individuals who acquired HIV as a result of intravenous drug use also have chronic hepatitis C [25]. By contrast, HCV infection occurs in less than 5% of men who acquired HIV through sexual contact with other men [26]. The long-term biological effects of coinfection are currently under active investigation. Initial studies suggested that progression of HCV-related liver disease is unchanged or even milder in HIV-positive patients [27]. Studies with longer follow-up, however, have shown that HCV behaves as an opportunistic infection in HIV-positive patients especially in the later stages of the disease. HCV-infected HIV-positive patients have a reduced likelihood of clearing the HCV infection and likely progress more rapidly to end-stage liver disease than do non-HIV-positive HCV-infected individuals [28–33]. The HCV effects are correlated with the severity of HIV-related immunosuppression. The development of HCV-related hepatocellular carcinoma also appears to be accelerated in HIV-positive individuals [34]. In addition, studies suggest that HCV coinfection accelerates progression to AIDS and death due to HIV [35, 36]. The degree to which this occurs appears to be HCV genotype dependent.

The histologic spectrum of changes seen in liver biopsies of patients with combined HCV liver disease and HIV positivity is wide and usually not specific. In many patients, the histologic findings do not differ from those observed in HIV-negative HCV-infected persons. However, in some, superimposed effects of drug injury may complicate the histologic picture. Several studies have demonstrated increased portal, periportal, and lobular inflammation and higher grades of activity in HIV/HCV-infected individuals (Fig. 4.2) [37–40]. In addition, the stage of fibrosis is often higher and cirrhosis develops more rapidly in coinfected patients, especially in the subgroup whose CD4 T lymphocyte counts are less than 200 cells/μl. Some studies have also shown that pericellular fibrosis is more common in coinfected patients [38, 41]. Occasionally, HIV/HCV-infected individuals may develop an autoimmune-like hepatitis (Fig. 4.3) [42].

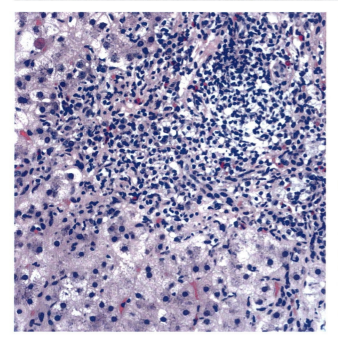

Fig. 4.2 HCV in HIV. The portal tract contains abundant chronic inflammatory cells with a lymphoid aggregate and marked interface activity

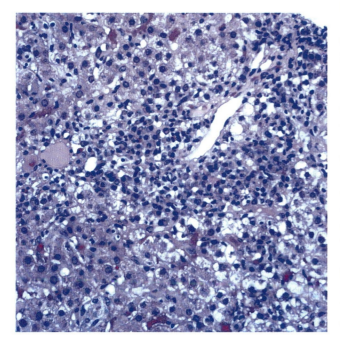

Fig. 4.3 Autoimmune-like hepatitis. This portal tract contains numerous plasma cells associated with marked interface activity and hepatocyte injury

Other Viral Infections

Cytomegalovirus

Reactivation of *Cytomegalovirus* infection is common in HIV-infected patients, but CMV rarely causes significant disease until CD4 lymphocyte counts decrease to less than 50 cells/µl. In general, hepatic disease due to parenchymal *Cytomegalovirus* infection is minimal [43]. In up to 10% of patients, liver biopsy shows rare *Cytomegalovirus* inclusions in hepatocytes, Kupffer cells and most commonly, endothelial cells. CMV inclusions may be associated with a small zone of necrosis or microabscess formation. Rarely, CMV infection may cause severe bile duct necrosis or a form of injury resembling sclerosing cholangitis.

Herpes Simplex Virus

Disseminated HSV infection is uncommon in patients with HIV. Those that do become infected, however, may present with liver failure. Autopsy studies have shown liver enlargement with hepatic necrosis affecting primarily zones 2 and 3, multinucleated hepatocytes, ground glass nuclear inclusions, and minimal inflammation [44].

Varicella–Zoster Virus

Varicella–zoster virus is a rare cause of fulminant hepatitis in immunocompromised patients including those who are HIV-positive [45]. Liver biopsy may reveal a severe acute hepatitis with confluent necrosis of hepatocytes. Typical herpes virus type nuclear inclusions are identified.

Epstein–Barr Virus

Epstein–Barr virus (EBV) is associated with lymphoproliferative disorders affecting many lymphoid organs in patients with HIV. The liver may sometimes be involved in this process. An EBV associated hemophagocytic syndrome has also been described [46].

Adenovirus

Adenovirus hepatitis occurs almost exclusively in HIV-positive children and occasionally young adults. Histologically, there is extensive zone 3 hepatocyte necrosis associated with little inflammation. Intranuclear viral inclusions are usually numerous [47, 48].

Bacterial Infections

Mycobacterium tuberculosis

Tuberculosis is highly prevalent among HIV-positive patients in Africa and India, and its incidence is increasing in industrialized countries [49]. In one African autopsy study [50], 50% of adults dying of AIDS had active tuberculosis. 85% of these patients have liver involvement. A similar study performed in India demonstrated that 41% of AIDS patients had tuberculosis involving the liver [51].

Grossly, the liver may demonstrate multiple miliary-type lesions or a single or multiple masses. The microscopic findings vary depending on the degree of immunosuppression of the affected patient. Histologically, typical caseating granulomas with or without giant cells may be seen in patients with

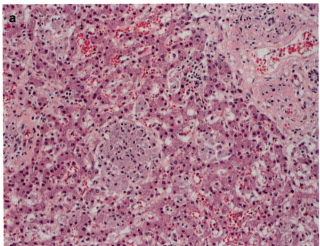

Fig. 4.4 Mycobacterium avium complex infection. (**a**) The portal tracts and lobular parenchyma contain numerous compact granulomas as well as less well-formed clusters of histiocytes. Sinusoidal histiocytic aggregates are also seen. (**b**) An acid-fast stain (Ziehl-Neelson) demonstrates large numbers of bacteria within the histiocytes

lesser degrees of immunocompromise. Among patients with end-stage HIV disease, histologic liver examination more commonly demonstrates foci of necrosis surrounded by degenerating macrophages containing large numbers of acid-fast bacilli [52].

Other *Mycobacterium* Species

The prevalence of Mycobacterium avium complex (MAC) infection among HIV-positive individuals varies geographically. It is rare in developing countries, and it occurs more commonly in patients with severe HIV-associated immunocompromise. MAC infection is commonly associated clinically with an elevated serum alkaline phosphatase level, most likely as a result of compression of the biliary tree by enlarged mycobacteria-containing lymph nodes. Microscopically, nonnecrotizing granulomas containing acid-fast bacilli may be seen (Fig. 4.4). In patients with more severe immunocompromise, hepatic parenchymal abscesses containing clusters of histiocytes and massive numbers of acid-fast bacilli may be seen. Rarely, disseminated *Mycobacterium kansasii* infection occurs in patients with end-stage HIV/AIDS [53]. The liver may sometimes be involved in such patients. Histologically, the liver contains numerous small intrahepatic granulomas containing acid-fast organisms.

Bacillary Angiomatosis

In HIV-positive patients, bacillary angiomatosis, characterized by the presence of multiple blood-filled cystic spaces of the liver (peliosis hepatis), is associated with infection with the bacterial organism *Bartonella henselae*. This organism causes both bacillary angiomatosis and cat scratch disease. The lesions of bacillary angiomatosis are visible as red spots underlying the capsule of the liver. The liver may be markedly enlarged. Histologically, numerous small blood-filled cysts (1–4 mm) are seen within the parenchyma of the liver. Some cysts may contain a partial endothelial lining. The adjacent sinusoids often appear ectatic. The bacteria are identifiable on Warthin–Starry stained sections.

Q Fever

Serologic studies suggest an infection with *Coxiella burnetii*, the organism associated with Q fever, is as many as three times more common among HIV-positive than among HIV-negative individuals [54]. The course of the disease and its treatment, however, do not differ depending on HIV status. Liver biopsy demonstrates granulomatous hepatitis.

Fungal Infection

Many disseminated fungal infections have been reported in AIDS patients. The most common organisms that are isolated include *Candida albicans, Cryptococcus neoformans, Histoplasma capsulatum, Coccidioides imitis,* and *Pneumocystis jiroveci*. Other fungal infections occur, but are uncommon.

Candida

Candida infection occurs commonly in HIV-positive patients. Liver involvement may occur in as many as 14% of patients in industrialized countries [12]. Histologically, small necrotizing abscesses containing yeast and pseudohyphal forms of the organism are identifiable.

Cryptococcus

In one study, *Cryptococcus* was identified in livers of 5% of Indian AIDS patients at autopsy [51]. The liver may be enlarged and microscopically there is a diffuse intracellular accumulation of fungi within Kupffer cells and portal macrophages.

Histoplasma

The frequency with which histoplasmosis occurs in HIV-infected patients depends on their geographic location. *Histoplasma* infection is rare in Europe, Asia, and Australia, but is relatively common in the USA [8, 55]. Liver involvement by *Histoplasma* has been reported in 1–4% of AIDS patients in the USA. Liver biopsy demonstrates multiple small granulomas dispersed throughout the hepatic parenchyma and portal tracts. Budding yeasts measuring 3–5 μ in diameter are identifiable with the use of fungal stains. Kupffer cells may also contain fungi.

Coccidioides

Coccidioidomycosis is restricted to the Americas and affects the liver as a part of disseminated disease in AIDS patients. Histologically, the liver contains granulomas containing the characteristic *Coccidioides* spherules.

Pneumocystis

Prior to the development of HAART, 85% of AIDS patients developed *Pneumocystis* pneumonia at some time during the course of their disease. Spread of the infection to extrapulmonary sites occurs when the CD4 T lymphocyte count drop to less than 50 cells/μl and is often associated with the use of nebulizer antibiotic therapy for *Pneumocystis* pneumonia. The liver is involved in up to 40% of such cases. Microscopically, focal areas of sinusoidal dilation and liver cell necrosis are present. These foci contain extracellular foamy pink material similar to that seen in the lungs of patients infected with *Pneumocystis*. Grocott staining demonstrates the characteristic cysts with folded membranes and a solid dark spot within the cytoplasm.

Protozoal Infection

Toxoplasmosis. Disseminated toxoplasmosis is not common in AIDS patients. Occasionally, however, hepatic lesions are encountered at autopsy in those patients who do become infected. *Toxoplasma* organisms may be identified within parasitized hepatocytes which are surrounded by scattered lymphocytes and neutrophils. Occasionally, larger necrotic lesions may occur [56].

Leishmaniasis. Like many other opportunistic infections in AIDS patients, the prevalence of leishmaniasis varies geographically. Most species of *Leishmania* are limited to southern Europe, South America, and Africa. The parasitic organisms, however, may remain dormant in the body for many years only to become reactivated as the patient becomes increasingly immunocompromised. Most HIV-positive patients with visceral leishmaniasis are intravenous drug abusers. These patients are typically European and are infected with *Leishmania infantum* [57]. Most affected patients already have AIDS and CD4+T lymphocyte counts less than 150 cells/μl. HIV-positive patients with visceral leishmaniasis may present clinically in atypical ways compared with HIV-negative patients. Hepatosplenomegaly is less common and antileishmanial serology is often negative [58]. Approximately 25% of patients die within one month presentation [59]. Liver biopsy demonstrates numerous amastigotes within Kupffer cells and portal macrophages. Occasionally, organisms are seen within endothelial cells [60–62]. Rarely, biopsy may show significant liver cell necrosis or nodular regenerative hyperplasia [63, 64].

Liver Tumors in HIV-Infected Patients

Kaposi's Sarcoma

Kaposi's sarcoma involving the liver is not an uncommon finding in HIV-positive patients living in industrialized countries. The incidence is lower in HIV-infected patients living in developing countries. The frequency with which Kaposi's sarcoma is identified, however, has declined in association with antiretroviral therapy [65]. Gross examination of the liver may show capsular deposits of tumor measuring 0.5–1 cm in diameter. The lesions are dark red in color. On cut section, multiple dark red spots may also be identifiable within the hepatic parenchyma. Histologically, the lesion is comprised of a bland spindle cell proliferation arising around bile ducts. The spindle cell proliferation produces slit-like spaces containing erythrocytes. Intracytoplasmic eosinophilic inclusions may be identified. Immunohistochemistry for HHV 8 is helpful in establishing the diagnosis.

Hepatocellular Carcinoma

The incidence of hepatocellular carcinomas in patients with HIV infection is increasing [65, 66]. Hepatocellular carcinoma arising in the setting of HIV almost invariably is associated with coinfection with hepatitis B or hepatitis C virus (Fig. 4.5). It is likely that the increased longevity currently seen in HIV/HCV or HIV/HBV-positive individuals due to HAART results in decreased mortality from AIDS, but an increase in development of end-stage liver disease and hepatocellular carcinoma [67].

Lymphoma

Liver involvement occurs in approximately 25% of HIV patients with lymphoma. It may be the primary site of

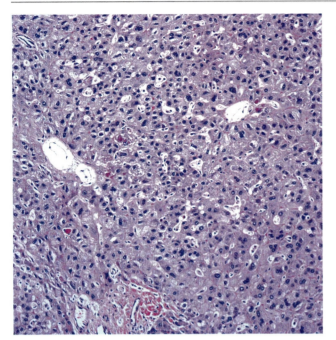 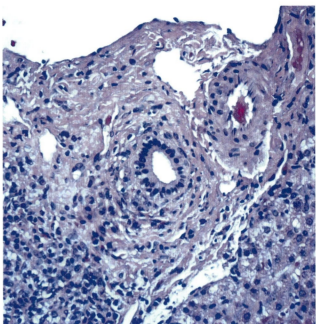

Fig. 4.5 Hepatocellular carcinoma. Moderately differentiated hepatocellular carcinoma in a patient with cirrhosis secondary to HIV and HCV infection

Fig. 4.6 Bile duct injury. The bile duct is infiltrated with lymphocytes (cholangitis) and the nuclei of epithelial cells are enlarged and overlap one another. There is associated periductal fibrosis

tumor [68]. Grossly, lymphomas often appear diffuse, but occasionally mass lesions may be seen. When mass lesions are present, they are often necrotic and can mimic tuberculosis or MAC infection. Primary bile duct lymphomas also occur, which may clinically and radiographically mimic sclerosing cholangitis [69]. Histologically, HIV-associated lymphomas are often centroblastic or immunoblastic in type and may contain cells with bizarre polylobated nuclei. Epstein–Barr viral infection is likely an important pathogenic factor in the development of HIV-associated lymphoma. HHV 8 infection may also play a role in lymphoma development [70].

HIV-Associated Biliary Disease

Cholangitis

Two types of cholangitis occur in HIV-positive patients: ascending bacterial cholangitis and HIV-associated sclerosing cholangitis. Bacterial cholangitis is usually associated with gram-negative bacilli and resembles the disease seen in non-HIV-infected patients. HIV-associated sclerosing cholangitis is increasingly recognized as a complication of advanced immunocompromised. The median CD4-positive T-lymphocyte count in patients with this disorder is 24 cells/μl [71]. The disease is characterized clinically by chronic abdominal pain, fever and cholestasis with dilation and irregularity of the bile ducts. Both intra- and extrahepatic bile ducts are affected (Fig. 4.6). The diagnosis is usually made by ERCP. HIV-associated sclerosing cholangitis has been associated with some infectious agents including *Cryptosporidium*, Microsporidia, and *Cytomegalovirus* [71–74].

Drug Toxicity in HIV Liver Disease

Drug reactions are increasingly an important cause of liver injury in patients with HIV infection. In industrialized countries, HIV-positive patients have access to many pharmaceutical agents, and as a result, the potential for drug interaction is high. Many of the antiretroviral and other drugs taken by these patients are hepatotoxic. HAART itself has significant hepatotoxicity and may result in severe liver damage, liver failure, and death. Histologic findings in patients with acute liver failure associated with antiretroviral therapy include microvesicular steatosis, confluent hepatocellular necrosis, inflammation, and cholestasis (Fig. 4.7) [75]. Recurrent HCV infection likely renders the liver more susceptible to toxic injury from antiretroviral therapy [76]. Some forms of antiretroviral therapy may additionally accelerate the development of fibrosis in HCV-infected patients [77].

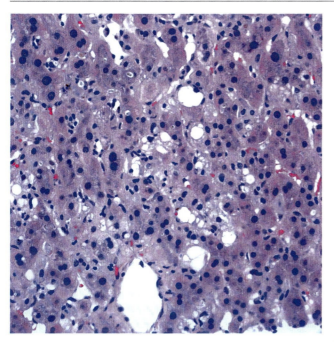

Fig. 4.7 HAART injury. The pericentral area shows marked hepatocytic and canalicular cholestasis associated with steatosis and scattered lymphocytes

References

1. Torre D, Speranza F, Martegani R. Impact of highly active antiretroviral therapy on organ specific manifestations of HIV-1 infection. HIV Med. 2005;6:66–78.
2. Thomas DL. Growing importance of liver disease in HIV-infected persons. Hepatology. 2006;43:S221–9.
3. Poles MA, Dieterich DT, Schwarz ED, et al. Liver biopsy findings in 501 patients infected with human immunodeficiency virus (HIV). J Acquir Immune Def Syndr Hum Retrovirol. 1996;11:170–7.
4. Sherman KE, Rouster SD, Chung RT, Rajicic N. Hepatitis C virus prevalence among patients infected with human immunodeficiency virus: a cross-sectional analysis of the US adult AIDS Clinical Trials Group. Clin Infect Dis. 2002;34:831–7.
5. Bodsworth N, Donovan B, Nightgale B. The effect of concurrent human immunodeficiency virus infection on chronic hepatitis B: A study of 150 homosexual men. J Infect Dis. 1989;160:577–82.
6. Eyster ME, Diamondstone LS, Lien JM, et al. The natural history of hepatitis C virus infection in multitransfused hemophiliacs: effect of coinfection with human immunodeficiency virus. J Acquir Immune Defic Syndr. 1993;6:602–10.
7. Soto B, Sanchez-Quijano A, Rodrigo L, et al. Reactivation of hepatitis B virus replication accompanied by acute hepatitis in patients receiving highly active antiretroviral therapy. J Hepatol. 1997;26:1–5.
8. Bonacini M. Hepatobiliary complications in patients with human immunodeficiency virus infection. Am J Med. 1992;92:404–11.
9. Lucas SB. Other viral and infectious disease and HIV-related liver disease. In: Burt AD, Portmann BC, Ferrell LD, editors. MacSween's pathology of the liver. 5th ed. Philadelphia, PA: Churchill Livingstone Elsevier; 2007. p. 443–91.
10. Centers for disease control and prevention. Revision of the CDC surveillance case definition for AIDS. MMWR. 1987;36:1S–15S
11. Buehler JW, Ward JW. A new case definition for AIDS surveillance. Ann Intern Med. 1993;118:390–2.
12. Klatt EC. Practical AIDS pathology. Chicago: ASCP press; 1992.
13. Vispo EA, Moreno AB, Maida IA, et al. Noncirrhotic portal hypertension in HIV-infected patients: unique clinical and pathological findings. AIDS. 2010;24:1171–6.
14. Dinh MH, Stosor V, Rao SM, Miller FH, Green RM. Cryptogenic liver disease in HIV-seropositive men. HIV Med. 2009;10:447–53.
15. Tolan DJ, Davies MH, Millson CE. The fibrosing cholestatic hepatitis after liver transplantation in a patient with hepatitis C and HIV infection. N Engl J Med. 2001;345:1781.
16. Cappell MS. Hepatobiliary manifestations of the acquired immune deficiency syndrome. Am J Gastroenterol. 1991;86:861–915.
17. Thio CL, Seaberg EC, Skolashky RL, et al. HIV-1, hepatitis B virus, and risk of liver-related mortality in the multicenter AIDS cohort study (MACS). Lancet. 2002;360:1921–6.
18. Konopnicki D, Mocroft A, De Wit S, et al. Hepatitis B and HIV: prevalence, AIDS progression, response to highly active antiretroviral therapy and increased mortality in the Euro-SIDA cohort. AIDS. 2005;19:593–601.
19. Otegbayo JA, Fasola FA, Abja A. Prevalence of hepatitis B surface and e antigens, risk factors for viral acquisition end of serum transaminase among blood donors in Ibadan, Nigeria. Trop Gastroenterol. 2003;24:196–7.
20. Bodsworth NJ, Cooper DA, Donovan B. The influence of human immunodeficiency virus type I infection on the development of hepatitis B virus carrier state. J Infect Dis. 1991;163:1138–40.
21. Waite J, Gilson RJ, Weller IV, et al. Hepatitis B virus reactivation or reinfection associated with HIV-1 infection. AIDS. 1988;2:443–8.
22. Goldin RD, Fish DE, Hay A, et al. Histological and immunohistochemical study of hepatitis B virus and human immunodeficiency virus infection. J Clin Pathol. 1990;43:203–5.
23. Rosenberg PM, Farrell JJ, Abraczinskas DR, Graeme-Cook FM, Dienstag JL, Chung RT. Rapidly progressive fibrosing cholestatic hepatitis – hepatitis C virus in HIV coinfection. Am J Gastroenterol. 2002;97:478–3.
24. Fang JW, Wright TL, Lau JY. Fibrosing cholestatic hepatitis in patients with HIV and hepatitis B. Lancet. 1993;342:1175.
25. Garfein RS, Doherty MC, Monterroso ER, et al. Prevalence and incidence of hepatitis C virus infection among young adult injection drug users. J Acquir Immunodef Syndr Hum Retrovirol. 1998;18 Suppl 1:S11–9.
26. Sulkowski MS, Thomas DL. Hepatitis C in the HIV-infected person. Ann Intern Med. 2003;138:197–207.
27. Vento S, Cruciani M, Di Perri G, et al. Hepatitis C virus with normal liver histology in symptomless HIV-1 infection. Lancet. 1992;340:1161.
28. Thomas DL, Astemborski J, Rai RM, et al. The natural history of hepatitis C virus infection: host, viral, and environmental factors. JAMA. 2000;284:450–6.
29. Garcia-Samaniego J, Soriano V, Castilla J, et al. Influence of hepatitis C virus genotypes and HIV infection on histological severity of chronic hepatitis C. The hepatitis/HIV Spanish study group. Am J Gastroenterol. 1997;92:1130–4.
30. Bierhoff E, Fischer HP, Willsch E, et al. Liver histopathology in patients with concurrent chronic hepatitis C and HIV infection. Virchows Arch [A]. 1997;430:271–7.
31. Dragoni F, Cafolla A, Gentile G, et al. HIV-HCV RNA loads and liver failure in coinfected patients with coagulopathy. Haematologica. 1999;A4:525–9.
32. Lesens O, Deschenes M, Steben M, Belanger G, Tsoukas CM. Hepatitis C virus is related to progressive liver disease in HIV+ve hemophiliacs and should be treated as an opportunistic infection. J Infect Dis. 1999;179:1254–8.

33. Ghany MG, Leissinger C, Lagier R, Sanchez-Pescador R, Lok AS. Effect of HIV infection of hepatitis C virus infection and hemophiliacs. Dig Dis Sci. 1998;17:167–70.
34. Garcia-Samaniego J, Rodriguez M, Berenguer J, et al. Hepatocellular carcinoma in HIV-infected patients with chronic hepatitis C. Am J Gastroenterol. 2001;96:179–83.
35. Sabin CA, Telfer P, Phillips AN, Bhagani S, Lee CA. The association between hepatitis C virus genotype and HIV disease progression in a cohort of hemophiliac men. J Infect Dis. 1997;175:164–8.
36. Piroth L, Duong M, Quantin C, et al. Does hepatitis C virus coinfection accelerate the clinical and immunological evolution of HIV-infected patients? AIDS. 1999;12:381–8.
37. Benhamou Y, Martino V, Bochet M, et al. Factors affecting liver fibrosis in human immunodeficiency virus and hepatitis C virus co-infected patients: Impacted of protease inhibitor therapy. Hepatology. 2001;34:283–7.
38. Marks K, Petrovic LM, Talal AH, et al. Histopathological findings and clinical characteristics associated with hepatic steatosis in patien's co-infected with HIV and hepatitis C virus. J Infect Dis. 2005;192:1943–9.
39. Allory Y, Charlotte F, Benhamou Y, et al. Impact of human immunodeficiency virus infection on the histological features of chronic hepatitis C: a case control study. Hum Pathol. 2000;31:69–74.
40. Bani-Sadr F, Carrat F, Bedossa P, et al. Hepatic steatosis in HIV/HCV co-infected patients: analysis of risk factors. AIDS. 2006;20:525–31.
41. McGovern BH, Ditelberg JS, Taylor LE, et al. Hepatic steatosis is associated with fibrosis, nucleoside analog use, and hepatitis C virus genotype 3 infection in HIV seropositive patients. Clin Infect Dis. 2006;43:365–72.
42. Petrovic LM. HIV/HCV co-infection: histopathologic findings, natural history, fibrosis, and impact of antiretroviral treatment: a review article. Liver Int. 2007;5:598–606.
43. Palmer M, Braly LF, Schaffner F. The liver in AIDS disease. Semin Liv Dis. 1987;7:192–202.
44. Zimmerli W, Bianchi L, Gudat F, et al. Disseminated herpes simplex type 2 and systemic *Candida* infection in a patient with previous asymptomatic HIV infection. J Infect Dis. 1988;157:597–8.
45. Lechiche C, Le Moing V, Francois Perrigault P, Reynes J. Fulminant varicella hepatitis in a human immunodeficiency virus infected patient: case report and review of the literature. Scand J Infect Dis. 2006;38:929–31.
46. Albrecht H, Schafer H, Stellbrink HJ, Greten H. Epstein–Barr-virus-associated hemophagocytic syndrome. A cause of fever of unknown origin in HIV infection. Arch Pathol Lab Med. 1997;121:853–8.
47. Janner D, Petru AM, Belchis D, Azimi PH. Fatal adenovirus infection in the child with acquired immunodeficiency syndrome. Pediatr Infec Dis J. 1990;9:434–6.
48. Krilov LR, Rubin LG, Frogel M, et al. Disseminated adenovirus infection with hepatic necrosis in patients with human immunodeficiency virus infection and other immunodeficiency states. Rev Infect Dis. 1990;12:303–7.
49. De Cock KM, Soro B, Coulibaly IM, Lucas SB. Tuberculosis and HIV infection in sub-Saharan Africa. JAMA. 1992;268:1581–7.
50. Lucas SB, Hounnou A, Peacock CS, et al. The mortality and pathology of HIV disease in a West African city. AIDS. 1993;7:1569–79.
51. Lanjewar DN, Rao RJ, Kulkarni S, Hira SK. Hepatic pathology in AIDS: a pathological study from mom Mumbai, India. HIV Med. 2004;5:253–7.
52. Nambuya A, Sewankambo NK, Mugerwa J, Goodgame RW, Lucas SB. Tuberculous lymphadenitis associated with human immunodeficiency virus (HIV) in Uganda. J Clin Pathol. 1988;41:93–6.
53. Smith MB, Molina CP, Schnadig VJ, et al. Pathologic features of *Mycobacterium kansasii* infection in patients with acquired immunodeficiency syndrome. Arch Pathol Lab Med. 2003;127:554–60.
54. Raoult D, Levy PY, Dupont HT, et al. Q fever and HIV infection. AIDS. 1993;7:81–6.
55. Freiman JP, Helfert KE, Hamrell MR, Stein DS. Hepatomegaly with severe steatosis in HIV-seropositive patients. AIDS. 1993;7:379–85.
56. Artigas J, Grosse G, Niedobitek F. Anergic disseminated toxoplasmosis in a patient with the acquired immunodeficiency syndrome. Arch Pathol Lab Med. 1993;117:540–1.
57. Albrecht H, Sobottka I, Emminger C, et al. Visceral leishmaniasis emerging as an important opportunistic infection in HIV-infected persons living in areas non-endemic for Leishmania donovani. Arch Pathol Lab Med. 1997;121:189–98.
58. Peters BS, Fish DF, Goldin R, et al. Visceral leishmaniasis in HIV infection and AIDS: clinical features and response to therapy. Q J Med. 1990;77:1101–11.
59. Lopez-Velez R, Perez-Molina JA, Guerrero A, et al. Clinicoepidemiologic characteristics, prognostic factors, in survival analysis of patients coinfection with HIV and leishmania in area of Madrid, Spain. Am J Trop Med Hyg. 1998;58:436–43.
60. Wilkins MJ, Lindley R, Doukaris SP, Goldin RD. Surgical pathology of the liver in HIV infection. Histopathology. 1991;18:459–64.
61. Hofman V, Marty P, Perrin C, et al. The histological spectrum of visceral leishmaniasis caused by Leishmania infantum MON-1 in AIDS. Hum Pathol. 2000;31:75–84.
62. Falk S, Helm EB, Hubner K, Stutte HJ. Disseminated visceral leishmaniasis (kala azar) in acquired immunodeficiency syndrome (AIDS). Path Res Pract. 1989;183:253–5.
63. Angarano G, Maggi P, Rollo MA, et al. Diffuse necrotic hepatic lesions due to visceral leishmaniasis in AIDS. J Infect Dis. 1998;36:167–9.
64. Fernandez-Miranda C, Colina F, Delgado JM, Lopez-Carriera M. Diffuse nodular regenerative hyperplasia of the liver associated with HIV and visceral leishmaniasis. Am J Gastroenterol. 1993;88:433–5.
65. Simard EP, Pfeiffer RM, Engels EA. Cumulative incidence of cancer among individuals with acquired immunodeficiency syndrome in the United States. Cancer. 2010; Epub ahead of print.
66. Giordano TP, Kramer JR, Souchek J, Richardson P, El-Serag HB. Cirrhosis and hepatocellular carcinoma in HIV-infected veterans with and without hepatitis C virus: A cohort study, 1992–2001. Arch Pathol Lab Med. 2004;164:2349–54.
67. Rosenthal E, Poiree M, Pradier C, et al. Mortality due to hepatitis C-related liver disease in HIV-infected patients in France (Mortavic 2001 study). AIDS. 2003;17:1803–9.
68. Caccamo D, Pervez NK, Marchevsky A. Primary lymphoma of the liver in the acquired immunodeficiency syndrome. Arch Pathol Lab Med. 1986;110:553–5.
69. Kaplan LD, Kahn J, Jacobson M, Bottles K, Cello J. Primary bile duct lymphoma in the acquired immunodeficiency syndrome (AIDS). Ann Intern Med. 1989;110:161–2.
70. Cesarman E, Knowles DM. The role of Kaposi's sarcoma associated herpes virus (KSHV/HHV 8) in lymphoproliferative diseases. Semin Canc Biol. 1999;9:165–74.
71. Forbes A, Blanshard C, Gazzard BG. Natural history of AIDS sclerosing cholangitis: a study of 20 cases. Gut. 1993;34:116–21.
72. McGowan I, Hawkins AS, Weller IV. The natural history of cryptosporidial diarrhoea in HIV-infected patients. AIDS. 1993;7:349–54.
73. Shadduck JA, Orenstein JM. Comparative pathology of microsporidiosis. Arch Pathol Lab Med. 1993;117:1215–9.

74. Schwartz DA, Sobottka I, Leitch GJ, Cali A, Visvesvara GS. Pathology of microsporidiosis. Arch Pathol Lab Med. 1996;120:173–88.
75. Akhtar MA, Mathieson K, Arey B, et al. Hepatic histopathology and clinical characteristics associated with anti-retroviral therapy in HIV patients without viral hepatitis. Eur J Gastroenterol Hepatol. 2008;20:1194–204.
76. Sulkowski MS, Thomas DL, Chaisson RE, Moore RD. Hepatotoxicity associated with anti-retroviral therapy in adults infected with HIV and the role of hepatitis C or B virus infection. JAMA. 2000;283:74–80.
77. Marcias J, Castellano V, Merchante N, et al. Effects of antiretroviral drugs on liver fibrosis in HIV-infected patients with chronic hepatitis C: harmful impact of nevirapine. AIDS. 2004;18:767–74.

Noninvasive Markers of Liver Injury and Fibrosis

Jenny O. Smith and Richard K. Sterling

Background

With the increasing use of highly active antiretroviral therapy (HAART) for human immunodeficiency virus (HIV) management and the subsequent decline in morbidity and mortality secondary to opportunistic infections, greater attention is being paid to the natural history of hepatitis C virus (HCV) among HIV–HCV coinfected patients. Graham et al. [1] have shown a combined adjusted relative risk in coinfected patients for developing histological cirrhosis of 2.07 with a relative risk of 6.14 for the development of decompensated liver disease compared to HCV monoinfected patients. Coinfected patients are also as likely to die from end-stage liver disease (ESLD) as they are from HIV/AIDS. Salmon-Ceron et al. [2] found that mortality related to ESLD in those coinfected with HCV was 31% and similar to the mortality from HIV/AIDS (29%).

Accurate determination of the presence and degree of hepatic fibrosis is essential for predicting prognosis and for planning treatment of patients with chronic HCV infection [3] as well as for patients with HCV and HIV coinfection. Percutaneous liver biopsy is considered the gold standard for assessing hepatic fibrosis, [4] and has traditionally been considered the key diagnostic tool in determining the degree of inflammation and fibrosis in chronic liver disease [5]. Liver biopsy also provides additional information regarding factors that might affect disease progression or response to anti-HCV therapy, such as steatosis. Understanding the degree of liver damage provides useful information in determining prognosis in chronic HCV infection, with a favorable prognosis given in the absence of moderate to significant inflammation and fibrosis [6, 7]. However, given the faster progression of fibrosis in those with coinfection, even those with mild disease can be considered for therapy.

Liver biopsy, however, is invasive and carries a complication rate ranging from 1 to 5%, with the risk of mortality ranging from 1 in 1,000 to 1 in 10,000 [8–10]. In addition, biopsy is subject to sampling error and interobserver variability [11, 12]. Because of the risks associated with liver biopsy, there have been attempts to identify other noninvasive tests or surrogate markers that could accurately predict liver histology. Single laboratory tests such as serum aspartate aminotransferase (AST) and alanine aminotransferase (ALT), prothrombin time, albumin, or bilirubin alone, however, are insensitive to accurately predict the degree of fibrosis.

A high proportion of coinfected patients can have a normal ALT at the time of liver biopsy, despite having significant histologic abnormalities. In one cohort, nearly 50% of patients with HIV–HCV coinfection had a normal ALT defined by local laboratory testing at the time of biopsy [13, 14] compared to 20–30% in HCV monoinfected individuals [15, 16]. In a study of patients with and without abnormal ALT, the histologic spectrum of liver disease was similar in coinfected patients compared to HCV controls [13]. When coinfected patients were stratified by normal or abnormal ALT, no significant differences were seen in hepatic activity index (HAI) or its inflammation or fibrosis components. The prevalence of advanced fibrosis, defined as bridging fibrosis or cirrhosis, was 26% in those with normal ALT. These results are similar to a study performed by Uberti-Foppa et al. [17], who compared clinical and histologic features of coinfected patients with persistently normal ALT values to patients with elevated ALT levels. Liver biopsy was performed on all subjects with subgroup analysis based on Ishak fibrosis scores. Clinically significant fibrosis was defined as having an Ishak fibrosis score ranging from 2 to 6. Sixty-nine percent of the group with elevated ALT values were found to have clinically significant fibrosis that would conventionally be considered for treatment, and 25% of patients

J.O. Smith (✉)
Virginia Commonwealth University Medical Center/Medical College of Virginia, Room 1492, 1200 East Broad St West Hospital, Richmond, VA 23298, USA
e-mail: jsmith5@mcvh-vcu.edu

Table 5.1 Examples of clinical characteristics and noninvasive tests used to assess fibrosis

Demographics	Biochemical tests
Used to assess fibrosis	
Age	
Gender	International Normalized Ratio (INR)
	Platelet count
	AST
	ALT
	GGT
	Bilirubin
	Serum cholesterol
	Albumin
	Glucose
	Alkaline phosphatase
	Delta-2-macroglobulin
	Alpha-2-macroglobulin
	Haptoglobin
	Apolipoprotein A1
	Procollagen III peptide (PIIIP)
	Hyaluronic acid (HA)
	YKL-40
	Collagen types I–IV
	7 S domain of type IV collagen (7 S-IV)
	HCV RNA
	Serum transforming growth factor-beta1 (TGF-beta1)
	Hepatic growth factor
	TIMP-1
	MMP

Table 5.2 Models and imaging methods used to assess fibrosis

Models	Imaging methods
AST to ALT ratio	Abdominal ultrasonography
APRI	Ultrasound elastography (transient elastography)
Forns	Single photon emission computed tomography (SPECT)
FIB-4	
SHASTA	
Hospital Gregorio Marañón index (HGM-1,2,3)	
Fibrotest	
Hepascore	
Fibrometer	

with persistently normal ALT values were found to have clinically significant fibrosis. This study also demonstrated on multivariate analysis that a CD4 count <500 in patients with persistently normal ALT values was independently associated with a hepatic fibrosis stage fulfilling histologic criteria for treatment of HCV. This finding highlights the importance of determining degree of hepatic fibrosis in this subset of coinfected individuals. It has also been determined that hepatic clearance of nonnucleoside reverse transcriptase inhibitors, particularly efavirenz, is impaired in patients with cirrhosis, further demonstrating the need for assessment of fibrosis to identify coinfected patients who would benefit from therapeutic drug monitoring [18].

In light of these concerns, investigators have sought other noninvasive markers of hepatic fibrosis. Various biochemical markers and imaging modalities (Table 5.1) have been evaluated in the HCV monoinfected population and a subset of these modalities have been examined in the HIV–HCV coinfected population. Predictive models including demographic measures, biochemical markers and models using these markers, and imaging methods studied in the coinfected population are summarized in Table 5.2.

Noninvasive Fibrosis Assessment Using Biochemical Markers

There have been several models developed to help differentiate mild-moderate from advanced fibrosis in HIV–HCV coinfected patients. These models utilize both routine and nonroutine laboratory tests. Routine laboratory tests include secondary markers of liver injury and fibrosis including serum AST, ALT, and albumin, as well as indirect markers including platelet count. Nonroutine tests include measures of hepatic metabolic activity, extracellular matrix remodeling proteins, collagen synthesis and degradation products, and enzymes involved in matrix degradation. The pathophysiology of fibrosis formation and the role these biomarkers play are detailed in Fig. 5.1. Many of these models were initially developed for the HCV monoinfected population, but it has been determined that the correlation between fibrosis markers with fibrosis stage and diagnostic performance of these tests is similar in HCV monoinfected and HCV–HIV coinfected patients [19]. The area under the ROC, which assesses the utility of a test, was similar for many but not all models in both HCV and HCV/HIV coinfected subjects. An excellent test has an AUROC of 0.9 or greater compared to a standard. An AUROC of 0.80 is considered minimally acceptable as a diagnostic test and anything less is considered unacceptable.

Models Utilizing Routine Laboratory Tests

Several models utilizing routine laboratory tests have been developed. These include AST to ALT ratio (AAR), AST to platelet ratio index (APRI), the Forns index, SHASTA, FIB-4, and the Hospital Gregorio Marañón (HGM) indices. Models derived from routine tests would be are appealing because they are both cost-effective and readily available. However, they must accurately predict the desired outcome.

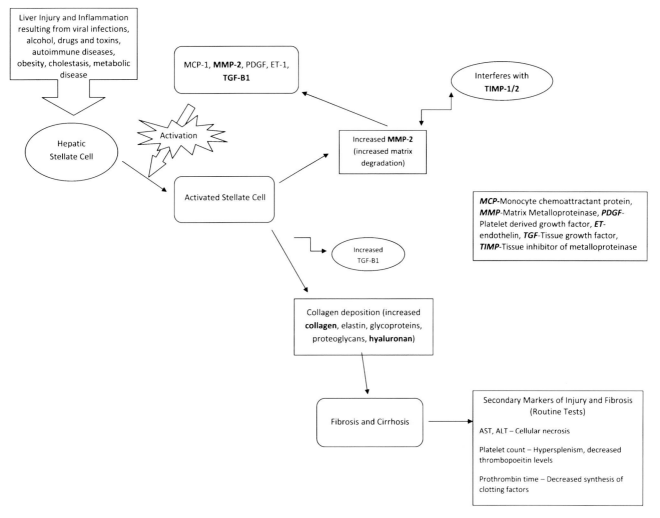

Fig. 5.1 Depicts stellate cell activation cascade. After injury cells become activated through the action of mediators including MCP-1, MMP-2, PDGF, ET-1, and TGF-B1. Increased MMP-2 interferes with TIMP-1,2 and continues the activation cascade, as does increased TGF-B1. The activated stellate cell also results increased collagen deposition by increasing collagen, elastin, glycoprotein, proteoglycan, and hyaluronan levels. This leads to fibrosis and cirrhosis. Secondary markers of liver injury and fibrosis include routine serum markers including AST, ALT, platelet count, prothrombin time, and albumin. *Bold* indicates the nonroutine markers and their role as discussed

AST to Platelet Ratiop Index (APRI)

The APRI is a formula that utilizes measurements of serum AST concentration and platelet count. Its value is determined by the formula [AST/(upper limit of normal)/platelet count $(10^9/L) \times 100$] [20]. APRI has been found to be accurate in estimating fibrosis in patients with HCV [21–23] and with HCV–HIV coinfection [24–26]. Al-Mohri et al. [24] demonstrated an AUROC of 0.847 for significant fibrosis in a coinfected cohort, with positive predictive value (PPV) of 100% for APRI >1.5 and 79% for APRI <0.5. Some studies, however, have reported that APRI cannot replace liver biopsy in the accurate staging of fibrosis in patients with hepatitis C monoinfection, with one study noting its inability to correctly classify 40–65% of patients with chronic HCV or HBeAg negative chronic hepatitis B [27]

Forns Index

The Forns index uses four common clinical measurements: patient age, serum concentrations of total cholesterol and gamma-glutamyl transpeptidase (GGT), and platelet count. This method can be used to differentiate patients with mild (F0–F1) fibrosis and those with severe (F2–F4) fibrosis (*AUROC 0.81*), but it is less accurate in distinguishing between patients with grades F2–F4. Forns should not be used in patients with genotype 3, however, due to varying serum cholesterol levels [28]. The Forns index has been validated in an HCV–HIV infected cohort of 357 patients with a PPV 94% for significant fibrosis, compared to 87% for APRI, and negative predictive value (NPV) 100% for cirrhosis [29].

SHASTA Index

The SHASTA index was also developed to stage mild and advanced fibrosis in coinfected patients, incorporating hyaluronic acid, albumin, and AST. Fibrosis was evaluated against AST, ALT, serum albumin, total bilirubin, the chitinase-like protein YKL-40, and hyaluronic acid (HA). This study found that fibrosis scores ≥F3 were found 27 times more often in patients with elevated HA levels (>86 ng/ml) and 5.5 times more often in persons with HA levels 41–86 ng/ml. Less substantial associations were detected when serum albumin was less than 3.5 g/dl (Odds Ratio (OR) 4.85), and serum AST was greater than 60 IU (OR 5.91) [30].

FIB-4 Index

Originally developed for use in HIV–HCV coinfection, FIB-4 also utilizes routine laboratory tests to differentiate Ishak fibrosis stages 0–3 (mild fibrosis) from stages 4–6 (advanced fibrosis). Based on multivariate logistic regression analysis, a simple index was developed: age ([year] × AST [U/L])/(Platelet count [10^9/L]) × (ALT [U/L] × 1/2). With a cutoff in the validation set of <1.45, NPV to exclude advanced fibrosis was 90% with a sensitivity of 70%, and a cutoff of >3.25 yielded a PPV of 65% and a specificity of 97%. Use of this index would correctly classify 87% of patients with FIB-4 values outside 1.45–3.25 and avoid biopsy in 71% of the validation set with AUROC 0.765, sensitivity 70%, specificity 97% for differentiating Ishak 0–3 from 4 to 6 [31]. FIB-4 has been compared to other noninvasive methods in comparative studies as discussed in that section and in Table 5.2.

Hospital Gregorio Marañón (HGM) Indices

Other models have also been developed to predict fibrosis in HCV–HIV coinfected patients, such as the Hospital Gregorio Marañón (HGM) index. Berenguer et al. [32] developed HGM-1 and HGM-2 to predict significant fibrosis (F≥2) and advanced fibrosis (F≥3), respectively, among HIV–HCV coinfected patients who were HCV treatment naïve. The HGM-1 index is based on platelet count, AST and glucose. The HGM-2 index is based on platelet count, INR, alkaline phosphatase (ALP), and AST. AUROCs of the HGM-1 index for the estimation group (EG) and the validation group (VG) were 0.807 and 0.712, respectively. The AUROCs of the HGM-2 index for the EG and the VG were 0.844 and 0.815 respectively. The NPV for HGM-1 index in the VG to exclude F≥2 was 54.5% and the PPV to confirm F≥2 was 93.3%. The NPV for HGM-2 index in the VG to exclude F≥3 was 92.3%, and the PPV to confirm F≥3 was 64.3%.

Models Utilizing Nonroutine Tests

Several noninvasive models have been developed for the evaluation of fibrosis in HCV and HCV–HIV coinfected patients, which include nonroutine measurements of extracellular matrix remodeling markers, such as amino-terminal propeptide of type III collagen (PIIIP), matrix metalloproteinase (MMP), tissue inhibitor of matrix metalloproteinase (TIMP), hyaluronic acid, and Type IV collagen (CL-4) alone or in combination with serum chemistries and HCV RNA.

Myers et al. [33] developed a noninvasive index that incorporated age, gender, alpha [2] microglobulin (A2M), haptoglobin, apolipoprotein A1 (ApoA1), and GGT. The main outcome measure was F2–F4 fibrosis by METAVIR scoring. The most useful markers, as determined by multivariate analysis, were A2M, Apo-A1, GGT, and gender. Using the five marker index, the AUROC was 0.856 with a PPV of 86% for scores greater than 0.60 and a NPV of 93% for scores of 0.20 or less, with the conclusion that these thresholds could reduce the necessity for liver biopsy by 55% while maintaining an accuracy of 89%. TIMP-1 and HA have also been shown to accurately predict fibrosis in HIV–HCV coinfected patients by Larrousse et al. [34] who have also evaluated these biomarkers in the coinfected population. MMP-1, MMP-2, procollagen III N peptide (PIIINP), and HA were obtained in a cohort of 119 chronic HCV patients with HIV coinfection at the time of liver biopsy and prior to initiation of HCV antiviral therapy. On multivariate analysis, TIMP-1 and HA>95 µg/dL were both shown to be independently associated with hepatic fibrosis. In discriminating mild (F0–F1) from significant (F2–F4) fibrosis, the AUROC was 0.84 using TIMP-1 and HA, with sensitivity of 72.9% and specificity of 83.1%. The HGM-3 includes both routine and nonroutine tests. It is an index including platelet count, ALP, hepatic growth factor, tissue inhibitor of matrix metalloproteinase (TIMP-1), and HA. The AUROC of HGM-3 for identification of F≥3 was 0.939, which was significantly higher than the AUROC for HGM-2, FIB-4, APRI, and Forns indices [35].

Biomarkers have also been analyzed in a cohort of coinfected patients where 90% have been currently treated with HAART. HA and transforming growth factor-beta1 (TGF-beta1) levels were collected in 69 patients undergoing liver biopsy. AST, ALT, and GGT levels were also measured, and were elevated in 81, 70, and 60% of patients, respectively. Serum HA was shown to have a statistically significant correlation with fibrosis stage with an AUROC of 0.83 for the discrimination of mild (F0–F2) from significant (F3–F4) fibrosis. Sensitivity and specificity for HA were 87% and 70%, respectively. TGF-beta1, however, was not predictive of fibrosis in this cohort [36].

Noninvasive Fibrosis Assessment Using Imaging Methods

Several methods utilizing radiographic techniques for the noninvasive assessment of hepatic fibrosis have also been evaluated in coinfected population. These include transient elastography and single photon emission computed tomography (SPECT).

Transient Elastography

Elastography or elastometry is a noninvasive method of measuring the mean stiffness of hepatic tissue with hepatic rigidity considered a marker of progressive fibrosis. Sandrin et al. [37] evaluated this method by obtaining in vivo liver elasticity measurements using the shear elasticity probe, a device based on one-dimensional (1D) transient elastography. With the ability for the transmitted elastic wave to be temporally separated from reflected elastic waves, the technique is less sensitive to boundary conditions than other elastographic techniques. The acquisition time is short (typically <100 ms), which enables measurements to be obtained from moving organs. This makes transient elastography (TE) well adapted to the study of the liver. A probe (Fibroscan) with an ultrasonic transducer transmits low frequency (50 MHz), low amplitude vibrations into the liver. These vibrations produce elastic shear waves that propagate throughout the liver. The probe also emits a pulse-echo ultrasound wave, which is used to determine the velocity of the shear wave. The velocity of the shear wave is directly related to liver stiffness (LS) [38]. Comparisons of TE with biopsy results have shown that cutoff values can be established to distinguish mild/moderate fibrosis from severe fibrosis/cirrhosis, with validation studies showing variable results and with greatest statistical significance being demonstrated in the differentiation of cirrhosis from mild fibrosis (*AUROC F = 4 0.94, sensitivity F ≥ 2 85%, specificity F ≥ 2 91%*) [38, 39]. Overall, advanced fibrosis is more likely with a higher cutoff [39–42].

Ziol et al. [43] evaluated elastography in a mixed cohort of 251 patients, including 13 patients with HIV–HCV coinfection. Elastography demonstrated AUROCs of 0.79, 0.91 and 0.91 for F ≥ 2, F ≥ 3, and F = 4 fibrosis, respectively. Kirk et al. [44] also evaluated TE in a cohort of HCV patients where 72% were coinfected with HIV. They found an AUROC of 0.87 for detection of both significant fibrosis and cirrhosis. Using cutoff values of 9.3 kPa for fibrosis and 12.3 kPa for cirrhosis, 79–83% of participants were correctly classified by liver stiffness measurement. It was noted, however, that accuracy appeared to be higher among HIV-uninfected participants than among HIV-infected participants.

Vergara et al. [45] evaluated elastography in an HIV–HCV cohort of 169 patients, demonstrating an AUROC of 0.87 for significant fibrosis and 0.95 for cirrhosis. Macias et al. [46] have also evaluated TE to validate cutoff values of liver stiffness to better discriminate F < 2 from F ≥ 2 fibrosis in coinfected patients. A cutoff value of 9.0 kPa yielded a PPV of 87% for F ≥ 2 and a cutoff of 6.0 kPa showed a NPV of 90% for F < 2. The NPV of LS ≤ 6.0 kPa for F ≥ 3 was 100% and NPV of LS ≥ 9.0 kPa for F = 0 was 100%.

A recent prospective study was conducted in a cohort of 13,369 examinations to determine the frequency and determinant of elastography failure and obtainment of unreliable results. Failure was define as no valid measurements and occurred in 3.1% of the examinations. Unreliable examinations had less than 10 valid measurements an interquartile range/liver stiffness measurement greater than 30% or a success rate less than 60%; this occurred in 15.8% of all examinations. Factors contributing to failure and/or unreliable measurements included body mass index >30 kg/m^2, operator inexperience, and age >52 years [47]. This study demonstrates the importance of appropriate patient selection and operator training to successfully use this modality. Other factors that may influence liver stiffness are hepatic inflammation, edema, and steatosis, which make this modality less than ideal.

Magnetic Resonance Elastography (MRE)

Magnetic resonance elastography (MRE) is another modality that has been evaluated in the viral hepatitis population but has not been tested in the HIV and/or HIV/HCV population. This modality has shown promising results with one study demonstrating AUROCs of 0.994 for F ≥ 2, 0.985 for F ≥ 3, and 0.998 for F = 4, which outperformed ultrasound elastography, APRI, and the combination of the two [48]. However, MRE requires special equipment and my not be available on all types of MRI scanners. Therefore, its use in clinical practice may be limited.

Single Photon Emission Computed Tomography (SPECT)

Single photon emission computed tomography (SPECT) has also been tested in HIV–HCV coinfected patients in an effort to correlate histologic severity of liver fibrosis with SPECT results. A number of SPECT parameters were associated with histologic changes, fibrosis, and cirrhosis. The minimum pixel count for spleen region of interest and maximum pixel count for right hepatic lobe correctly correlated 39 of 46 SPECT scans with biopsy results. Larger studies are needed, however, to validate these results [49].

Correllation Among Noninvasive Modalities

Other studies have compared various biochemical measures and indices as well as between biochemical measures and imaging modalities in HIV–HCV coinfected patients to discern the optimal method for the noninvasive determination of liver fibrosis.

De Ledinghen et al. [50] evaluated the use of liver stiffness measurement in coinfected patients utilizing transient elastography, and also compared elastography with platelet count, AST:ALT ratio, AST:APRI ratio, and FIB-4. They found a statistically significant correlation of liver stiffness with fibrosis stage. The AUROC for stiffness was 0.72 for $F \geq 2$ and 0.97 for $F = 4$. For the diagnosis of cirrhosis, AUROC of liver stiffness were significantly higher than those for platelet count, AST to ALT ratio, and FIB-4. Masaki et al. [51] also evaluated a cohort of 57 hemophiliac patients with HCV, 33 of which had HIV–HCV coinfection. In this study, patients were categorized into four stages by abdominal ultrasound: 1-normal or fatty liver, 2-mild, 3-moderate, and 4-severe chronic liver disease. Liver stiffness was found to be significantly increased as ultrasound stages increased. Stiffness was also significantly correlated with platelet count and 7 S domain of Type IV collagen in the non-HIV and HIV groups. This study compared fibroscan, abdominal ultrasound, platelet counts, Type IV collagen, procollagen type III, and hyaluronic acid. In the coinfected cohort, fibroscan results correlated with type IV-collagen, ultrasound, procollagen type III, platelet count, and hyaluronic acid. Sanchez-Conde et al. [52] has also recently compared TE with serum assessments (APRI, Forns, FIB-4 and HGM-2) of liver fibrosis in 100 coinfected patients. The AUROC for TE was 0.80 for discriminating $F \leq 1$ from $F > 2$, 0.93 for discriminating $F \leq 2$ from $F > 3$ and 0.99 for discriminating $F \leq 3$ from F4. Using best cutoff values [$F \leq 1$ (<7 kPa), $F \geq 3$ (≥ 11 kPa) and F4 (≥ 14 kPa)], the NPV and PPV were 81.1 and 70.2% for $F \leq 1$, 96.3 and 60% for $F \geq 3$ and 100 and 57.1% for F4, respectively. They concluded that TE accurately predicted liver fibrosis and outperformed other simple noninvasive indexes in HIV–HCV-coinfected patients.

Shaheen and Myers [53] have also previously performed a systematic review of the diagnostic accuracy of fibrosis marker panels in this population, with only five studies meeting inclusion criteria and including four fibrosis measures (APRI, Forns, FibroTest, and SHASTA) with the finding that these panels have acceptable performance for the identification of significant fibrosis and cirrhosis, but cautioned that these tests were not yet adequate to replace liver biopsy.

Maor et al. [54] evaluated a cohort of 132 hemophilia patients with HCV, 27 of which were coinfected with HIV, utilizing fibrotest, APRI, Forns, age-platelet index, and hyaluronic acid. They found that fibrotest accurately identified minimal or advanced liver disease, and a concordance of fibrotest with APRI and/or Forns can be used to avoid liver biopsy. Cacoub et al. [55] also evaluated a coinfected population in the fibrovic study – ANRS HCO_2. In this study, fibrotest (FT), Hepascore (HS), fibrometer (FM), SHASTA, APRI, Forns, and FIB-4 were examined to determine the accuracy of these tests in the differentiation between mild to moderate (F2) and advanced fibrosis (F4). The AUROCs were 0.78, 0.84, and 0.89 for F2 for FT, HS, and FM, respectively. The other tests were only able to well classify fibrosis in 37–61% of patients and with lower accuracies. Of note, FM, HS, and FT in combination did not significantly increase the accuracy of each test individually. Loko et al. [56] have also assessed four noninvasive indexes (FIB-4, APRI, Forns, and platelet count) in HIV–HCV coinfected patients, examining 200 coinfected patients from the ANRS-CO3 Aquitaine cohort who underwent liver biopsy. For predicting significant fibrosis ($F \geq 2$), APRI, Forns index, and FIB-4 had AUROCs of 0.77, 0.75, and 0.79, with 39, 25, and 70% of patients correctly identified, respectively. For predicting severe fibrosis ($F \geq 3$), FIB-4 had an AUROC of 0.77 with 56% of patients correctly identified. For predicting cirrhosis (F4), FIB-4, APRI, and platelet count had AUROCs of 0.80, 0.79, and 0.78, with 59, 60, and 76% of patients correctly identified, respectively. FIB-4, APRI, Forns, and platelet count did not differ significantly for fibrosis and cirrhosis, but could save liver biopsies in up to 56–76% of cases.

Another study evaluated APRI, FORNS, and FIB-4, alone or combined, with the finding that the three tests demonstrated similar accuracy in identifying F2/F3. When the lowest cutoff values of all three tests were used to rule out F3 for greater fibrosis, the sensitivity of the tests was 79–84% and NPVs were 87–91%. When F3 or greater fibrosis was identified with highest cutoff values, the specificity was 90–96% and PPVs were 63–73%. This demonstrated that these tests were able to accurately determine degree of fibrosis in greater than 50% of the coinfected population [57]. This has also been echoed in an additional study analyzing APRI and Forns in coinfected patients under "real-life" conditions, as opposed to validation studies. In the 120 members of the cohort who had a liver biopsy available and ≥ 15 mm in length, the PPV was 85% for APRI and 81% for Forns. Used individually, it was determined that liver biopsy could be avoided in 22% of patients, and when used sequentially, this number increased to 30% [58].

Other Uses of Noninvasive Markers of Hepatic Fibrosis

Other studies have examined additional potential uses for the noninvasive biomarkers of hepatic fibrosis in the coinfected population to extend their utility beyond that of fibrosis determination alone. With the wide use of HAART in this population as well as the lack of information about the longitudinal effects of HAART on the progression of hepatic fibrosis, Al-Mohri et al. [59] evaluated APRI with regard to its predictive value for liver-related complications in HIV patients with and without HCV coinfection. Coinfected patients had a higher baseline APRI. The baseline natural logarithm of APRI (lnAPRI) was predictive of hepatic complications, as was coinfection with HCV. HAART was not found to be protective against hepatic complications, but correlated with progression of APRI scores. As the lnAPRI varied over time in the coinfected population, it was felt that APRI may prove useful for longitudinal determination of liver disease progression in the coinfected population.

With regard to potential hepatic complications, liver stiffness measurements (LSM) have also been evaluated in a mixed cirrhotic population to predict the presence of esophageal varices. LSM was strongly correlated with a diagnosis of esophageal varices, with mean LSM 42.7 in patients with esophageal varices and 19.1 in patients without esophageal varices [60]. The AUROC was 0.818 (95% CI, 0.732–0.904) for predicting the presence of EV, and an LSM value of 19.7 kPa was predictive of the presence of EV with a sensitivity of 87%, a specificity of 70%, a PPV of 89%, and a NPV of 66%. However, there was a weak correlation between LSM and the size of EV.

Nunes et al. [61] prospectively evaluated a cohort of HCV infected patients with and without HIV coinfection to determine if noninvasive biomarkers could accurately predict liver related mortality. APRI and FIB-4, both derived indices of fibrosis, as well as HA and YKL-40, markers of extracellular matrix metabolism, were compared to Child–Turcotte–Pugh (CTP) and Model for End-Stage Liver Disease (MELD) scores. The cohort consisted of 303 patients, 207 of which were HIV positive, and was followed for a mean of 3.1 years. There were 33 liver-related deaths in the cohort. The ability to predict 3-year mortality was expressed as an AUROC, with the following results: HA 0.92, CPT 0.91, APRI 0.88, FIB-4 0.87, and MELD 0.84. HA, APRI, and FIB-4 were all found on multivariate analysis to be independent predictors of mortality when included with MELD or CPT in statistical models. This study demonstrates the utility of these models not only in fibrosis determination but also in predicting liver related mortality in the coinfected population. However, until further studies, noninvasive models should not replace MELD or CPT in clinical practice.

Summary

Liver biopsy is considered to be the gold standard for the histopathologic assessment of hepatic tissue, as it is considered to be the most accurate modality for assessing severity and etiology of liver disease as well as monitoring response to therapy. Biopsy, however, carries inherent risks including bleeding, pain, hypotension, and the potential for organ perforation. Multiple studies have been performed to evaluate the accuracy of noninvasive methods of determination of the degree of liver fibrosis in the HCV monoinfected, hepatitis B, alcoholic, posttransplant, and other chronic liver disease populations. Attention is now turned to the subset population of HIV–HCV coinfected patients who have longer life expectancies and subsequent increased progression of liver disease in the era of HAART (Table 5.3).

This coinfected population often requires more frequent biopsies due to the almost unpredictable nature of their fibrosis progression. It has been shown that up to 25% of patients with normal ALT can have significant fibrosis, [17] and that HIV anti-viral medications can have impaired clearance in the coinfected patient, potentially requiring therapeutic drug monitoring [18]. These issues represent unique challenges in the coinfected population and reiterate the need for validation of noninvasive methods of fibrosis analysis in this population, as liver biopsy is not without the aforementioned risks.

Given these risks, there has been a drive to develop noninvasive measures of hepatic fibrosis and to validate these in the coinfected population. Numerous modalities including serum measurements and imaging modalities have been developed, but a significant portion of these has not yet been validated in the HIV population.

The ideal method of assessing fibrosis would involve the utilization of a readily available test that accurately discriminates between minimal/mild (Metavir F0–F2) and advanced fibrosis (Metavir F3–4). Systematic review of noninvasive models of assessing liver fibrosis has previously been performed for HCV monoinfected patients with promising results, [62] and several indices and models have also been developed for or tested in the coinfected population including APRI, Forns, SHASTA, FIB-4, and the HGM indices. Systematic review and meta-analysis of noninvasive marker panels has demonstrated acceptable performance of these models for fibrosis assessment in the HIV–HCV coinfected population [53]. Shire et al. have [63] recently compared 5 models (AST/ALT Ratio, age-platelet idex, APRI, FIB-4, and Bonacini index) in 173 coinfected subjects participating in ACTG 5178. In this cohort, 31% had advanced fibrosis (bridging fibrosis or cirrhosis). Among the models, FIB-4 had the best performance (88% specificity for cirrhosis and greater than 86%

Table 5.3 Summary of studies including coinfected patients

Biochemical methods

Author, year (ref)	Patient population	Test	Correlation coefficient	AUROC	Sensitivity	Specificity	PPV	NPV	Accuracy
Myers et al. 2003 [33]	N=130, HCV/HIV	Index of age, sex, A2M, ApoA1, GGT, haptoglobin, bilirubin					5 marker index 86% for score >0.60	93% for scores ≤0.20	89%
Al-Mohri et al. 2005 [24]	N=46, HCV/HIV	APRI		0.847±0.057 for significant fibrosis	APRI >1.5: 53% APRI <0.5: 82%	APRI >1.5: 100% APRI <0.5: 46%	APRI >1.5: 100% APRI <0.5: 79%	APRI >1.5: 45% APRI <0.5: 50%	
Larrousse et al. 2005 [34]	N=119, HCV/HIV	MMP-1, MMP-2, TIMP-1,PIIIP, HA	TIMP-1 (r=0.6), TIMP-1/MMP-1 ratio (r=0.5), TIMP-1/MMP-2 ratio (r=0.3, MMP-2 (r=0.2), PIIINP (r=0.4), and HA (r=0.5)	To discriminate mild (F0–F1) from significant (F2–F4) fibrosis: using TIMP-1 and HA: 0.84	72.9%	83.1%			
Macias et al. 2006 [29]	N=357, HCV/HIV	Forns					Forns 94%, APRI 87% for significant fibrosis	Forns 100% for cirrhosis	
Sterling et al. 2006 [31]	N=832, HCV/HIV	FIB-4		AUROC 0.765 for differentiating Ishak 0–3 from 4–6	Cutoff of <1.45: 70%	Cutoff of >3.25: 97%	Cutoff of >3.25: 65%	Cutoff of <1.45: 90%	
Shastry et al. 2007 [26]	N=50, HCV/HIV	APRI					APRI >0.6: 100% for F3/F4	APRI ≤0.6: 100% for excluding F3/F4	
Berenguer et al. 2007 [32]	N=296, HCV/HIV	HGM-1, HGM-2		HGM-1 for F≥2: estimation group (EG): 0.807, validation group (VG): 0.712; HGM-2 for F≥3: 0.844 (EG) and 0.815 (VG)			HGM-1 (VG) to confirm F≥2: 93.3%; HGM-2 (VG) to confirm F≥3: 64.3%	HGM-1 (VG) to exclude F≥2: 54.5%; HGM-1 (VG) to exclude F≥3: 92.3%	
Carvalho-Filho et al. 2008 [25]	N=111, HCV/HIV	APRI		0.774±0.045 for significant fibrosis			APRI ≥1.8: 75% for significant fibrosis	APRI <0.6: 87%	
Sanvisens et al. 2009 [36]	N=69, HCV/HIV	TGF-beta-1 and HA	HA (r=0.56). No correlation between TGF-beta1 and fibrosis	For discriminating mild (F0–F2) from significant (F3–F4) fibrosis, HA: 0.83	HA: 87%	HA: 70%			
Resino et al. 2010 [35]	N=195, HCV/HIV	HGM-3		0.939 for identification of F≥3					

Imaging methods

Author, year (ref)	Patient population	Method	Correlation coefficient	AUROC	Sensitivity	Specificity	PPV	NPV
Shiramizu et al. 2003 [49]	N=38, HIV/HCV	SPECT			For differentiating F1/F2 for F3–F6: 86%	83.3%	86%	86%
Ziol et al. 2005 [43]	N=251, HCV only – 215; HIV/HCV – 13; HBV/HCV – 5; EtOH/HCV – 18	Elastography	0.55	F≥2: 0.79 F≥3: 0.91 F=4: 0.91	F≥2: 56% F≥3: 86% F=4: 86%	F≥2: 91% F≥3: 85% F=4: 96%	F≥2: 88% F≥3: 71% F=4: 78%	F≥2: 56% F≥3: 93% F=4: 97%
Vergara et al. 2007 [45]	N=169, HIV–HCV	Elastography		0.87 (fibrosis) 0.95 (cirrhosis)			88% (F) 86% (C)	75% (F) 94% (C)
Kirk et al. 2009 [44]	N=192, HCV/HIV – 139	Elastography		0.87 for significant fibrosis and cirrhosis				

Comparative studies

Author, year (ref)	Patients population	Tests	Comments
Nunes et al. 2005 [19]	N=97, HCV/HIV – 40; HCV alone – 57	INR, platelet, AST/ALT, APRI, Forns, procoll III, hyaluronic acid, YKL-40	Diagnostic performance of noninvasive markers similar in mono- and coinfected patients
Kelleher et al. 2005 [30]	N=137, HCV/HIV	SHASTA, ALT, AST, APRI, albumin, bilirubin, HA, YKL-40	HA, albumin, and AST accurately staged mild and advanced fibrosis
de Ledinghen et al. 2006 [50]	N=72, HCV/HIV	Elastography, platelet count, AST/ALT, FIB-4	Liver stiffness significantly correlated with fibrosis stage; AUROC of stiffness was 0.72 for F≥2 and 0.97 for F=4. For the diagnosis of cirrhosis, AUROCs of liver stiffness were significantly higher than those for platelet count, AST/ALT, APRI, and FIB-4
Masaki et al. 2006 [51]	N=57, HCV/HIV – 33; HCV alone – 24	Fibroscan, abdominal ultrasound (US), platelet counts, type IV collagen, procollagen type III, hyaluronic acid	In coinfected group, Fibroscan correlated with IV-coll, US, PIIIP, PLT and HA. In non-HIV group, Fibroscan correlated with US, platelet count, and IV-coll
Maor et al. 2006 [54]	N=132, HCV/HIV – 27; HCV alone – 105	Fibrotest, APRI, Forns index, age-platelet index, hyaluronic acid	Concordance of Fibrotest with APRI and/or Forns can be used to avoid biopsy. Fibrotest accurately identified advanced or minimal liver disease
Cacoub et al. 2008 [55]	N=272, HCV/HIV	Fibrotest, hepascore, fibrometer, SHASTA, APRI, Forns, FIB-4	AUROC for FT, HS, and FM were 0.78, 0.84, and 0.89, respectively
Loko et al. 2008 [56]	N=200, HCV/HIV	FIB-4, APRI, Forns, and platelet count	For significant fibrosis (F≥2), APRI, Forns index, and FIB-4 had AUROCs of 0.77, 0.75, and 0.79. For severe fibrosis (F≥3), FIB-4 had AUROC of 0.77. For cirrhosis (F4), FIB-4, APRI, and platelet count had AUROCs of 0.80, 0.79, and 0.78
Tural et al. 2009 [57]	N=324, HCV/HIV	APRI, Forns, FIB-4	F≥2: APRI, FORNS, and FIB-4 had AUROCs of 0.72, 0.67, and 0.72, respectively. F≥3: AUROCs of 0.75, 0.73, and 0.78, respectively
Sanchez-Conde et al. 2009 [52]	N=100, HCV/HIV	TE, APRI, Forns, FIB-4, HGM-2	AUROC for TE was 0.80 for discriminating F≤1 from F2 or greater and 0.99 for F≤3 from F4; TE outperformed other markers
Macias et al. 2010 [58]	N=519, HCV/HIV	APRI, Forns	AUROC for both APRI and Forns was 0.67. Applying both models sequentially, 30% of patients could be spared liver biopsy

HA hyaluronic acid, *HGM* hospital gregoric marañon *SPECT* single photon emission computed tomography *HCV* hepatitis C virus, *ApoA1* apolipoprotein A-1, *GGT* gamma-glutamyl transferase, *PPV* positive predictive value, *NPV* negative predictive value, *APRI* AST-to-platelet ratio index, *MMP* matrix metallopeptidase, *TIMP* tissue Inhibitor of metalloproteinases, *PIIIP* procollagen III peptide, *HA* hyaluronic acid, *PIIINP* N-terminal propeptide of collagen type III, *HGM* hospital gregorio marañón, *AUROCs* area under the receiver operating characteristic curves, *TGF-Beta* transforming growth factor-beta, *SPECT* single photon emission computed tomography, *ALT* alanine aminotransferase, *AST* aspartate aminotransferase, *YKL-40* human cartilage glycoprotein 39

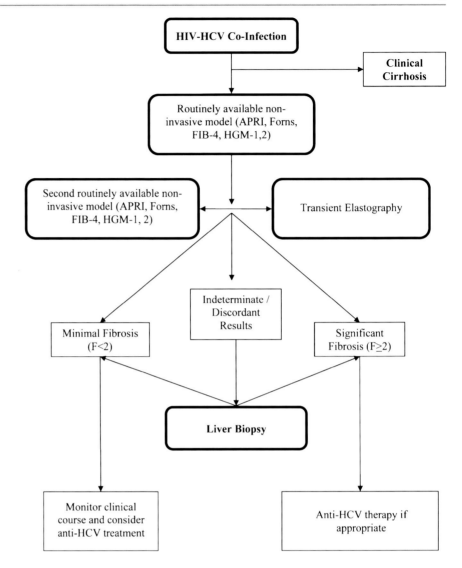

Fig. 5.2 Algorithm for noninvasive fibrosis assessment

negative predictive value for advanced fibrosis). However, the AUROC was low (0.56) for advanced fibrosis. Ordinal regression models of patient specific data improved the AUROC (0.85), which classified 77% of patients correctly highlighting the difficulty in applying these types of algorithms to diverse coinfected patient populations.

Other models utilizing nonroutine measurements of extracellular matrix remodeling markers (PIIIP, MMP, TIMP, HA, and Type IV collagen) have also been developed and have been compared to serum chemistries and HCV RNA. Fibrotest, a composite measurement of several serum proteins, as well as Actitest, a modified Fibrotest that includes ALT, has been developed and evaluated in the monoinfected population, but are not validated in the coinfected population. However, the components of these models utilizing nonroutine tests are not readily available and are very expensive, limiting their widespread use.

Various imaging tests including transient elastography and SPECT have been evaluated in the co-infected population. SPECT imaging has demonstrated the ability to differentiate normal from cirrhotic livers and has been tested in the coinfected population, but is not readily available and also does not show more diagnostic capability than other readily available tests. Transient elastography has shown promising results in the diagnosis of advanced fibrosis and cirrhosis and has also been tested in the coinfected population. TE also appears easy to perform and will likely be readily available in the near future. However, its use has been shown to be limited in morbidly obese patients and requires experienced operators for optimal utility and accurate results.

Ultrasound is also readily available and is used for hepatocellulcar carcinoma screening, but unenhanced Doppler ultrasound is not reliable in the discrimination of varying degrees of fibrosis. MRE been shown to differentiate mild from moderate or advanced fibrosis in the monoinfected population, but is not validated in the coinfected population. MR studies also have limitations including cost and availability.

With the primary objective of determining the optimal method of diagnosing advanced fibrosis and cirrhosis in the coinfected population in mind, it is recommended to use readily available modalities for initial evaluation in the patients. The nonroutine markers such as the extracellular matrix markers have been shown to be accurate in diagnosis of fibrosis, but do not increase performance in the discrimination between minimal and significant fibrosis. When liver biopsy is not feasible, we recommend using a serum marker index such as APRI, Forns, or FIB-4 for initial evaluation (Fig. 5.2). SHASTA has shown acceptable diagnostic accuracy as well, but incorporates YKL-40 and HA, which are not readily available. We then recommend performing confirmatory testing with either a second of these tests or transient elastography, if available. Multiple studies have shown increased diagnostic accuracy with the combination of tests in various chronic liver disease populations [38–41, 64].

In conclusion, accurate determination of the degree of hepatic fibrosis is essential to determining the need for anti-HCV therapy, for determining the potential for complications and liver-related mortality, and for determining the need for therapeutic drug monitoring in the HIV–HCV coinfected population. Liver biopsy is still considered to be the gold standard for making this determination, but great strides are being made in the development of accurate noninvasive methods for determination of severity of fibrosis. These methods, including routine and nonroutine serum markers and radiographic examinations, are also now being validated in the coinfected population with further studies ongoing.

References

1. Graham CS, Baden LR, Yu E, et al. Influence of human immunodeficiency virus infection on the course of hepatitis C virus infection: a meta-analysis. Clin Infect Dis. 2001;33(4):562–9.
2. Salmon-Ceron D, Lewden C, Morlat D, et al. Liver disease as a major cause of death among HIV infected patients: role of hepatitis C and B viruses and alcohol. J Hepatol. 2005;42(6):799–805.
3. Schlichting P, Fauerholdt L, Christensen E, et al. Clinical relevance of restrictive morphological criteria for the diagnosis of cirrhosis in liver biopsies. Liver. 1981;1(1):56–61.
4. Bravo AA, Sheth SG, Chopra S. Liver biopsy. New Engl J Med. 2001;344(7):495–500.
5. Sterling RK. Role of liver biopsy in the evaluation of hepatitis C virus infection in HIV coinfection. Clin Infect Dis. 2005;40 Suppl 5:S270–5.
6. Yano M, Kumada H, Kage M, et al. The long-term pathological evolution of chronic hepatitis C. Hepatology. 1996;23(6):1334–40.
7. Ghany MG, Kleiner DE, Alter H, et al. Progression of fibrosis in chronic hepatitis C. Gastroenterology. 2003;124(1):97–104.
8. Froehlich F, Lamy O, Fried M, et al. Practice and complications of liver biopsy. Results of a nationwide survey in Switzerland. Dig Dis Sci. 1993;38(8):1480–4.
9. Thampanitchawong P, Piratvisuth T. Liver biopsy: complications and risk factors. World J Gastroenterol. 1999;5(4):301–4.
10. Lindor KD, Bru C, Jorgensen RA, et al. The role of ultrasonography and automatic-needle biopsy in outpatient percutaneous liver biopsy. Hepatology. 1996;23(5):1079–83.
11. Abdi W, Millan JC, Mezey E. Sampling variability on percutaneous liver biopsy. Arch Intern Med. 1979;139(6):667–9.
12. Maharaj B, Bhoora IG. Complications associated with percutaneous needle biopsy of the liver when one, two or three specimens are taken. Postgrad Med J. 1992;68(806):964–7.
13. Sterling RK, Contos MJ, Sanyal AJ, et al. The clinical spectrum of hepatitis C virus in HIV coinfection. J Acquir Immune Defic Syndr. 2003;32(1):30–7.
14. Pol S, Hepatitis C. virus and human immunodeficiency virus co-infection. Gastroenterol Clin Biol. 2001;25(4 Suppl):B152–6.
15. Martinot-Peignoux M, Boyer N, Cazals-Hatem D, et al. Prospective study on anti-hepatitis C virus-positive patients with persistently normal serum alanine transaminase with or without detectable serum hepatitis C virus RNA. Hepatology. 2001;34(5):1000–5.
16. Shiffman ML, Stewart CA, Hofmann CM, et al. Chronic infection with hepatitis C virus in patients with elevated or persistently normal serum alanine aminotransferase levels: comparison of hepatic histology and response to interferon therapy. J Infect Dis. 2000;182(6):1595–601.
17. Uberti-Foppa C, De Bona A, Galli L, et al. Liver fibrosis in HIV-positive patients with hepatitis C virus. J Acquir Immune Defic Syndr. 2006;41(1):63–7.
18. Barreiro P, Rodriguez-Novoa S, Labarga P, et al. Influence of liver fibrosis stage on plasma levels of antiretroviral drugs in HIV-infected patients with chronic hepatitis c. J Infect Dis. 2007;195(7):973–9.
19. Nunes D, Fleming C, Offner G, et al. HIV infection does not affect the performance of noninvasive markers of fibrosis for the diagnosis of hepatitis C virus-related liver disease. J Acquir Immune Defic Syndr. 2005;40(5):538–44.
20. Wai CT, Greenson JK, Fontana RJ, et al. A simple noninvasive index can predict both significant fibrosis and cirrhosis in patients with chronic hepatitis C. Hepatology. 2003;38(2):518–26.
21. Snyder N, Gajula L, Xiao SY, et al. APRI: an easy and validated predictor of hepatic fibrosis in chronic hepatitis C. J Clin Gastroenterol. 2006;40(6):535–42.
22. Yu ML, Lin SM, Lee CM, et al. A simple noninvasive index for predicting long-term outcome of chronic hepatitis C after interferon-based therapy. Hepatology. 2006;44(5):1086–97.
23. Snyder N, Nguyen A, Gajula L, et al. The APRI may be enhanced by the use of the FIBROSpect II in the estimation of fibrosis in chronic hepatitis C. Clin Chem Acta. 2007;381(2):119–23.
24. Al-Mohri H, Cooper C, Murphy T, et al. Validation of a simple model for predicting liver fibrosis in HIV/hepatitis C virus-coinfected patients. HIV Med. 2005;6(6):375–8.
25. Carvalho-Filho RJ, Schiavon LL, Narciso-Schiavon JL, et al. Optimized cutoffs improve performance of the aspartate aminotransferase to platelet ratio index for predicting significant liver fibrosis in human immunodeficiency virus/hepatitis C virus co infection. Liver Int. 2008;28(4):486–93.
26. Shastry I, Wilson T, Lascher S, et al. The utility of aspartate aminotransferase/platelet ratio index in HIV/hepatitis C-co-infected patients. AIDS. 2007;21(18):2541–3.
27. Chrysanthos NV, Papatheodoridis GV, Savvas S, et al. Aspartate aminotransferase to platelet ratio index for fibrosis evaluation in chronic viral hepatitis. Eur J Gastroenterol Hepatol. 2006;18(4):389–96.
28. Forns X, Ampurdanès S, Llovet JM, et al. Identification of chronic hepatitis C patients without hepatic fibrosis by a simple predictive model. Hepatology. 2002;36(4 Pt 1):986–92.
29. Macías J, Girón-González JA, González-Serrano M, et al. Prediction of liver fibrosis in human immunodeficiency virus/hepatitis C virus coinfected patients by simple non-invasive indexes. Gut. 2006;55(3):409–14.
30. Kelleher TB, Mehta SH, Bhaskar R, Sulkowski M, Astemborski J, Thomas DL, et al. Prediction of hepatic fibrosis in HIV/HCV co-infected patients using serum fibrosis markers: the SHASTA index. J Hepatol. 2005;43:78–84.

31. Sterling RK, Lissen E, Clumeck N, et al. Development of a simple noninvasive index to predict significant fibrosis in patients with HIV/HCV coinfection. Hepatology. 2006;43(6):1317–25.
32. Berenguer J, Bellón JM, Miralles P, et al. Identification of liver fibrosis in HIV/HCV-coinfected patients using a simple predictive model based on routine laboratory data. J Viral Hepat. 2007;14(12):859–69.
33. Myers RP, Benhamou Y, Imbert-Bismut F, Thibault V, Bochet M, Chlotte F, et al. Serum biochemical markers accurately predict liver fibrosis in HIV and hepatitis C virus co-infected patients. AIDS. 2003;17:721–5.
34. Larrousse M, Laguno M, Segarra M, et al. Noninvasive diagnosis of hepatic fibrosis in HIV/HCV-coinfected patients. J Acquir Immune Defic Syndr. 2007;46(3):304–11.
35. Resino S, Micheloud D, Miralles P, et al. Diagnosis of advanced fibrosis in hiv and hepatitis c virus-coinfected patients via a new noninvasive index: The hgm-3 index. HIV Med. 2010;11(1):64–73.
36. Sanvisens A, Serra I, Tural C, et al. Hyaluronic acid, transforming growth factor-beta1 and hepatic fibrosis in patients with chronic hepatitis c virus and human immunodeficiency virus coinfection. J Viral Hepat. 2009;16(7):513–8.
37. Sandrin L, Fourquet B, Hasquenoph JM, et al. Transient elastography: a new noninvasive method for assessment of hepatic fibrosis. Ultrasound Med Biol. 2003;29(12):1705–13.
38. Coco B, Oliveri F, Maina AM, et al. Transient elastography: a new surrogate marker of liver fibrosis influenced by major changes of transaminases. J Viral Hepat. 2007;14(5):360–9.
39. Gómez-Domínguez E, Mendoza J, Rubio S, et al. Transient elastography: a valid alternative to biopsy in patients with chronic liver disease. Aliment Pharmacol Ther. 2006;24(3):513–8.
40. Kettaneh A, Marcellin P, Douvin C, et al. Features associated with success rate and performance of FibroScan measurements for the diagnosis of cirrhosis in HCV patients: a prospective study of 935 patients. J Hepatol. 2007;46(4):628–34.
41. Ogawa E, Furusyo N, Toyoda K, et al. Transient elastography for patients with chronic hepatitis B and C virus infection: Non-invasive, quantitative assessment of liver fibrosis. Hepatol Res. 2007;37(12):1002–10.
42. Takeda T, Yasuda T, Nakayama Y, et al. Usefulness of noninvasive transient elastography for assessment of liver fibrosis stage in chronic hepatitis C. World J Gastroenterol. 2006;12(48):7768–73.
43. Ziol M, Handra-Luca A, Kettaneh A, et al. Noninvasive assessment of liver fibrosis by measurement of stiffness in patients with chronic hepatitis C. Hepatology. 2005;41(1):48–54.
44. Kirk GD, Astemborski J, Mehta SH, et al. Assessment of liver fibrosis by transient elastography in persons with hepatitis c virus infection or HIV-hepatitis c virus coinfection. Clin Infect Dis. 2009;48(7):963–72.
45. Vergara S, Macías J, Rivero A, et al. The use of transient elastometry for assessing liver fibrosis in patients with HIV and hepatitis C virus coinfection. Clin Infect Dis. 2007;45(8):969–74.
46. Macias J, Recio Eva, Vispo E, et al. Application of transient elastometry to differentiate mild from moderate to severe liver fibrosis in hiv/hcv co-infected patients. J Hepatol. 2009;49(6):916–22.
47. Castera L, Foucher J, Bernard PH, et al. Pitfalls of liver stiffness measurement: a 5-year prospective study of 13,369 examinations. Hepatology. 2010;51(3):828–35.
48. Huwart L, Sempoux C, Vicaut E, et al. Magnetic resonance elastography for the noninvasive staging of liver fibrosis. Gastroenterology. 2008;135(1):32–40.
49. Shiramizu B, Theodore D, Bassett R, et al. Correlation of single photon emission computed tomography parameters as a noninvasive alternative to liver biopsies in assessing liver involvement in the setting of HIV and hepatitis C virus coinfection: a multicenter trial of the Adult AIDS Clinical Trials Group. J Acquir Immune Defic Syndr. 2003;33(3):329–35.
50. de Ledinghen V, Douvin C, Kettaneh A, Ziol M, Roulot D, Marcellin P, et al. Diagnosis of hepatic fibrosis and cirrhosis by transient elastography in HIV/Hepatitis C virus coinfected patients. J Acquir Immune Defic Syndr. 2006;41:175–9.
51. Masaki N, Imamura M, Kikuchi Y, et al. Usefulness of elastometry in evaluating the extents of liver fibrosis in hemophiliacs coinfected with hepatitis C virus and human immunodeficiency virus. Hepatol Res. 2006;35(2):135–9.
52. Sanchez-Conde M, Montes-Ramirez, ML, Miralles P et al. Comparison of transient elastography and liver biopsy for the assessment of liver fibrosis in hiv/hepatitis c virus-coinfected patients and correlation with noninvasive serum markers. *Journal of viral hepatitis* 2009 Sept 2. [Epub ahead of print]
53. Shaheen AA, Myers RP. Systematic review and meta-analysis of the diagnostic accuracy of fibrosis marker panels in patients with hiv/hepatitis c coinfection. HIV Clin Trials. 2008;9(1):43–51.
54. Maor Y, Bashari D, Kenet G, et al. Non-invasive biomarkers of liver fibrosis in haemophilia patients with hepatitis C: can you avoid liver biopsy? Haemophilia. 2006;12(4):372–9.
55. Cacoub P, Carrat F, Bédossa P, et al. Comparison of non-invasive liver fibrosis biomarkers in HIV/HCV co-infected patients: the fibrovic study–ANRS HC02. J Hepatol. 2008;48(5):765–73.
56. Loko M-A et al. Validation and comparison of simple noninvasive indexes for predicting liver fibrosis in HIV–HCV-coinfected patients: ANRS CO3 Aquitaine cohort. Am J Gastroenterol. 2008;103(8):1973–80.
57. Tural C, Tor J, Sanvisens A, et al. Accuracy of simple biochemical tests in identifying liver fibrosis in patients co-infected with human immunodeficiency virus and hepatitis c virus. Clin Gastro and Hep. 2009;7:339–45.
58. Macias J, Gonzalez J, Ortega E et al. Use of simple noninvasive biomarkers to predict liver fibrosis in HIV/HCV coinfection in routine clinical practice. HIV Med 2010 Feb 17. [Epub ahead of print]
59. Al-Mohri H, Murphy T, Lu Y, Lalonde RG, Klein MB. Evaluating liver fibrosis progression and the impact of antiretroviral therapy in HIV and hepatitis C coinfection using a non-invasive mark. J Acquir Immune Defic Syndr. 2007;44(4):463–9.
60. Jung HS, Kim YS, Kwon OS, et al. Usefulness of liver stiffness measurement for predicting the presence of esophageal varices in the patients with liver cirrhosis. Korean J Hepatol. 2008;14(3):342–50.
61. Nunes D, Fleming C, Offner G et al. Noninvasive markers of liver fibrosis are highly predictive of liver-related death in a cohort of HCV-infected individuals with and without HIV infection. Am J Gastro 2010 Feb 23. [Epub ahead of print]
62. Smith JO, Sterling RK. Systematic review: noninvasive models of fibrosis analysis in chronic hepatitis C. Aliment Pharmacol Ther. 2009;30(6):557–76.
63. Shire NJ, Rao MB, Succop P, et al. Improving noninvasive methods of assessing liver fibrosis in patients with hepatitis C/human immunodeficiency virus co-infection. Clin Gastroenterol Hepatol. 2009;7:471–80.
64. Boursier J, Vergniol J, Sawadogo A, et al. The combination of a blood test and Fibroscan improves the non-invasive diagnosis of liver fibrosis. Liver Int. 2009;29(10):1507–15.

Mechanisms of Alcoholic Steatosis/Steatohepatitis

Zhanxiang Zhou, Ross E. Jones, and Craig J. McClain

Introduction

Despite extensive research, alcohol remains one of the most common causes of both acute and chronic liver disease in the USA. In Western countries, up to 50% of cases of end-stage liver disease have alcohol as a major etiologic factor. Excessive alcohol consumption is the third leading preventable cause of death in the USA. Alcohol-related deaths, excluding accidents/homicides, accounted for 22,073 deaths in the USA in 2006 with 13,000 of those specifically attributed to alcoholic liver disease (ALD). Given these grim statistics, the mortality of this liver disease is more than that of many major forms of cancer, such as breast, colon and prostate. Importantly, there is no Food and Drug Administration (FDA)-approved therapy for any stage of ALD.

This review heavily focuses on the initial phase of alcoholic liver disease, fatty liver, or steatosis. Almost everyone who drinks heavily for 2–3 weeks will develop hepatic steatosis. However, with abstinence this is rapidly reversible. A small subset (<25%) of patients who continue to drink will develop alcoholic steatohepatitis (AH), and even smaller numbers will ultimately develop cirrhosis and possibly even hepatocellular carcinoma. This article reviews the effects of alcohol on fat metabolism in the liver and mechanisms for alcohol-induced steatosis. We then review the interactions of the microbiome, altered gut permeability, endotoxin, and cytokines in the transition from alcoholic fatty liver to AH and cirrhosis.

Alcoholic Steatosis

As noted above, alcoholic steatosis (fatty liver) is one of the earliest pathological changes in alcoholic liver disease [1]. Alcoholic steatosis is characterized by accumulation of macro- and micro-lipid droplets, which contain triglyceride and cholesterol, in the cytoplasm of hepatocytes, namely, macrovesicular and microvesicular steatosis. Accumulation of lipid in the hepatocyte makes the liver susceptible to inflammatory mediators or other toxic agents ("second hits"-reviewed subsequently), leading to further progression to hepatitis and eventually fibrosis [2]. Alcoholic steatosis is a reversible stage of liver damage and reduction of steatosis will likely halt or slow the progression of alcoholic liver disease.

Hepatic lipid metabolism involves multiple pathways including de novo lipogenesis, lipid uptake, fatty acid oxidation, and lipid export. Alterations of lipid metabolic pathways have been repeatedly reported in patients with alcoholic steatosis and animal models [3, 4]. Alcohol exposure has been shown to cause an imbalance between lipid income and outcome, i.e., increased lipogenesis and lipid uptake, and decreased fatty acid β(beta)-oxidation and very low density lipoproteins (VLDL) secretion. Obviously, these alcohol-induced changes in lipid metabolic pathways favor lipid accumulation in the liver. Mechanistic studies suggest that dysregulation of multiple factors, both intrahepatic and extrahepatic, may affect alcohol metabolic pathways, including transcription factors, oxidative stress, adipokines, and malnutrition.

Alcohol-Induced Disorders in Hepatic Lipid Metabolism

De Novo Lipogenesis

The role of alcohol on liver de novo fatty acid synthesis has long been a research focus related to the pathogenesis of alcoholic fatty liver. Alcohol exposure has been repeatedly

Z. Zhou (✉)
Department of Nutrition, University of North Carolina Greensboro,
500 Laureate Way, Ste 4226, Kannapolis, NC 40202, USA
e-mail: z.zhou@uncg.edu

reported to upregulate fatty acid synthesis genes, including fatty acid synthase (FAS), acetyl-Co A carboxylase (ACC), stearoyl-CoA desaturase (SCD), ATP citrate lyase (ACL), and malic enzyme [5–7]. These lipogenesis genes are regulated by the transcription factor, sterol regulatory element binding proteins (SREBPs) [8]. Activation of SREBPs has been suggested as a major mechanism of alcohol-stimulated fatty acid synthesis in the liver [5, 9, 10]. However, detection of fatty acid synthesis using ^3H_2O incorporation method demonstrated controversial data. A human study showed that the ^3H incorporation to fatty acids in liver slices is significantly lower in patients with alcoholic steatosis in comparison with normal subjects [11]. Chronic alcohol feeding to rats significantly decreases fatty acid synthesis in the liver as indicated by reduced ^3H incorporation to fatty acids and triglycerides after ^3H_2O administration, which agreed well with the results of enzyme activities involved in fatty acid synthesis [12, 13]. Dietary components such as fat level may have impact on hepatic lipogenesis under alcohol exposure. Low-fat/high-carbohydrate diet is likely to promote hepatic de novo lipogenesis in animals chronically fed alcohol [14].

Fatty Acid Oxidation

Fatty acid oxidation occurs in the mitochondria, peroxisomes, or microsomes [15]. Mitochondrial β-oxidation is primarily involved in the oxidation of short-chain, medium-chain, and long-chain fatty acids, while peroxisomal β-oxidation is responsible for the metabolism of very long chain fatty acids. Fatty acids are also oxidized by the microsomal ω(omega)-oxidation system by cytochrome P450 4A enzymes (CYP4A). Decreased hepatic fatty acid oxidation has been suggested as an important mechanism in the development of alcoholic steatosis [9, 10, 14–16]. Early reports with isolated hepatocytes, liver slices, perfused liver, and in vivo showed that the mitochondrial fatty acid oxidation was diminished in the liver after alcohol exposure [17–20]. Rats chronically fed alcohol showed a persistent impairment of mitochondrial β-oxidation of fatty acids to CO_2, although the oxidation of fatty acids to acetyl-CoA is not decreased [20]. Alcohol metabolism is known to reduce NAD^+ to NADH, leading to a reduced ratio of $NAD^+/NADH$ [21]. Because NAD^+ is required for tricarboxylic acid cycle and β-oxidation of fatty acid, reduction of NAD^+ will certainly impair mitochondrial fatty acid β-oxidation. However, peroxisomal fatty acid β-oxidation was reported to be increased alcohol-fed rats as indicated by increased β-oxidation of palmitoyl CoA [22]. Cytochrome P450-dependent lauric acid ω-hydroxylation was also increased as indicated by an increase in microsomal fatty acid ω-oxidation [22, 23]. Acetyl-CoA dehydrogenase medium chain (MCAD), long chain (LCAD), or very long chain (VLCAD) enzymes are important enzymes involved in fatty acid oxidation. Chronic alcohol exposure in mice decreased the mRNA levels of MCAD and LCAD [24]. PPAR-α (alpha) is a key regulator of these fatty acid oxidation genes, and inactivation of PPAR-α transcriptional activity has been suggested as a major molecular mechanism of alcohol-impaired fatty acid oxidation [9, 10, 25].

VLDL Secretion

Triglyceride and cholesterol synthesized in the liver are exported to the peripheral organs in the form of VLDL. The VLDL secretion rate from the liver is commonly assessed by measuring increase in blood lipid after administration of lipoprotein lipase inhibitor, Triton WR-1339. By using this method, the VLDL secretion rate as well as the contents of cholesterol and triacylglycerol of VLDL was found to be reduced in alcohol-fed rats [26]. A 16% reduction of VLDL-triglyceride secretion from isolated hepatocyte was also found in alcohol-fed rats [27]. Recent studies showed that acceleration of hepatic VLDL secretion is one of the protective mechanisms underlying reduction of alcohol-induced hepatic lipid accumulation by betaine or zinc [28, 29]. Microsomal triglyceride transfer protein (MTTP) plays a central role in the assembly of VLDL. Chronic alcohol exposure to rats decreased the mRNA level and the activity of Mttp in association with lipid accumulation in the liver [30, 31]. Administration of hepatocyte growth factor attenuated alcoholic fatty liver in association with upregulation of MTTP [32]. On the contrary, the main structural protein of VLDL, apolipoprotein B 100 (Apo B), also critically regulates VLDL secretion. Alcohol exposure to rats dramatically reduced the ApoB in the liver and VLDL in serum [33]. PPAR-α and hepatocyte nuclear factor-4α (HNF-4α) are transcription factors involved in regulation of lipid export genes such as Mttp and ApoB. Chronic alcohol exposure has shown to inhibit the DNA binding activity of PPAR-α and HNF-4α [24, 29]. In addition, increased ApoB protein was associated with reduction of hepatic lipid after treatment of hepatocyte growth factor or a PPAR-γ (gamma) agonist [32, 34].

Fatty Acid Uptake

Increased fatty acid uptake by hepatocytes due to reverse transport from adipose tissue has been suggested to contribute to the development of alcoholic steatosis [3, 4]. An in vitro study with HepG2 cells showed that alcohol exposure increased fatty acid uptake (^3H-oleic acid) in a dose-dependent manner [35]. Primary hepatocyte culture studies also showed that the fatty acid uptake (^3H-oleic acid) in rats chronically fed alcohol was increased by 2.6-fold in comparison with pair-fed controls [36]. One dose alcohol exposure to rats increased the incorporation of ^{14}H-palmitate to the liver triglyceride by 50% [37]. Chronic alcohol feeding to rats induced a twofold increase in the incorporation of ^{3}H-palmitate to triglyceride or total lipid [38]. These results suggest that increased fatty acid uptake may play an important role in the development of alcoholic fatty liver. In support of these observations, alcohol exposure has been shown to cause excess lipolysis of the adipose tissue, and the released fatty acids are likely a major source of hepatic lipid [3, 4].

Clinical studies demonstrated that alcoholics may have a significantly lower body weight and lower fat mass than controls [39, 40]. Importantly, most of the alcoholics were shown to have fatty liver, suggesting a negative correlation between liver fat and body fat mass. Alcohol feeding to rats for 2–4 weeks showed a time-dependent decrease in epididymal adipose mass by up to −31% [29, 41]. The effects of alcohol on fatty acid mobilization from the adipose tissue and hepatic uptake have been determined in animal study [42]. This study utilized ^{14}C-palmitate to in situ-label the gonadal adipose depots, followed with acute alcohol administration. The release of labeled fatty acid from the gonadal adipose depots measured 16 h later showed that the mobilization of ^{14}C-palmitate-labeled gonadal adipose depots were 2.3-fold higher than saline control. In accordance with these findings, the incorporation of the mobilized ^{14}C in the liver was 2.7-fold higher in the alcohol-treated rats vs. the saline controls [42]. This study clearly showed a link between alcohol-induced adipose tissue lipolysis and hepatic fatty acid uptake. Dietary zinc supplementation has been shown to reverse hepatic lipid accumulation in mice chronically fed alcohol. Interestingly, zinc also partially attenuated alcohol-reduced white adipose mass. These data suggest that fatty acid release from the adipose tissue may have significant impact on the development of alcoholic steatosis.

Molecular Mechanisms of Alcohol Actions on Lipid Metabolism

Several transcription factors have shown to critically regulate lipid metabolic genes, including PPAR-α, SREBPs, HNF-4α. Generally speaking, PPAR-α and HNF-4α regulate lipid utilization and export, while SREBPs regulate lipid synthesis. However, alcohol exposure has been shown to differentially modulate these transcription factors, inhibiting PPAR-α/HNF-4α and stimulating SREBPs. Multiple mechanisms have been suggested to mediate alcohol effects on these transcriptional factors, including adiponectin deficiency, inhibition of adenosine monophosphate-dependent protein kinase (AMPK) signaling pathway, oxidative stress, and zinc deficiency.

PPAR-α

PPAR-α is a member of nuclear hormone receptor family and plays crucial role in regulation of hepatic lipid metabolism [9, 10, 43]. PPAR-α critically regulates genes involved in fatty acid transport into mitochondria such as carnitine palmitoyl-transferase-I (CPT-I) and genes of fatty acid oxidation such as ACAD. PPAR-α also regulates genes involved in hepatic lipid export such as Mttp and ApoB. Knockout of PPAR-α in mice led to progressive dyslipidemia and steatosis [44]. PPAR-α-Knockout mice were also more susceptible to methionine-choline deficiency-induced steatohepatitis [45]. PPAR-α is one of the most well recognized transcription factors in mechanistic studies on the pathogenesis of alcoholic steatosis [25, 43]. Although the data on PPAR-α mRNA and protein levels are controversial, chronic alcohol exposure in mice has been repeatedly reported to suppress the DNA binding activity of PPAR-α [14, 29]. Treatment with the PPAR-α agonist, WY14,643, has been shown to stimulate fatty acid β-oxidation and attenuated hepatic lipid accumulation in mice chronically fed alcohol [24]. WY14,643 increased PPAR-α protein by 1.5-fold and DNA binding activity by threefold. Accordingly, PPAR-α target genes; in particular, the fatty acid β-oxidation-related genes were upregulated by WY14,643. Treatment with other PPAR-α agonists, fenofibrate and clofibrate, in chronic alcohol-fed rats also remarkably reduced alcoholic steatosis [46, 47]. Restoration of PPAR-α activity was also associated with the reversal effect of zinc on alcoholic steatosis in mice chronically fed alcohol [29]. These studies clearly demonstrated that dysfunction of PPAR-α is an etiologic factor in the development of alcoholic steatosis.

HNF-4α

HNF-4α is a member of the nuclear receptor superfamily and a master regulator of hepatic gene expression [48], and it has been shown to bind to the reporters of more than 1,200 genes involved in most aspects of hepatocyte function [49]. Liver-specific conditional knockout of HNF-4α in adult mice led to severe steatosis in association with disruption of expression of genes involved in VLDL secretion [50]. Mice lacking HNF4 exhibited decreases in gene expression of Mttp, ApoB, ApoAII, ApoCII, and ApoCIII [50]. Therefore, HNF-4α is likely a major regulator of genes involved in the control of lipid export from the liver. Blunted lipid export has been well documented in alcohol-induced liver steatosis [26–29]. Mechanistic studies showed that alcohol has inhibitory effects on Mttp activity, and ApoB secretion in hepatoma cells [30], and on the synthesis of apolipoproteins in the liver of rats chronically fed alcohol [30, 33, 51]. However, the role of HNF-4α in regulation of VLDL synthesis and secretion is poorly understood in the pathogenesis of alcoholic steatosis. A recent study demonstrated that chronic alcohol exposure in mice did not affect the mRNA and protein levels of HNF-4α protein, but decreased the DNA binding activity of HNF-4α [29]. In accordance, chronic alcohol exposure downregulated Mttp and ApoB genes and reduced VLDL secretion rate from the liver. Reactivation of HNF-4α by zinc supplementation was accompanied by upregulation of genes involved in both VLDL secretion (Mttp, Apob) and fatty acid β-oxidation (LCAD). These results suggest that inactivation of HNF-4α, at least partially, accounts for alcohol-induced suppression of VLDL secretion and fatty acid oxidation.

SREBPs

SREBPs are transcription factors involved in the synthesis of fatty acids, triglycerides, and cholesterol. SREBP-1c and SREBP-2 predominately distribute in the liver and regulate hepatic genes involved in triglyceride and cholesterol synthesis, respectively [5, 9, 10, 43]. Usually found in endoplasmic reticulum as inactive molecules, these proteins undergo activation through exposure to ethanol [5, 43]. SREBP-1c critically regulates genes involved in de novo lipogenesis such as ACC, FAS, fatty acid elongase 6, and SCD-1. Feeding mice a low-fat diet with ethanol for 4 weeks resulted in a significant increase in steady-state levels of the mature (active) form of SREBP-1 [5]. Activation of SREBP-1 by ethanol feeding was associated with increased expression of hepatic lipogenic genes as well as the accumulation of triglyceride in the livers [5]. This ethanol-induced activation is believed to be secondary to ethanol's inhibition of AMPK, a regulatory protein that responds to cellular stress such as oxidative stress or reduced energy states [5, 43]. Additional studies have also implicated the stimulatory effects of alcohol on MAPK, which in turn activates the SREBPs [5]. Mice lacking genes expressing SREBP-1 were found to be protected from the effects of chronic alcohol feeding [52]. Furthermore, decreased steatosis development and inhibition of SREBPs was observed in mice pretreated with TNF-α blocking agents [53]. Accumulation of acetaldehydes and inhibition of AMPK have been suggested as mechanisms of alcohol-induced activation of SREBPs [43].

AMPK

AMPK is a crucial regulator in energy metabolism in the liver [43, 54]. AMPK signal transduction stimulates energy-generating pathways such as fatty acid oxidation but inhibits energy-requiring pathways such as fatty acid and triglyceride synthesis, thereby negatively impacting on hepatic lipid concentration [43, 54]. Inhibition of AMPK activity has been reported in association with reduction of CPT1, activation of ACC and accumulation of malonyl-CoA in animals chronically fed alcohol [55]. A proposed mechanism involves decreased AMPK activation after ethanol exposure resulting in upregulation of SREBPs and sequential downregulation of PPAR-α [14]. Administration of AICAR, an AMPK activator, to rats chronically fed alcohol restored AMPK activity, decreased SREBP-1c, and reduced FAS expression, leading to suppression of alcoholic steatosis [56]. Resveratrol, a dietary polyphenol, has been identified as a potent activator of AMPK. Resveratrol treatment has been shown to reduce lipid synthesis, increase fatty acid oxidation, and prevent alcoholic liver steatosis in mice [57]. The protective action of resveratrol is in whole or in part mediated through the upregulation of AMPK signaling in the liver. Activation of AMPK in association with a reduction of lipid synthesis and increase in fatty acid oxidation was also associated with the beneficial effects of metadoxine/garlic oil on alcohol-induces hepatic steatosis in a rats [58]. This downregulation of AMPK by ethanol was suggested to be the toxic effect of acetaldehyde, but now is also thought to be secondary to circulating levels of adiponectin [43, 59].

Adiponectin

Increasing evidence suggests that adiponectin, an adipokine secreted exclusively from adipocytes, critically regulate lipid metabolism, stimulating fatty acid oxidation and suppressing lipogenesis [52, 59]. Two major adiponectin receptors have been identified on plasma membrane, adiponectin receptor 1 (AdipoR1) and adiponectin receptor 2 (AdipoR2), and adipoR2 is the predominate subtype in the liver. Activation of adiponectin receptor-mediated signaling is known to activate AMPK, leading to inhibition of fatty acid synthesis via inhibition of SREBP-1c [59]. Conversely, adiponectin signaling in the liver also stimulates fatty acid β-oxidation via activating PPAR-α and PGC-1α [52]. Thus, the consequence of adiponectin signal transduction in the liver is reduction of lipid accumulation. Dysregulation of adiponectin and hepatic adiponectin receptors has been reported in animal model of alcoholic steatosis. Alcohol exposure reduced the mRNA and protein expression of adiponectin in adipose tissues, leading to reduction of serum adiponectin level [57, 60, 61]. Chronic alcohol exposure also downregulated the mRNA and protein levels of adiponectin receptors in the liver [6, 57, 61]. Delivery of recombinant adiponectin has been reported to dramatically alleviate alcoholic steatosis as well as inflammation and the elevated levels of serum alanine aminotransferase [62]. Elevation of circulating adiponectin level was associated with the beneficial effects of dietary supplementation with resveratrol, S-adenosylmethionine, taurine, saturated fat, and rosiglitazone (a PPAR-γ agonist) on alcoholic steatosis [6, 57, 63–65]. Resveratrol administration also enhanced mRNA expression of hepatic adiponectin receptors (AdipoR1/R2) [57]. Similarly, rosiglitazone treatment upregulated the mRNA and protein levels of adiponectin and its receptors in adipose tissue and liver, respectively [65].

Oxidative Stress

Oxidative stress is a fundamental cellular disorder in alcohol-induced liver disease [21]. Alcohol is metabolized in the liver via alcohol dehydrogenase (ADH) and the microsomal cytochrome P450 2E1 (CYP2E1). The K_m for ethanol oxidation by the microsomal CYP2E1 is about 10 mM, which was about an order of magnitude greater than the K_m for ethanol by ADH. Chronic alcohol exposure is well known to upregulate hepatic CYP2E1 rather than ADH [66–69]. Alcohol metabolism via CYP2E1 generates reactive oxygen species, and CYP2E1 has been suggested to be highly responsible for alcohol-induced oxidant stress [70]. While oxidative stress is well known to induce cell injury, increasing evidence suggests that oxidative stress is also a causal factor in the development of alcoholic steatosis.

Overexpression of CYP2E1 in the liver not only exaggerated alcohol-induced oxidative stress, but also dramatically increased lipid accumulation in CYP2E1 transgenic mice chronically fed alcohol [71, 72]. Conversely, CYP2E1 deficiency in the liver normalized alcohol-induced triglyceride accumulation in CYP2E1-knockout mice chronically fed alcohol [73]. Similarly, treatment with CYP2E1 inhibitor, chlormethiazole, attenuated alcoholic steatosis in association with inhibition of oxidative stress [73]. In addition, introduction of CYP2E1 to CYP2E1-knockout mice via an adenovirus restored macrovesicular fat accumulation. Interestingly, PPAR-α activation and upregulated PPAR-α targeted genes such as acyl-CoA oxidase were associated with attenuation of oxidative stress due to CYP2E1 knockout/inhibition [73]. These data indicate a possible link between oxidative stress and PPAR-α inactivation in the development of alcoholic steatosis.

Zinc Deficiency

Zinc is the send abundant trace element in the body next to iron. While zinc is well known to act as a cofactor in more than 300 metalloenzymes, zinc also plays important role in cellular functions such as signal transduction and gene expression. Increasing evidence suggests that zinc plays a critical role in regulation of hepatic lipid metabolism. A lower hepatic zinc level was associated with steatosis in leptin receptor deficiency rats [74]. Feeding rats with a zinc-deficient diet (a single nutrient deficiency) causes hepatic lipid accumulation in association with dysregulation of a large number of genes involved in lipid metabolism [75, 76]. Zinc deficiency is one of the most consistently observed nutritional/biochemical manifestations in alcoholic liver disease [77]. Clinical studies demonstrated that zinc concentrations in both serum and liver were significantly reduced in patients with alcoholic steatosis, hepatitis and cirrhosis [78–80].

Dietary supplementation with zinc in mice reverses alcoholic steatosis in the presence of alcohol exposure [29]. Reactivation of HNF-4α and PPAR-α was involved in zinc action on hepatic fatty acid β-oxidation and VLDL secretion. Inhibition of oxidative stress and acceleration of alcohol metabolism were associated with zinc action on alcoholic steatosis and liver injury. Cell culture studies further identified the zinc depletion significantly suppressed the DNA-binding activities of HNF-4α and PPAR-α, without affecting their protein levels, indicating a requirement of zinc coordination for HNF-4α and PPAR-α function [29]. HNF-4α and PPAR-α are zinc-finger transcription factors, and elimination of zinc coordination by oxidative stress from the zinc finger will disassemble the secondary structure of these proteins, leading to defective DNA binding and decreased transcription of target genes [81]. Therefore, the mechanistic link between oxidative stress and zinc deficiency, at least partially, accounts for alcohol-induced inactivation of PPAR-α and HNF-4α and hepatic lipid dyshomeostasis.

Gut–Liver Axis in Progression of ALD

Almost everyone who drinks heavily for at least 1–2 weeks will develop fatty liver, the first histological stage of ALD. A much smaller subset of subjects who continue to drink regularly will go on to develop AH. A baseline of fatty liver transitions to more severe inflammation, injury, and fibrosis through a series of insults or "second hits" (Fig. 6.1). We have thus far reviewed mechanisms of altered lipid metabolism in ALD and mechanisms for the development of initial alcoholic steatosis. We now focus on the interactions of the microbiome, gut permeability, endotoxin, and proinflammatory cytokines as one pathway for driving steatosis to steatohepatitis and cirrhosis.

It has been recognized for over a half century that the gut flora and gut-derived toxins play a critical role in the development of both liver disease and certain complications such as hepatic or portal systemic (PSE) encephalopathy [82–91]. Indeed, over 50 years ago, it was shown that germ free rodents or rodents treated with antibiotics to "sterilize the gut" were resistant to nutritional and toxin-induced liver injury. Elegant studies by Broitman and coworkers showed that rats fed a choline-deficient diet developed cirrhosis

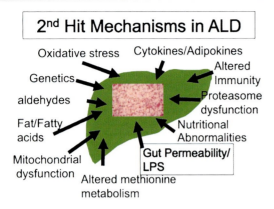

Fig. 6.1 Chronic alcohol feeding and a fatty liver sensitizes the liver to multiple second hits, which can cause progression to inflammation/injury and fibrosis

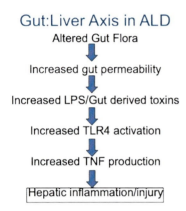

Fig. 6.2 Alcohol-induced alterations in gut flora/permeability can lead to activation of Tolls and subsequent hepatic inflammation/injury

which could be prevented by oral neomycin. However, when endotoxin was added to the water supply, neomycin was no longer able to prevent the development of liver injury and fibrosis [86]. Subsequently, it was been shown that alcohol alters gut flora and intestinal permeability. Alterations and permeability allow gut-derived toxins to cross the intestinal barrier and activate Kupffer cells, which are "primed" to overproduce inflammatory cytokines, which in turn cause liver inflammation/injury (Fig. 6.2). Mechanisms for intestinal permeability changes include acetaldehyde generation from alcohol, nitric oxide production, alterations in nutrition such as zinc deficiency, and others. Gut-derived toxins that cross the barrier include not only endotoxins or LPS but also other gut-derived products such as peptidoglycan.

Later, studies showed that antibiotics, prebiotics, and probiotics all prevented the development of experimental alcohol-induced liver injury [92–95]. Increased plasma/hepatic concentrations of proinflammatory cytokines such as tumor necrosis factor (TNF) were noted in rodent models of alcoholic liver disease (ALD), and mice given anti-TNF antibodies or mice lacking TNFR1 were protected against the development of experimental ALD [96, 97]. Moreover, chronic alcohol feeding was shown to sensitize to the hepatotoxicity induced by gut-derived endotoxin and TNF, and specific components of the TLR4 pathway responsible for alcohol-related liver injury are being defined [98, 99]. Indeed, TLR4 activation by endotoxin results in recruitment of the adaptor molecules MyD88 and Toll/interleukin-1 receptor (TIR) domain-containing adapter-inducing interferon-β (TRIF), which each activate separate downstream signaling cascades. Recent data suggest that the MyD88-independent pathway (TRIF) is more important in the development of ALD, whereas nonalcoholic steatohepatitis appears to signal through the MyD88-dependent pathway [99].

Concomitant studies in patients with alcoholic hepatitis (AH) and/or cirrhosis showed increased gut permeability and endotoxemia. Over 20 years ago, we first reported that patients with AH had increased basal and endotoxin-stimulated monocyte TNF production, and subsequent studies showed that plasma and monocyte proinflammatory cytokines correlated with the clinical course of AH and survival [100, 101]. Unfortunately, recent human studies have not demonstrated therapeutic efficacy for biologics such as anti-TNF antibody/TNF soluble receptors in AH [102, 103]. Thus, it appears that complete TNF blockade is not a viable therapeutic option in ALD, possibly because of the necessary role for a basal level of TNF in liver regeneration [104, 105]. However, compelling data suggest that gut-derived toxins play an etiologic role in the development/progression of ALD, and new therapeutic approaches for this target are necessary. Similar to alcohol, HIV (especially early in the course of infection) can disrupt gut barrier and cause endotoxemia. Microbial/toxin translocation is associated with systemic immune inflammation, which plays a role in certain HIV complications such as neurological degeneration [106]. The role of alcohol in aggravating HIV effects/complications has not been well defined. In theory, some of the factors that may improve gut barrier function following alcohol abuse may be of benefit in HIV infections/complications.

Therapy for ALD and Conclusions

Major advances have been made in our understanding of the mechanisms for the development and progression of ALD, and we have reviewed many of the mechanisms leading to initial steatosis. In experimental animals, one can block fatty liver and initial liver injury by blocking TNF/proinflammatory cytokine production, inhibiting oxidative stress, or altering the clotting cascade. Moreover, many of these pathways are highly interactive; for example, there are major interactions between oxidative stress and proinflammatory cytokine production. Unfortunately, these seemingly straightforward mechanisms for ALD have not translated into effective therapy for human ALD [107–109].

There are multiple potential reasons for this apparent lack of translation of therapeutic efficacy into humans. In most experimental models (both in vitro and in vivo), the experimental design focuses on preventing the development of liver disease rather than treating already-developed liver injury. In the clinical situation, patients present with AH or cirrhosis and treatment instead of prevention is required.

Next, clinical trials have shown that small biologic molecules, such as anti-TNF, appear to be ineffective in acute AH [110]. Such therapy is highly effective at preventing experimental ALD, but it may be less effective treating established disease. A "baseline" low concentration of TNF appears to be required for liver regeneration, while excess TNF can be hepatotoxic. Thus, inhibiting all TNF activity with biologic therapy may not be an appropriate strategy for treatment of AH. Rather, drugs such as pentoxifylline and corticosteroids that downregulate TNF production may be a more effective therapeutic approach. Indeed, two randomized clinical trials have shown therapeutic efficacy of pentoxifylline in severe AH. The first trial compared pentoxifylline against placebo and the second compared it against corticosteroids [111, 112]. The dose of pentoxifylline, a nonspecific phosphodiesterase inhibitor, was 400 mg tid in both studies. Pentoxifylline was especially beneficial in blocking hepatorenal syndrome. Multiple meta-analyses have documented benefits of corticosteroids in patients with severe AH who do not have factors that would contraindicate corticosteroid therapy [113]. Standard therapy for severe AH is 40 mg prednisone/day to be tapered after about 1 month of therapy. Importantly, the early change in bilirubin level accurately predicts who will not respond to steroid therapy. Thus, if there is no drop in the serum bilirubin over 1 week, steroids should be stopped [114]. Both of these agents work by dampening the proinflammatory immune system (and possibly through other mechanisms).

Doses and formulations of agents may also play an important role in therapeutic efficacy, especially in antioxidant therapy. Drugs such as vitamin E may impact terminal processes in oxidative stress and may not be potent enough to be effective. Potentially stimulating the body's own endogenous antioxidant systems may be more beneficial than providing exogenous antioxidants. Moreover, we need to monitor therapeutic endpoints. Thus, if patients are receiving antioxidant therapy, is this therapy effective in decreasing biomarkers of oxidative stress? Such monitoring was not performed in the past.

Lastly, as noted above, most large clinical trials have focused on therapeutic intervention for acute alcoholic hepatitis which is a more advanced and often lethal component in the spectrum of ALD. Limited clinical studies have focused earlier stages of ALD. Extensive studies in animals have shown that probiotics and prebiotics (such as oats) improved gut barrier function and endotoxemia [69, 93, 94]. Moreover, supplementation certain nutrients such as zinc also improves gut barrier function and endotoxemia in early ALD [115, 116]. We have shown that patients hospitalized for detoxification and psychosis due to alcohol abuse have altered gut flora, and they had more rapid correction of their liver enzymes with probiotic therapy. Thus, there is great promise for this type of gut oriented therapy in ALD, and it could in theory also benefit patients who are HIV positive with altered gut flora/barrier function.

Summary

We have markedly expanded our understanding of all phases of ALD, and we highlight early steatosis in this review. This knowledge now needs to be translated into the development of effective therapy, and this will require close interactions between basic scientists, clinicians, and industry. We have an improved understanding of mechanisms for fatty liver in ALD, the role of the gut–liver axis in disease progression, and the possible role of potential therapeutic interventions that modulate gut bacteria or barrier function. The linkage between HIV-associated increases in gut permeability, alcohol, and liver injury also remains to be elucidated.

References

1. Hall P. Pathological spectrum of alcoholic liver disease. In: Hall P, editor. Alcoholic liver disease. 2nd ed. London: Edward Arnold; 1995. p. 41–88.
2. Purohit V, Russo D, Coates PM. Role of fatty liver, dietary fatty acid supplements, and obesity in the progression of alcoholic liver disease: introduction and summary of the symposium. Alcohol. 2004;34:3–8.
3. Lakshman MR. Some novel insights into the pathogenesis of alcoholic steatosis. Alcohol. 2004;34:45–8.
4. Baraona E, Lieber CS. Effects of ethanol on lipid metabolism. J Lipid Res. 1979;20(3):289–315.
5. You M, Fischer M, Deeg MA, Crabb DW. Ethanol induces fatty acid synthesis pathways by activation of sterol regulatory element-binding protein (SREBP). J Biol Chem 2002;277(32):29342–7.
6. Esfandiari F, You M, Villanueva JA, et al. S-adenosylmethionine attenuates hepatic lipid synthesis in micropigs fed ethanol with a folate-deficient diet. Alcohol Clin Exp Res. 2007;31(7):1231–9.
7. Yin HQ, Je YT, Kim M, et al. Analysis of hepatic gene expression during fatty liver change due to chronic ethanol administration in mice. Toxicol Appl Pharmacol. 2009;235(3):312–20.
8. Shimano H. Sterol regulatory element-binding protein family as global regulators of lipid synthetic genes in energy metabolism. Vitam Horm. 2002;65:167–94.
9. You M, Crabb DW. Recent advances in alcoholic liver disease II. Minireview: molecular mechanisms of alcoholic fatty liver. Am J Physiol Gastrointest Liver Physiol. 2004;287(1):G1–6.
10. Purohit V, Gao B, Song BJ. Molecular mechanisms of alcoholic fatty liver. Alcohol Clin Exp Res. 2009;33(2):191–205.

11. Venkatesan S, Leung NW, Peters TJ. Fatty acid synthesis in vitro by liver tissue from control subjects and patients with alcoholic liver disease. Clin Sci (Lond). 1986;71(6):723–8.
12. Tijburg LB, Maquedano A, Bijleveld C, et al. Effects of ethanol feeding on hepatic lipid synthesis. Arch Biochem Biophys. 1988;267(2):568–79.
13. Simpson KJ, Venkatesan S, Peters TJ. Fatty acid synthesis by rat liver after chronic ethanol feeding with a low-fat diet. Clin Sci (Lond). 1994;87(4):441–6.
14. You M, Matsumoto M, Pacold CM, et al. The role of AMP-activated protein kinase in the action of ethanol in the liver. Gastroenterology. 2004;127(6):1798–808.
15. Reddy JK, Hashimoto T. Peroxisomal-oxidation and peroxisome proliferator-activated receptor: an adaptive metabolic system. Annu Rev Nutr. 2001;21:193–230.
16. Sozio M, Crabb DW. Alcohol and lipid metabolism. Am J Physiol Endocrinol Metab. 2008;295(1):E10–6.
17. Lieber CS, Lefevre A, Spritz N, et al. Difference in hepatic metabolism of long and medium-chain fatty acids: the role of fatty acid chain length in the production of alcoholic fatty liver. J Clin Invest. 1967;46:1451–60.
18. Blomstrand R, Kager L, Lantto O. Studies on the ethanol-induced decrease of fatty acid oxidation in rat and human liver slices. Life Sci. 1973;13:1131–41.
19. Ontko JA. Effects of ethanol on the metabolism of free fatty acids in isolated liver cells. J Lipid Res. 1973;14:78–85.
20. Cederbaum AI, Lieber CS, Beattie DS, Rubin E. Effect of chronic ethanol ingestion on fatty acid oxidation by hepatic mitochondria. J Biol Chem. 1975;250(13):5122–9.
21. Lieber CS. Ethanol metabolism, cirrhosis and alcoholism. Clin Chim Acta. 1997;257:59–84.
22. Orellana M, Rodrigo R, Valdés E. Peroxisomal and microsomal fatty acid oxidation in liver of rats after chronic ethanol consumption. Gen Pharmacol. 1998;31(5):817–20.
23. Ma X, Baraona E, Lieber CS. Alcohol consumption enhances fatty acid omega-oxidation, with a greater increase in male than in female rats. Hepatology. 1993;18(5):1247–53.
24. Fischer M, You M, Matsumoto M, Crabb DW. Peroxisome proliferator-activated receptor alpha (PPARalpha) agonist treatment reverses PPARalpha dysfunction and abnormalities in hepatic lipid metabolism in ethanol-fed mice. J Biol Chem. 2003;278(30):27997–8004.
25. Crabb DW, Galli A, Fischer M, You M. Molecular mechanisms of alcoholic fatty liver: role of peroxisome proliferator-activated receptor alpha. Alcohol. 2004;34(1):35–8.
26. Venkatesan S, Ward RJ, Peters TJ. Effect of chronic ethanol feeding on the hepatic secretion of very-low-density lipoproteins. Biochim Biophys Acta. 1988;960(1):61–6.
27. García-Villafranca J, Guillén A, Castro J. Desensitization of cyclic GMP-mediated regulation of fatty acid metabolism in hepatocytes from ethanol-fed rats. Int J Biochem Cell Biol. 2005;37(3):655–64.
28. Kharbanda KK, Todero SL, Ward BW, et al. Betaine administration corrects ethanol-induced defective VLDL secretion. Mol Cell Biochem. 2009;327(1–2):75–8.
29. Kang X, Zhong W, Liu J, et al. Zinc supplementation reverses alcohol-induced steatosis in mice through reactivating hepatocyte nuclear factor-4alpha and peroxisome proliferator-activated receptor-alpha. Hepatology. 2009;50(4):1241–50.
30. Lin MC, Li JJ, Wang EJ, et al. Ethanol down-regulates the transcription of microsomal triglyceride transfer protein gene. FASEB J. 1997;11(13):1145–52.
31. Sugimoto T, Yamashita S, Ishigami M, et al. Decreased microsomal triglyceride transfer protein activity contributes to initiation of alcoholic liver steatosis in rats. J Hepatol. 2002;36(2):157–62.
32. Tahara M, Matsumoto K, Nukiwa T, Nakamura T. Hepatocyte growth factor leads to recovery from alcohol-induced fatty liver in rats. J Clin Invest. 1999;103(3):313–20.
33. Lau PP, Cahill DJ, Zhu HJ, Chan L. Ethanol modulates apolipoprotein B mRNA editing in the rat. J Lipid Res. 1995;36(10):2069–78.
34. Tomita K, Azuma T, Kitamura N, et al. Pioglitazone prevents alcohol-induced fatty liver in rats through up-regulation of c-Met. Gastroenterology. 2004;26(3):873–85.
35. Zhou SL, Gordon RE, Bradbury M, et al. Ethanol up-regulates fatty acid uptake and plasma membrane expression and export of mitochondrial aspartate aminotransferase in HepG2 cells. Hepatology. 1998;27(4):1064–74.
36. Berk PD, Zhou S, Bradbury MW. Increased hepatocellular uptake of long chain fatty acids occurs by different mechanisms in fatty livers due to obesity or excess ethanol use, contributing to development of steatohepatitis in both settings. Trans Am Clin Climatol Assoc. 2005;116:335–44.
37. Abrams MA, Cooper C. Quantitative analysis of metabolism of hepatic triglyceride in ethanol-treated rats. Biochem J. 1976;156(1):33–46.
38. Baraona E, Lieber CS. Effects of chronic ethanol feeding on serum lipoprotein metabolism in the rat. J Clin Invest. 1970;49(4):769–78.
39. Addolorato G, Capristo E, Greco AV, et al. Energy expenditure, substrate oxidation, and body composition in subjects with chronic alcoholism: new findings from metabolic assessment. Alcohol Clin Exp Res. 1997;21(6):962–7.
40. Leggio L, Malandrino N, Ferrulli A, et al. Is cortisol involved in the alcohol-related fat mass impairment? A longitudinal clinical study. Alcohol. 2009;44(2):211–5.
41. Kang L, Chen X, Sebastian BM, et al. Chronic ethanol and triglyceride turnover in white adipose tissue in rats: inhibition of the antilipolytic action of insulin after chronic ethanol contributes to increased triglyceride degradation. J Biol Chem. 2007;282(39):28465–73.
42. Kessler JI, Yalovsky-Mishkin S. Effect of ingestion of saline, glucose, and ethanol on mobilization and hepatic incorporation of epididymal pad palmitate-1-14C in rats. J Lipid Res. 1966;7(6):772–7.
43. Crabb DW, Liangpunsakul S. Alcohol and lipid metabolism. J Gastroenterol Hepatol. 2006;21 Suppl 3:S56–60.
44. Costet P, Legendre C, More J, et al. Peroxisome proliferator-activated receptor alpha-isoform deficiency leads to progressive dyslipidemia with sexually dimorphic obesity and steatosis. J Biol Chem. 1998;273:29577–85.
45. Kersten S, Seydoux J, Peters JM, et al. Peroxisome proliferator-activated receptor alpha mediates the adaptive response to fasting. J Clin Invest. 1999;103:1489–98.
46. Tsutsumi A, Takase S. Effect of fenofibrate on fatty liver in rats treated with alcohol. Alcohol Clin Exp Res. 2001;25:75S–9.
47. Nanji AA, Dannenberg AJ, Jokelainen K, Bass NM. Alcoholic liver injury in the rat is associated with reduced expression of peroxisome proliferator-alpha (PPARalpha)-regulated genes and is ameliorated by PPARalpha activation. J Pharmacol Exp Ther. 2004;310(1):417–24.
48. Watt AJ, Garrison WD, Duncan SA. HNF4: a central regulator of hepatocyte differentiation and function. Hepatology. 2003;37:1249–53.
49. Odom DT, Zizlsperger N, Gordon DB, et al. Control of pancreas and liver gene expression by HNF transcription factors. Science. 2004;303:1378–81.
50. Hayhurst GP, Lee YH, Lambert G, et al. Hepatocyte nuclear factor 4alpha (nuclear receptor 2A1) is essential for maintenance of hepatic gene expression and lipid homeostasis. Mol Cell Biol. 2001;21:1393–403.
51. Lakshman MR, Chirtel SJ, Chambers LC. Hepatic synthesis of apoproteins of very-low-density and high density lipoproteins in perfused rat liver: Influence of chronic heavy and moderate doses of ethanol. Alcohol Clin Exp Res. 1989;13:554–9.
52. You M, Rogers CQ. Adiponectin: a key adipokine in alcoholic fatty liver. Exp Biol Med. 2009;234:850–9.
53. Endo M, Masaki T, Seike M, Yoshimatsu H. TNF-beta inces hepatic steatosis in mice by enhancing gene expression of sterol regulatory element binding protein-1c (SREBP-1c). Exp Biol Med. 2007;232:614–21.

54. Misra P. AMP activated protein kinase: a next generation target for total metabolic control. Expert Opin Ther Targets. 2008;12:91–100.
55. García-Villafranca J, Guillén A, Castro J. Ethanol consumption impairs regulation of fatty acid metabolism by decreasing the activity of AMP-activated protein kinase in rat liver. Biochimie. 2008;90:460–6.
56. Tomita K, Tamiya G, Ando S, et al. AICAR, an AMPK activator, has protective effects on alcohol-induced fatty liver in rats. Alcohol Clin Exp Res. 2005;29:240S–5.
57. Ajmo JM, Liang X, Rogers CQ, et al. Resveratrol alleviates alcoholic fatty liver in mice. Am J Physiol Gastrointest Liver Physiol. 2008;295(4):G833–42.
58. Ki SH, Choi JH, Kim CW, Kim SG. Combined metadoxine and garlic oil treatment efficaciously abrogates alcoholic steatosis and CYP2E1 induction in rat liver with restoration of AMPK activity. Chem Biol Interact. 2007;169:80–90.
59. Kadowaki T, Yamauchi T. Adiponectin and adiponectin receptors. Endocr Rev. 2005;26:439–51.
60. Chen X, Sebastian BM, Nagy LE. Chronic ethanol feeding to rats decreases adiponectin secretion by subcutaneous adipocytes. Am J Physiol Endocrinol Metab. 2007;292:E621–8.
61. Song Z, Zhou Z, Deaciuc I, et al. Inhibition of adiponectin production by homocysteine: a potential mechanism for alcoholic liver disease. Hepatology. 2008;47:867–79.
62. Xu A, Wang Y, Keshaw H, et al. The fat-derived hormone adiponectin alleviates alcoholic and nonalcoholic fatty liver diseases in mice. J Clin Invest. 2003;112(1):91–100.
63. Chen X, Sebastian BM, Tang H, et al. Taurine supplementation prevents ethanol-induced decrease in serum adiponectin and reduces hepatic steatosis in rats. Hepatology. 2009;49:1554–62.
64. You M, Considine RV, Leone TC, et al. Role of adiponectin in the protective action of dietary saturated fat against alcoholic fatty liver in mice. Hepatology. 2005;42:568–77.
65. Shen Z, Liang X, Rogers CQ, et al. Involvement of adiponectin-SIRT1-AMPK signaling in the protective action of rosiglitazone against alcoholic fatty liver in mice. Am J Physiol Gastrointest Liver Physiol. 2010;298(3):G364–74.
66. Morimoto M, Zern MA, Hagbjork AL, et al. Fish oil, alcohol, and liver pathology: role of cytochrome P450 2E1. Proc Soc Exp Biol Med. 1999;207:197–205.
67. Nanji AA, Zhao S, Sadrzadeh SM, et al. Markedly enhanced cytochrome P450 2E1 induction and lipid peroxidation is associated with severe liver injury in fish oil–ethanol-fed rats. Alcohol Clin Exp Res. 1994;18:1280–5.
68. Tsukamoto H, Horne W, Kamimura S, et al. Experimental liver cirrhosis induced by alcohol and iron. J Clin Invest. 1995;96:620–30.
69. Zhou Z, Wang L, Song Z, et al. Zinc supplementation prevents alcoholic liver injury in mice through attenuation of oxidative stress. Am J Pathol. 2005;166(6):1681–90.
70. Wu D, Cederbaum AI. Oxidative stress and alcoholic liver disease. Semin Liver Dis. 2009;29(2):141–54.
71. Bardag-Gorce QX, Yuan J, Li BA, et al. The effect of ethanol-induced cytochrome p4502E1 on the inhibition of proteasome activity by alcohol. Biochem Biophys Res Commun. 2000;279:23–9.
72. Butura A, Nilsson K, Morgan K, et al. The impact of CYP2E1 on the development of alcoholic liver disease as studied in a transgenic mouse model. J Hepatol. 2009;50(3):572–83.
73. Lu Y, Zhuge J, Wang X, et al. Cytochrome P450 2E1 contributes to ethanol-induced fatty liver in mice. Hepatology. 2008;47(5):148314–94.
74. Tomita K, Azuma T, Kitamura N, et al. Leptin deficiency enhances sensitivity of rats to alcoholic steatohepatitis through suppression of metallothionein. Am J Physiol Gastrointest Liver Physiol. 2004;287:G1078–85.
75. tom Dieck H, Döring F, Fuchs D, et al. Changes in rat hepatic gene expression in response to zinc deficiency as assessed by DNA arrays. J Nutr. 2003;133:1004–10.
76. Dieck H, Döring F, Roth HP, Daniel H. Transcriptome and proteome analysis identifies the pathways that increase hepatic lipid accumulation in zinc-deficient rats. J Nutr. 2005;135:199–205.
77. McClain CJ, Antonow DR, Cohen DA, Shedlofsky S. Zinc metabolism in alcoholic liver disease. Alcohol Clin Exp Res. 1986;10:582–9.
78. Kiilerich S, Dietrichson O, Loud FB, et al. Zinc depletion in alcoholic liver diseases. Scand J Gastroenterol. 1980;15:363–7.
79. Bode JC, Hanisch P, Henning H, Koenig W, et al. Hepatic zinc content in patients with various stages of alcoholic liver disease and in patients with chronic active and chronic persistent hepatitis. Hepatology. 1988;8:1605–9.
80. Rodríguez-Moreno F, González-Reimers E, Santolaria-Fernández F, et al. Zinc, copper, manganese, and iron in chronic alcoholic liver disease. Alcohol. 1997;14:39–44.
81. Webster KA, Prentice H, Bishopric NH. Oxidation of zinc finger transcription factors: physiological consequences. Antioxid Redox Signal. 2001;3:535–48.
82. Nolan JP. The role of intestinal endotoxin in liver injury: a long and evolving history. Hepatology. 2010;52(5):1829–35.
83. McClain CJ, Song Z, Barve SS, Hill DB, Deaciuc I. Recent advances in alcoholic liver disease. IV. Dysregulated cytokine metabolism in alcoholic liver disease. Am J Physiol Gastrointest Liver Physiol. 2004;287(3):G497–502.
84. Leach BE, Forbes JC. Sulfonamide drugs as protective agents against carbon tetrachloride poisoning. Proc Soc Exp Biol Med. 1941;48:361–3.
85. Rutenburg AM, Sonnenblick E, Koven I, et al. The role of intestinal bacteria in the development of dietary cirrhosis in rats. J Exp Med. 1957;106(1):1–14.
86. Broitman SA, Gottlieb LS, Zamcheck N. Influence of neomycin and ingested endotoxin in the pathogenesis of choline deficiency cirrhosis in the adult rat. J Exp Med. 1964;119:633–42.
87. Nolan JP. The contribution of gut-derived endotoxins to liver injury. Yale J Biol Med. 1979;52(1):127–33.
88. Gabuzda GJ. Hepatic coma: clinical considerations, pathogenesis, and management. Adv Intern Med. 1962;11:11–73.
89. Purohit V, Bode JC, Bode C, et al. Alcohol, intestinal bacterial growth, intestinal permeability to endotoxin, and medical consequences: summary of a symposium. Alcohol. 2008;42(5):349–61.
90. Zieve L. Pathogenesis of hepatic coma. Arch Intern Med. 1966;118(3):211–23.
91. McClain CJ, Zieve L. Portal systemic encephalopathy: recognition and variations. In: Davidson CS, editor. Problems in liver diseases. New York: Stratton Intercontinental Medical Book Corp; 1979. p. 162–72.
92. Adachi Y, Moore LE, Bradford BU, et al. Antibiotics prevent liver injury in rats following long-term exposure to ethanol. Gastroenterology. 1995;108(1):218–24.
93. Keshavarzian A, Choudhary S, Holmes EW, et al. Preventing gut leakiness by oats supplementation ameliorates alcohol-induced liver damage in rats. J Pharmacol Exp Ther. 2001;299(2):442–8.
94. Nanji AA, Khettry U, Sadrzadeh SM. Lactobacillus feeding reduces endotoxemia and severity of experimental alcoholic liver (disease). Proc Soc Exp Biol Med. 1994;205(3):243–7.
95. McClain CJ, Song Z, Barve SS, et al. Recent advances in alcoholic liver disease. IV. Dysregulated cytokine metabolism in alcoholic liver disease. Am J Physiol Gastrointest Liver Physiol. 2004;287(3):G497–502.
96. Iimuro Y, Gallucci RM, Luster MI, et al. Antibodies to tumor necrosis factor alfa attenuate hepatic necrosis and inflammation caused by chronic exposure to ethanol in the rat. Hepatology. 1997;26(6):1530–7.

97. Yin M, Wheeler MD, Kono H, et al. Essential role of tumor necrosis factor alpha in alcohol-induced liver injury in mice. Gastroenterology. 1999;117(4):942–52.
98. Honchel R, Ray MB, Marsano L, et al. Tumor necrosis factor in alcohol enhanced endotoxin liver injury. Alcohol Clin Exp Res. 1992;16(4):665–9.
99. Szabo G, Bala S. Alcoholic liver disease and the gut-liver axis. World J Gastroenterol. 2010;16(11):1321–9.
100. McClain CJ, Cohen DA. Increased tumor necrosis factor production by monocytes in alcoholic hepatitis. Hepatology. 1989;9(3):349–51.
101. Khoruts A, Stahnke L, McClain CJ, et al. Circulating tumor necrosis factor, interleukin-1 and interleukin-6 concentrations in chronic alcoholic patients. Hepatology. 1991;13(2):267–76.
102. Naveau S, Chollet-Martin S, Dharancy S, et al. A double-blind randomized controlled trial of infliximab associated with prednisolone in acute alcoholic hepatitis. Hepatology. 2004;39(5):1390–7.
103. Boetticher NC, Peine CJ, Kwo P, et al. A randomized, double-blinded, placebo-controlled multicenter trial of etanercept in the treatment of alcoholic hepatitis. Gastroenterology. 2008;135(6):1953–60.
104. Markiewski MM, DeAngelis RA, Lambris JD. Liver inflammation and regeneration: two distinct biological phenomena or parallel pathophysiologic processes? Mol Immunol. 2006;43(1–2):45–56.
105. Fausto N. Involvement of the innate immune system in liver regeneration and injury. J Hepatol. 2006;45(3):347–9.
106. Haynes BF. Gut microbes out of control in HIV infection. Nat Med. 2006;12(12):1351–2.
107. Carithers RI, McClain CJ. Chapter 81: Alcoholic liver disease. In: Feldman M, Friedman LS, Brant LJ, editors. Sleisenger & Fordtran's gastrointestinal and liver disease, vol. 2. Philadelphia: Elsevier; 2006. p. 1771–92.
108. Bergheim I, McClain CJ, Arteel GE. Chapter 28: Treatment of alcoholic liver disease. In: Singer M, Brenner DA, editors. Alcohol and the gastrointestinal tract. Basel, Switzerland: Karger AG; 2006. p. 196–213.
109. Barve A, Khan R, Marsano L, et al. Treatment of alcoholic liver disease. Ann Hepatol. 2008;7(1):5–15.
110. Akriviadis E, Botla R, Briggs W, et al. Pentoxifylline improves short-term survival in severe acute alcoholic hepatitis: a double-blind, placebo-controlled trial. Gastroenterology. 2000;119(6):1637–48.
111. De BK, Gangopadhyay S, Dutta D, et al. Pentoxifylline versus prednisolone for severe alcoholic hepatitis: a randomized controlled trial. World J Gastroenterol. 2009;15(1):1613–9.
112. Mathurin P, Mendenhall CL, Carithers Jr RL, et al. Corticosteroids improve short-term survival in patients with severe alcoholic hepatitis (AH): individual data analysis of the last three randomized placebo controlled double blind trials of corticosteroids in severe AH. J Hepatol. 2003;36:480–7.
113. Mathurin P, Abdelnour M, Ramond MJ, et al. Early change in bilirubin levels is an important prognostic factor in severe alcoholic hepatitis treated with prednisolone. Hepatology. 2003;38:1363–9.
114. Tang Y, Forsyth CB, Banan A, et al. Oats supplementation prevents alcohol-induced gut leakiness in rats by preventing alcohol-induced oxidative tissue damage. J Pharmacol Exp Ther. 2009;329(3):952–8.
115. Zhong W, McClain CJ, Cave M, Kang YJ, Zhou Z. The role of zinc deficiency in alcohol-induced intestinal barrier dysfunction. Am J Physiol Gastrointest Liver Physiol. 2010;298(5):G625–33.
116. Kirpich IA, Solovieva NV, Leikhter SN, et al. Probiotics restore bowel flora and improve liver enzymes in human alcohol-induced liver injury: a pilot study. Alcohol. 2008;42(8):675–82.

Immunopathogenesis of Liver Injury

Mohamed Tarek M. Shata

Introduction

The liver is the largest organ in the body with many vital metabolic functions. It occupies a key position between the gastrointestinal tract and systemic venous circulations. A healthy liver receives 70–75% of its blood form the portal vein (Fig. 7.1). The mesenteric veins of the intestinal tracts as well as the splenic vein are main sources of blood for the portal vein. Additionally, about 30% of the total blood passes through the liver every minute [1], carrying about 10^{10} lymphocytes in 24 h [2].

Therefore, the immune cells in liver are continuously exposed to foreign antigens from the gut including foods antigens, potential microbial antigens and toxins. The liver has complex mechanisms to recognize nonharmful antigens such as food antigens and induce tolerance to these antigens. The liver also identifies virulent organisms such as bacteria and viruses and develops protective immune responses to these damaging organisms. To explore these mechanisms, this chapter describes the structure of the liver and the functions of intrahepatic cells in the immune responses, and how the immune cells in the liver adapt different mechanisms in response to foreign antigens and how the liver sustains damage during these responses.

Liver Structure

Liver consists of the following cell types (Fig. 7.2):

M.T.M. Shata (✉)
Department Viral Immunology Lab/Div Digestive Diseases,
University of Cincinnati, 231 Albert B. Sabin Way, MSB6360,
Cincinnati, OH 45267, USA
e-mail: ShataMT@ucmail.uc.edu

Hepatocytes

They constitute two thirds of total cells in the liver. While the importance of their metabolic functions is well established their roles in the immune responses are under active investigation. Recent data suggest that cytokines such as IL-28B secreted by hepatocytes may play important roles in viral resistance [3]. Also, the role of hepatocytes in induction of tolerance is discussed.

Stellate Cells

They are small number of cells in normal healthy liver localized in the subendothelial space of Disse. They synthesize extracellular matrix proteins, including collagen types 1 and 4, laminin, and heparin sulfate proteoglycan [4] upon stimulation, and are responsible for initiation of liver fibrosis and cirrhosis.

Biliary Epithelial Cells

They represent about 5% of nonhepatocytes and make the intrahepatic and extrahepatic biliary ducts. They secrete chemokines and cytokines and participate in immune responses by expression of costimulatory molecules [4, 5].

Lymphocytes

The average human liver contains about 10^{10} lymphocytes, which makes it one of the largest reservoirs in the body for lymphocytes. Different subsets of lymphocytes are present, including the following.

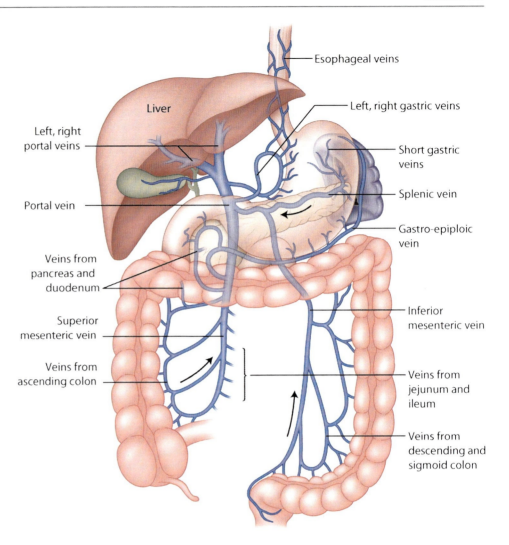

Fig. 7.1 Structure and composition of the immune cells in the liver

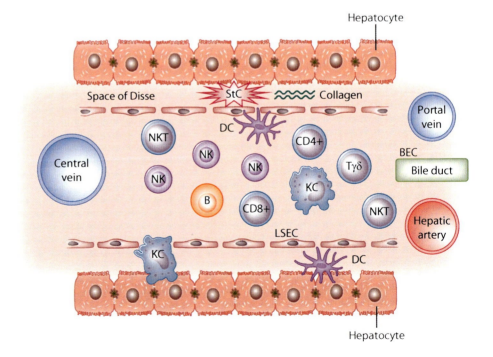

Fig. 7.2 Portal circulation. The portal vein carries blood to the liver from veins that drain the gut and the major splanchnic organs

Conventional α/β T Cells (CD4 and CD8)

These T cells express a diverse repertoire of T cell receptors with α and β chains. They recognize antigens in the context of Class I and Class I molecules on the surface of antigen-presenting cells (APCs). The liver has higher frequency of CD8 (15–30%) and memory T cells (20–30%) than in the peripheral blood (8–10% and 10–15% respectively) [6].

Unconventional γ/δ T Cells

The liver is the richest sources of γ/δ T cells. They represent 15–25% of all intrahepatic lymphocytes. They recognize a limited range of antigens.

B Cells

The number of B cells in the liver is small compared to the peripheral blood and represent less than 6% of the total intrahepatic lymphocytes.

Natural Killer Cells

They are at higher frequency in the liver than in the peripheral blood. They represent about 30% of the total lymphocytes in the liver. They have strong cytotoxic and antiviral activity.

NKT Cells

They recognize antigen in the context of CD1d molecule. They are at a higher frequency in the liver than in other organs and can reach up to 30% of the intrahepatic lymphocytes. Upon stimulation, they secrete large quantities of IFN-γ and IL-4 and may play a role in the regulation of the immune responses in the liver.

Antigen-Presenting Cells

Liver Sinusoidal Endothelial Cells

They represent 50% of the nonparenchymal cells in the liver. They line sinusoids and form fenestrated surfaces, which allow direct connection between lymphocytes and hepatocytes. They are highly efficient in antigen presentation [7].

Kupffer Cells

They are resident hepatic macrophages and represent approximately 80–90% of tissue-fixed macrophages of the body [8] and 20% of nonparenchymal cells in the liver [9]. They are responsible for recognizing and elimination of microbes by phagocytosis. They represent heterogeneous populations of macrophages that reside in the periportal zone of liver lobule (43%) and to a lesser extent in the midzone (28%) and central areas (29%) [10] of the hepatic lobule. Three subsets of Kupffer cells have been identified: (1) Small Kupffer cells with no phagocytic activity but responsible for secretion of TNF-α and immune regulation, (2) Intermediate Kupffer cells with high phagocytic activity, and (3) Large Kupffer cells with intermediate phagocytic activity. Both the intermediate and large Kupffer cells secrete IL-6 and IL-10 and exert antimicrobial and anti-inflammatory functions [10]. They attach to the liver sinusoidal endothelial cell (LSEC) layer and are activated by endotoxin-type stimuli, including bacterial lipopolysaccharides (LPS) and superantigens with the release of acute phase proteins and cytokines.

Hepatic Dendritic Cells

They are predominantly immature dendritic cells that are tolerogenic in the noninflammatory microenvironment condition in the liver. But during infection, they may migrate to regional lymph nodes and mature to induce effective immune responses.

Immune Responses in Liver

Induction of Immune Responses

Innate Immune Responses

NK, NKT cells and Kupffer cells represent about 35% of nonhepatocytes in the liver [9], and play important role in innate immunity. Kupffer cells are important in initiation of the innate immune responses to infection. For example, Kupffer cells secrete IL-12 and IL-18 in responses to infection. These cytokines promote local expansion and stimulation of NK and NKT cells to secrete IFN-γ [11], which suppresses viral replication. Additionally, Kupffer cells secrete other cytokines such as IL-1β, IL-6, and TNF-α, which stimulate infiltration of the neutrophil and increase their microbicidal activity (Fig. 7.3) [12].

NK cells regulate the immune responses by balancing the production of proinflammatory cytokines of Th1 and the anti-inflammatory cytokines of Th2 through regulation of their stimulatory and inhibitory receptors [13–15]. In the absence of inhibitory receptors and the presence of certain cytokines such as Type I IFN, NK will be activated to secrete IFN-γ and lyse infected cells [16]. IFN-γ also stimulates hepatocytes and LSEC to recruit T cells to the liver [16]. IL-12 secreted by Kupffer cells activates NKT cells to kill infected cells through Fas-mediated cell lysis, and to secret large quantities of IFN-γ and IL-4 [17, 18]. Regulation of the balance between these two cytokines play important role in polarizing the immune response to either Th1 or Th2 responses. There is strong evidence that NKT cells play important role in liver infection, because NKT deficient mice are more susceptible to viral [19] and bacterial infection [20, 21] and activation of NKT downregulates HBV viral infection in the transgenic mice model [22].

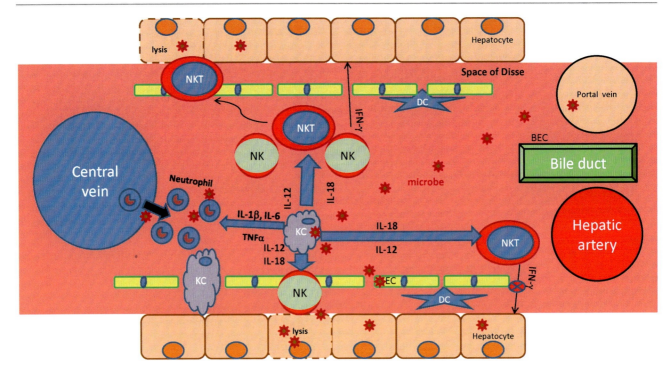

Fig. 7.3 Stimulation of the innate immune responses of the liver

Ag-Specific Immune Responses

To induce effective Ag-specific immune responses, T cells needs two signals; the first signal is provided through peptide-MHC-TCR complex, and the second signal is through costimulatory molecules present in professional APCs in the presence of proinflammatory conditions (Fig. 7.4) [23].

In the microenvironment of the liver, most of the Ag presentations lack the second signal, and, therefore, are unable to induce effective Ag-specific immune responses; instead, they produce tolerance [24].

However, in case of microbial infection with associated inflammation and killing of hepatocytes, Kupffer cells and professional immature hepatic dendritic cells (DCs) in the liver engulf the dead cells and migrate to the regional lymph nodes where they become mature DCs. Mature DCs efficiently cross-present the infected cells and the foreign Ags to naïve T cells in the presence of costimulatory second signal. The stimulated Ag-specific T cells immigrate to the liver to secrete cytokines or kill the infected cells [25].

Induction of Tolerance

Kupffer cells respond to bacterial LPS, and superantigens present in the portal circulation by secretion of TNF-α and IL-10 [26, 27]. These cytokines downregulate Ag-uptake and MHC class II expression by LSECs and DCs and decrease T cell activation [27]. Kupffer cells also produce nitric oxide and reactive oxygen intermediate, which suppress T cell activation [28]. Additionally, lack of second signal in Kupffer cells and DCs in the healthy noninflammatory liver leads to the induction of tolerance in T cells upon presentation of the surrounding Ags (Fig. 7.5) [29]. In fact, tolerance in the liver depends on Kupffer cells because depletion of Kupffer cells in the mice model leads to impairment of tolerance [30].

Furthermore, LSEC-mediated presentation of antigens to naïve T cells results in secretion of IL-4 and IL-10 (Th2 type) rather than IL-2 and IFN-γ [26, 31]. The dominance of IL-10 in the liver downregulates chemokine receptors on DC and inhibits their migration to draining lymph nodes [32]. Consequently, priming T cells in the presence of IL-10 leads to decreased effector functions and cytokine secretions by T cells [27].

Induction of Apoptosis

Hepatocytes are less susceptible to cell death in comparison to other primary cells. In normal primary cells, Fas ligation alone induces the activation of caspases and apoptosis (type 1 cell). By contrast, hepatocytes require the amplification of the apoptotic Fas/FasL signal thorough the mitochondria (type II cell), equivalent to many tumor cells. Three main mechanisms are involved in apoptosis of hepatocytes; FasL, TNFα, and Tumor necrosis factor (TNF)-related apoptosis-inducing

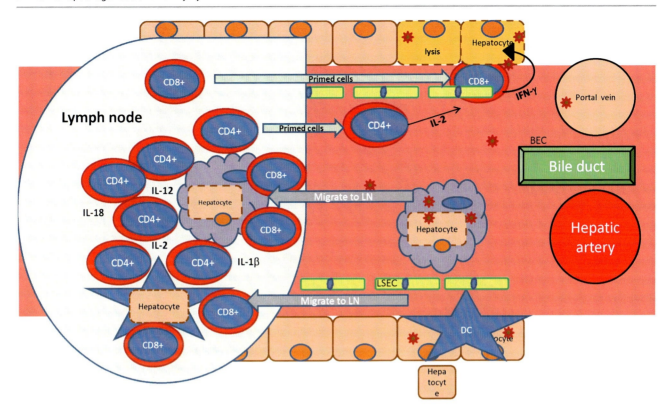

Fig. 7.4 Stimulation of Ag-specific immune response in the liver

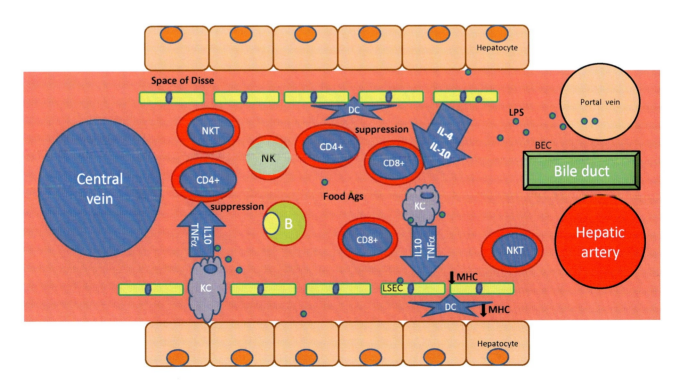

Fig. 7.5 Induction of tolerance in the liver

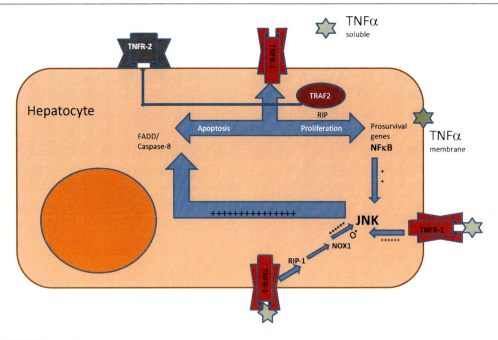

Fig. 7.6 TNF-α/TNF-R interactions

ligand (TRAIL) [33]. The following section reviews the three mechanisms of apoptosis and their regulation.

Fas/FasL Interaction

Fas-induced apoptosis is the most important pathways involved in liver injury. Under normal physiological conditions, Fas receptors are expressed on hepatocytes, Kupffer cells, stellate cells (STC), LSECs, whereas FasL is normally expressed on NK, NKT and activated T cells [34]. Binding of Fas receptors on hepatocytes to FasL on activated NK, NKT and T cells may lead to death of hepatocytes. Fas-mediated cell death is important for the removal of viral infected or transformed hepatocytes [35]. It is also a common final pathway for liver injury in acetaminophen overdose [36–38], alcohol [39–41], and cholestatic liver damage [42, 43].

TNF-α/TNF-αR Interaction

TNFα is a proinflammatory cytokine secreted in the liver mainly by activated Kupffer cells, and also to lesser extent by NK, LSECs, and STC [44]. TNFα is present in two forms; soluble and membrane-bound forms (Fig. 7.6). The biological role of TNFα in the liver is highly regulated. TNFα can bind to two main receptors on hepatocytes; TNFR-1 and TNFR-2 [45]. TNFR-1 stimulation can induce both proliferation and apoptosis, while TNFR-2 does not contains death or proliferation domains and its main function is to amplify the effect of TNFR-1 in promoting apoptosis. TNFR-1 signals through recruitment of TNFR-associated protein (TRAF2) and receptor-interacting protein (RIP), which leads to activation of NF-κB and prosurvival genes and induction of cell proliferation. The apoptotic pathway occurs through activation of Fas-associated death domain protein (FADD)/caspase 8-dependent pathway. TNFR2 receptors amplify the apoptotic pathway by its ability to attract the TRAF2, therefore inhibiting the TNFR-1 proliferation pathway.

Additionally, NF-κB controls the activation of another important regulator, the Jun Kinase pathway (JNK). Transient and modest activation of JNK is associated with proliferation, while prolonged and strong JNK activations induce apoptosis and cell death.

Moreover, TNFR-1 activation leads to the recruitment of RIP-1, and activation of Nox1 and formation of reactive oxygen species which leads to sustained activation of JNK and consequently activation of the apoptotic pathway [46].

Tumor Necrosis Factor-Related Apoptosis-Inducing Ligand Pathway

It was initially thought that Tumor necrosis factor (TNF)-related apoptosis-inducing ligand (TRAIL) activation induces apoptosis and cell death only in tumor cells and not primary cells, however, recent data suggest that TRAIL sensitivity in primary cells is under strict control and can only be activated under pathological conditions [47].

TRAIL and TRAIL-R are expressed on normal hepatocytes and NK cells but at a low level. During viral infection, inflammation, drug toxicity, or fatty liver, TRAIL-R expression on hepatocytes is upregulated and the sensitivity of hepatocytes to TRAIL-induced apoptosis increases [48]. Additionally, in proinflammatory microenvironment and in the presence of cytokines such as IFNs, TRAIL expressions in intrahepatic lymphocytes and NK cells increase, which lead to selective killing of the infected hepatocytes by lymphocytes and NK cells [49]. TRAIL pathways also collaborate with other apoptotic pathways in the liver [33].

Immunopathogenesis and Liver Injury in HCV Infection

Immune Responses and Tolerance

The mechanisms that determine the balance between the immune responses and tolerance to foreign antigens are still speculative [50]. Different hypotheses have been suggested. One of the hypotheses suggests that the presence of proinflammatory conditions in the liver maturates the intrahepatic APCs and upregulates the secondary signals [51]. These mature APCs induce effective antigen presentation and activation of T cells [52]. The inflammatory microenvironment is mainly induced by stimulation of innate immune responses by microorganisms and massive production of proinflammatory cytokines which overcomes the hyporesponses induced by LPS to intrahepatic DCs, and LSECs [53, 54].

Another hypothesis depends on the sites of priming the immune responses. If priming occurs with professional APCs in the lymph nodes, effective immune responses are elicited. However, if priming occurs by the immature DCs in the liver or hepatocytes, T cell tolerance is likely to ensure [29]. Additionally, it has been suggested that the levels of Ag expression in the liver are important. The presence of high Ag concentration in the liver favors T cell depletion and tolerance induction [55].

In most hepatotropic viruses, there are successful and effective immune responses to remove the viral infection [9, 56]. However, in HCV-infected individuals more than half of the patients become chronically infected. The reasons for the persistent HCV infection are unclear but probably different factors are involved including; the high replication and mutation rates of HCV [57, 58], the effect of HCV core protein on immune function [59–61], the initial presentation of HCV Ags by the hepatocytes and intrahepatic immature DCs with the induction of tolerance to HCV Ags [25, 31, 62], and the induction of Th2 responses due to the presentation of HCV Ags by intrahepatic immature DCs, and LSECs [25]. There are also some data that suggest that the frequency of chronically HCV-infected patients may be overestimated and there are unrecognized previously HCV-infected patients who cleared the infection with cell-mediated immune responses without serological markers of infection [63–67].

Apoptosis

The role of Fas/FasL in HCV infection is still controversial. During HCV infection, Fas and FasL are upregulated on infected hepatocytes, and activated T cell respectively [68]. These upregulations are induced by viral proteins and cytokines and correlate with the severity of the damage [69, 70]. Alternatively, HCV infection could protect hepatocytes from Fas-mediated apoptosis by repressing the release of cyotchrome c from the mitochondria [70, 71], the secondary signal necessary to induce apoptosis in hepatocytes. Therefore, HCV inhibits apoptosis to allow for persistent infection and chronicity.

HCV viral infection also sensitizes the hepatocytes to TRAIL-induced apoptosis by upregulations of TRAIL-R on hepatocytes and increases the expression of TRAIL on intrahepatic lymphocytes and NK cells [72], leading to death of hepatocytes. The ultimate outcomes of apoptosis in HCV infection depends on the balances among these different mechanisms.

Hepatocyte Responses to Infection

Hepatocytes have intrinsic capacity to inhibit viral replication through induction of interferons (IFNs). Three groups of IFNs have been identified. Type II (IFN-γ) is mainly secreted by immune cells, whereas Type I (IFNs-α and β) and Type III (IFNs-λ) IFNs are secreted by hepatocytes and other nucleated cells. IFNs bind to distinct transmembrane receptors to induce potent antiviral responses [73, 74]. The three newly identified IFNs – λ1, λ2, λ3 proteins (also termed IL-28A, IL-28B, and IL-29) – bind to a heterodimeric receptor composed of a previously unknown IFN-λR1 subunit and IL-10R2, which also serves as the second chain of the IL-10R [3].

The antiviral activity of IFNs is mediated through the activation of the JAK-STAT (IFN-αs, IFN-γs, and IFN-λs) and MAPK (IFN αs and IFN-λs) pathways [3]. These IFNs play an important role in the inhibition of viral infections in hepatocytes.

Recent genome wide association studies (GWAS) links variation in IFN-λ3 (IL-28B) gene to chronic HCV infection and failure to treatment [75, 76], as well as response to therapy [77–80] and spontaneous HCV clearance [80]. Moreover, in vitro study suggested that IFN-λ1 (IL-29) and IFN-λ2 (IL-28A) block HCV replication in human hepatocyte cell lines [81, 82]. IFN-λ has been tested in phase 1B as a treatment of chronic hepatitis C. The drug had a robust activity against HCV with limited toxicity due to the reduced tissue expression of the IFN-λ receptor to the hepatocytes compared with IFN-α/β receptors.

Immunopathogenesis and Liver Injury in HIV Infection

HCV and HIV infections are common among injection drug users (IDUs) with approximately 80–90% of HIV-infected IDUs are coinfected with HCV [83]. Furthermore, these HCV–HIV coinfected patients are at a higher risk of progressing to end-stage liver disease and cirrhosis [84–86]. Liver disease in HCV–HIV coinfected patients is characterized by inflammation and cell-death [87–89]. Recent studies suggest that the HIV envelope protein gp120 may induce apoptosis and inflammation in hepatocytes through increased Fas expression in hepatocytes, and induction of IL-8 [90–92]. Recently, Th17 cells, a subset of CD4 T helper cells, have been described. Th17 appears to be critical for regulating gut mucosal immune responses against extracellular microbial pathogens and may serve as a link between innate and adaptive immune responses. Th17 cells are permissive to HIV infection and appear to play important role in HIV pathogenesis. Th17 cells are depleted from the gut of HIV-infected individuals and their depletion is associated with microbial translocation, which is a cause for chronic immune activation and disease progression [93, 94]. A pronounced loss of mucosal Th17 cells in the simian immunodeficiency virus-infected rhesus macaque model of AIDS is linked to impaired immune responses in the gut mucosa [93, 95]. Microbial translocation is associated with increased LPS in the liver and chronic stimulation of intrahepatic lymphocytes (Fig. 7.7). Kupffer cells, which clear most of microbial translocation products, can be infected by HIV, and their numbers decrease in HIV-infected patients [96], which augments the deleterious effect of microbial translocation on the liver. Microbial translocation may also alter the cytokine production in the microenvironment in the liver [97]. It favors Th2 production and induction of tolerance [98] and is associated with progression of hepatic fibrosis [96].

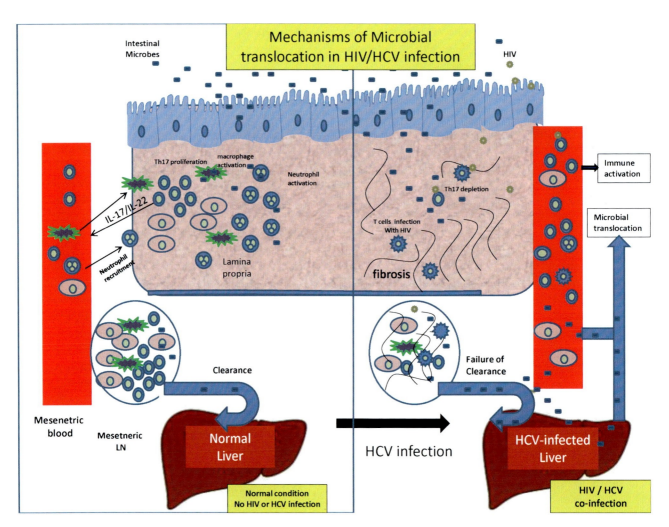

Fig. 7.7 Mechanisms of microbial translocation in HIV/HCV Infection

Summary

The liver is a site for both immune tolerance and effective immune responses. Different factors affect the outcome of liver responses to foreign antigens. These factors include the presence of inflammatory cytokines in the microenvironment and the induction of innate immune responses. Additionally, the site of priming the immune cells either in the lymph nodes or the intrahepatic environment might affect the outcome. Hepatocyte injury and repair is a consequence of immune clearance and modulation of apoptotic pathways. In HCV and HIV infections, both the immune responses and apoptosis inductions are altered by viral infection and/or viral proteins.

References

1. Sheth K, Bankey P. The liver as an immune organ. Curr Opin Crit Care. 2001;7(2):99–104.
2. Wick MJ, Leithauser F, Reimann J. The hepatic immune system. Crit Rev Immunol. 2002;22(1):47–103.
3. Li M, Liu X, Zhou Y, Su SB. Interferon-lambdas: the modulators of antivirus, antitumor, and immune responses. J Leukoc Biol. 2009;86(1):23–32.
4. Kita H, Mackay IR, Van De Water J, Gershwin ME. The lymphoid liver: considerations on pathways to autoimmune injury. Gastroenterology. 2001;120(6):1485–501.
5. Reynoso-Paz S, Coppel RL, Mackay IR, Bass NM, Ansari AA, Gershwin ME. The immunobiology of bile and biliary epithelium. Hepatology. 1999;30(2):351–7.
6. Yan J, Greer JM, Hull R, O'Sullivan JD, Henderson RD, Read SJ, et al. The effect of ageing on human lymphocyte subsets: comparison of males and females. Immun Ageing. 2010;7:4.
7. Steffan AM, Gendrault JL, McCuskey RS, McCuskey PA, Kirn A. Phagocytosis, an unrecognized property of murine endothelial liver cells. Hepatology. 1986;6(5):830–6.
8. Lloyd CM, Phillips AR, Cooper GJ, Dunbar PR. Three-colour fluorescence immunohistochemistry reveals the diversity of cells staining for macrophage markers in murine spleen and liver. J Immunol Methods. 2008;334(1–2):70–81.
9. Mackay IR. Hepatoimmunology: a perspective. Immunol Cell Biol. 2002;80(1):36–44.
10. Nemeth E, Baird AW, O'Farrelly C. Microanatomy of the liver immune system. Semin Immunopathol. 2009;31(3):333–43.
11. Lauwerys BR, Garot N, Renauld JC, Houssiau FA. Cytokine production and killer activity of NK/T-NK cells derived with IL-2, IL-15, or the combination of IL-12 and IL-18. J Immunol. 2000;165(4):1847–53.
12. Gregory SH, Wing EJ. Neutrophil-Kupffer-cell interaction in host defenses to systemic infections. Immunol Today. 1998;19(11):507–10.
13. Moretta A, Vitale M, Sivori S, Bottino C, Morelli L, Augugliaro R, et al. Human natural killer cell receptors for HLA-class I molecules. Evidence that the Kp43 (CD94) molecule functions as receptor for HLA-B alleles. J Exp Med. 1994;180(2):545–55.
14. Moretta L, Ciccone E, Poggi A, Mingari MC, Moretta A. Ontogeny, specific functions and receptors of human natural killer cells. Immunol Lett. 1994;40(2):83–8.
15. Salazar-Mather TP, Orange JS, Biron CA. Early murine cytomegalovirus (MCMV) infection induces liver natural killer (NK) cell inflammation and protection through macrophage inflammatory protein 1alpha (MIP-1alpha)-dependent pathways. J Exp Med. 1998;187(1):1–14.
16. Itoh Y, Morita A, Nishioji K, Fujii H, Nakamura H, Kirishima T, et al. Time course profile and cell-type-specific production of monokine induced by interferon-gamma in Concanavalin A-induced hepatic injury in mice: comparative study with interferon-inducible protein-10. Scand J Gastroenterol. 2001;36(12):1344–51.
17. Bendelac A, Rivera MN, Park SH, Roark JH. Mouse CD1-specific NK1 T cells: development, specificity, and function. Annu Rev Immunol. 1997;15:535–62.
18. Kumagai K, Takeda K, Hashimoto W, Seki S, Ogasawara K, Anzai R, et al. Interleukin-12 as an inducer of cytotoxic effectors in anti-tumor immunity. Int Rev Immunol. 1997;14(2–3):229–56.
19. Grubor-Bauk B, Simmons A, Mayrhofer G, Speck PG. Impaired clearance of herpes simplex virus type 1 from mice lacking CD1d or NKT cells expressing the semivariant V alpha 14-J alpha 281 TCR. J Immunol. 2003;170(3):1430–4.
20. Behar SM, Dascher CC, Grusby MJ, Wang CR, Brenner MB. Susceptibility of mice deficient in CD1D or TAP1 to infection with *Mycobacterium tuberculosis*. J Exp Med. 1999;189(12):1973–80.
21. Kumar H, Belperron A, Barthold SW, Bockenstedt LK. Cutting edge: CD1d deficiency impairs murine host defense against the spirochete, *Borrelia burgdorferi*. J Immunol. 2000;165(9):4797–801.
22. Kakimi K, Guidotti LG, Koezuka Y, Chisari FV. Natural killer T cell activation inhibits hepatitis B virus replication in vivo. J Exp Med. 2000;192(7):921–30.
23. Gonzalo JA, Delaney T, Corcoran J, Goodearl A, Gutierrez-Ramos JC, Coyle AJ. Cutting edge: the related molecules CD28 and inducible costimulator deliver both unique and complementary signals required for optimal T cell activation. J Immunol. 2001;166(1):1–5.
24. Bertolino P, McCaughan GW, Bowen DG. Role of primary intrahepatic T-cell activation in the 'liver tolerance effect'. Immunol Cell Biol. 2002;80(1):84–92.
25. Racanelli V, Rehermann B. The liver as an immunological organ. Hepatology. 2006;43(2 Suppl 1):S54–62.
26. Knolle PA, Loser E, Protzer U, Duchmann R, Schmitt E, zum Buschenfelde KH, et al. Regulation of endotoxin-induced IL-6 production in liver sinusoidal endothelial cells and Kupffer cells by IL-10. Clin Exp Immunol. 1997;107(3):555–61.
27. Groux H, Bigler M, de Vries JE, Roncarolo MG. Interleukin-10 induces a long-term antigen-specific anergic state in human CD4+ T cells. J Exp Med. 1996;184(1):19–29.
28. Roland CR, Walp L, Stack RM, Flye MW. Outcome of Kupffer cell antigen presentation to a cloned murine Th1 lymphocyte depends on the inducibility of nitric oxide synthase by IFN-gamma. J Immunol. 1994;153(12):5453–64.
29. Bowen DG, Zen M, Holz L, Davis T, McCaughan GW, Bertolino P. The site of primary T cell activation is a determinant of the balance between intrahepatic tolerance and immunity. J Clin Invest. 2004;114(5):701–12.
30. Roland CR, Mangino MJ, Duffy BF, Flye MW. Lymphocyte suppression by Kupffer cells prevents portal venous tolerance induction: a study of macrophage function after intravenous gadolinium. Transplantation. 1993;55(5):1151–8.
31. Knolle PA, Schmitt E, Jin S, Germann T, Duchmann R, Hegenbarth S, et al. Induction of cytokine production in naive CD4(+) T cells by antigen-presenting murine liver sinusoidal endothelial cells but failure to induce differentiation toward Th1 cells. Gastroenterology. 1999;116(6):1428–40.
32. Takayama T, Morelli AE, Onai N, Hirao M, Matsushima K, Tahara H, et al. Mammalian and viral IL-10 enhance C-C chemokine receptor 5 but down-regulate C-C chemokine receptor 7 expression by myeloid dendritic cells: impact on chemotactic responses and in vivo homing ability. J Immunol. 2001;166(12):7136–43.

33. Corazza N, Badmann A, Lauer C. Immune cell-mediated liver injury. Semin Immunopathol. 2009;31(2):267–77.
34. Malhi H, Gores GJ. Cellular and molecular mechanisms of liver injury. Gastroenterology. 2008;134(6):1641–54.
35. Takahashi T, Tanaka M, Brannan CI, Jenkins NA, Copeland NG, Suda T, et al. Generalized lymphoproliferative disease in mice, caused by a point mutation in the Fas ligand. Cell. 1994;76(6): 969–76.
36. Liu ZX, Kaplowitz N. Role of innate immunity in acetaminophen-induced hepatotoxicity. Expert Opin Drug Metab Toxicol. 2006;2(4):493–503.
37. Liu ZX, Han D, Gunawan B, Kaplowitz N. Neutrophil depletion protects against murine acetaminophen hepatotoxicity. Hepatology. 2006;43(6):1220–30.
38. Tagami A, Ohnishi H, Hughes RD. Increased serum soluble Fas in patients with acute liver failure due to paracetamol overdose. Hepatogastroenterology. 2003;50(51):742–5.
39. Batey RG, Cao Q, Gould B. Lymphocyte-mediated liver injury in alcohol-related hepatitis. Alcohol. 2002;27(1):37–41.
40. Batey RG, Wang J. Molecular pathogenesis of T lymphocyte-induced liver injury in alcoholic hepatitis. Front Biosci. 2002;7: d1662–1675.
41. Tagami A, Ohnishi H, Moriwaki H, Phillips M, Hughes RD. Fas-mediated apoptosis in acute alcoholic hepatitis. Hepatogastroenterology. 2003;50(50):443–8.
42. Faubion WA, Guicciardi ME, Miyoshi H, Bronk SF, Roberts PJ, Svingen PA, et al. Toxic bile salts induce rodent hepatocyte apoptosis via direct activation of Fas. J Clin Invest. 1999;103(1): 137–45.
43. Miyoshi H, Rust C, Roberts PJ, Burgart LJ, Gores GJ. Hepatocyte apoptosis after bile duct ligation in the mouse involves Fas. Gastroenterology. 1999;117(3):669–77.
44. Hatano E. Tumor necrosis factor signaling in hepatocyte apoptosis. J Gastroenterol Hepatol. 2007;22 Suppl 1:S43–44.
45. MacEwan DJ. TNF receptor subtype signalling: differences and cellular consequences. Cell Signal. 2002;14(6):477–92.
46. Wullaert A, Heyninck K, Beyaert R. Mechanisms of crosstalk between TNF-induced NF-kappaB and JNK activation in hepatocytes. Biochem Pharmacol. 2006;72(9):1090–101.
47. Zheng SJ, Wang P, Tsabary G, Chen YH. Critical roles of TRAIL in hepatic cell death and hepatic inflammation. J Clin Invest. 2004;113(1):58–64.
48. Mundt B, Kuhnel F, Zender L, Paul Y, Tillmann H, Trautwein C, et al. Involvement of TRAIL and its receptors in viral hepatitis. FASEB J. 2003;17(1):94–6.
49. Shigeno M, Nakao K, Ichikawa T, Suzuki K, Kawakami A, Abiru S, et al. Interferon-alpha sensitizes human hepatoma cells to TRAIL-induced apoptosis through DR5 upregulation and NF-kappa B inactivation. Oncogene. 2003;22(11):1653–62.
50. Bowen DG, McCaughan GW, Bertolino P. Intrahepatic immunity: a tale of two sites? Trends Immunol. 2005;26(10):512–7.
51. Crispe IN. Hepatic T cells and liver tolerance. Nat Rev Immunol. 2003;3(1):51–62.
52. Salazar-Mather TP, Hokeness KL. Calling in the troops: regulation of inflammatory cell trafficking through innate cytokine/chemokine networks. Viral Immunol. 2003;16(3):291–306.
53. De Creus A, Abe M, Lau AH, Hackstein H, Raimondi G, Thomson AW. Low TLR4 expression by liver dendritic cells correlates with reduced capacity to activate allogeneic T cells in response to endotoxin. J Immunol. 2005;174(4):2037–45.
54. Uhrig A, Banafsche R, Kremer M, Hegenbarth S, Hamann A, Neurath M, et al. Development and functional consequences of LPS tolerance in sinusoidal endothelial cells of the liver. J Leukoc Biol. 2005;77(5):626–33.
55. Mehal WZ. Intrahepatic T cell survival versus death: which one prevails and why? J Hepatol. 2003;39(6):1070–1.
56. Mackay IR, Popper H. Immunopathogenesis of chronic hepatitis: a review. Aust N Z J Med. 1973;3(1):79–88.
57. Koff RS. Problem hepatitis viruses: the mutants. Am J Med. 1994;96(1A):52S–56.
58. Pawlotsky JM. Hepatitis C virus population dynamics during infection. Curr Top Microbiol Immunol. 2006;299:261–84.
59. Eisen-Vandervelde AL, Yao ZQ, Hahn YS. The molecular basis of HCV-mediated immune dysregulation. Clin Immunol. 2004;111(1): 16–21.
60. Moorman JP, Joo M, Hahn YS. Evasion of host immune surveillance by hepatitis C virus: potential roles in viral persistence. Arch Immunol Ther Exp (Warsz). 2001;49(3):189–94.
61. Yao ZQ, Ray S, Eisen-Vandervelde A, Waggoner S, Hahn YS. Hepatitis C virus: immunosuppression by complement regulatory pathway. Viral Immunol. 2001;14(4):277–95.
62. Knolle PA, Germann T, Treichel U, Uhrig A, Schmitt E, Hegenbarth S, et al. Endotoxin down-regulates T cell activation by antigen-presenting liver sinusoidal endothelial cells. J Immunol. 1999; 162(3):1401–7.
63. Al-Sherbiny M, Osman A, Mohamed N, Shata MT, Abdel-Aziz F, Abdel-Hamid M, et al. Exposure to hepatitis C virus induces cellular immune responses without detectable viremia or seroconversion. Am J Trop Med Hyg. 2005;73(1):44–9.
64. Freeman AJ, Ffrench RA, Post JJ, Harvey CE, Gilmour SJ, White PA, et al. Prevalence of production of virus-specific interferon-gamma among seronegative hepatitis C-resistant subjects reporting injection drug use. J Infect Dis. 2004;190(6):1093–7.
65. Semmo N, Barnes E, Taylor C, Kurtz J, Harcourt G, Smith N, et al. T-cell responses and previous exposure to hepatitis C virus in indeterminate blood donors. Lancet. 2005;365(9456):327–9.
66. Kamal SM, Amin A, Madwar M, Graham CS, He Q, Al Tawil A, et al. Cellular immune responses in seronegative sexual contacts of acute hepatitis C patients. J Virol. 2004;78(22):12252–8.
67. Koziel MJ, Wong DK, Dudley D, Houghton M, Walker BD. Hepatitis C virus-specific cytolytic T lymphocyte and T helper cell responses in seronegative persons. J Infect Dis. 1997;176(4): 859–66.
68. Hiramatsu N, Hayashi N, Katayama K, Mochizuki K, Kawanishi Y, Kasahara A, et al. Immunohistochemical detection of Fas antigen in liver tissue of patients with chronic hepatitis C. Hepatology. 1994;19(6):1354–9.
69. Bode JG, Brenndorfer ED, Haussinger D. Hepatitis C virus (HCV) employs multiple strategies to subvert the host innate antiviral response. Biol Chem. 2008;389(10):1283–98.
70. Chou AH, Tsai HF, Wu YY, Hu CY, Hwang LH, Hsu PI, et al. Hepatitis C virus core protein modulates TRAIL-mediated apoptosis by enhancing Bid cleavage and activation of mitochondria apoptosis signaling pathway. J Immunol. 2005;174(4):2160–6.
71. Sacco R, Tsutsumi T, Suzuki R, Otsuka M, Aizaki H, Sakamoto S, et al. Antiapoptotic regulation by hepatitis C virus core protein through up-regulation of inhibitor of caspase-activated DNase. Virology. 2003;317(1):24–35.
72. Lan L, Gorke S, Rau SJ, Zeisel MB, Hildt E, Himmelsbach K, et al. Hepatitis C virus infection sensitizes human hepatocytes to TRAIL-induced apoptosis in a caspase 9-dependent manner. J Immunol. 2008;181(7):4926–35.
73. Sheppard P, Kindsvogel W, Xu W, Henderson K, Schlutsmeyer S, Whitmore TE, et al. IL-28, IL-29 and their class II cytokine receptor IL-28R. Nat Immunol. 2003;4(1):63–8.
74. Kotenko SV, Gallagher G, Baurin VV, Lewis-Antes A, Shen M, Shah NK, et al. IFN-lambdas mediate antiviral protection through a distinct class II cytokine receptor complex. Nat Immunol. 2003;4(1):69–77.
75. Rauch A, Kutalik Z, Descombes P, Cai T, Di Iulio J, Mueller T, et al. Genetic variation in IL28B is associated with chronic hepatitis C and treatment failure: a genome-wide association study. Gastroenterology. 2010;138(4):1338–45.

76. Imazeki F, Yokosuka O, Omata M. Impact of IL-28B SNPs on control of hepatitis C virus infection: a genome-wide association study. Expert Rev Anti Infect Ther. 2010;8(5):497–9.
77. Tanaka Y, Nishida N, Sugiyama M, Kurosaki M, Matsuura K, Sakamoto N, et al. Genome-wide association of IL28B with response to pegylated interferon-alpha and ribavirin therapy for chronic hepatitis C. Nat Genet. 2009;41(10):1105–9.
78. Suppiah V, Moldovan M, Ahlenstiel G, Berg T, Weltman M, Abate ML, et al. IL28B is associated with response to chronic hepatitis C interferon-alpha and ribavirin therapy. Nat Genet. 2009;41(10):1100–4.
79. Ge D, Fellay J, Thompson AJ, Simon JS, Shianna KV, Urban TJ, et al. Genetic variation in IL28B predicts hepatitis C treatment-induced viral clearance. Nature. 2009;461(7262):399–401.
80. Thomas DL, Thio CL, Martin MP, Qi Y, Ge D, O'Huigin C, et al. Genetic variation in IL28B and spontaneous clearance of hepatitis C virus. Nature. 2009;461(7265):798–801.
81. Robek MD, Boyd BS, Chisari FV. Lambda interferon inhibits hepatitis B and C virus replication. J Virol. 2005;79(6):3851–4.
82. Zhu H, Butera M, Nelson DR, Liu C. Novel type I interferon IL-28A suppresses hepatitis C viral RNA replication. Virol J. 2005;2:80.
83. Thomas DL. Hepatitis C and human immunodeficiency virus infection. Hepatology. 2002;36(5 Suppl 1):S201–209.
84. Sulkowski MS, Thomas DL. Hepatitis C in the HIV-infected patient. Clin Liver Dis. 2003;7(1):179–94.
85. Mrus JM, Sherman KE, Leonard AC, Sherman SN, Mandell KL, Tsevat J. Health values of patients coinfected with HIV/hepatitis C: are two viruses worse than one? Med Care. 2006;44(2):158–66.
86. Graham CS, Baden LR, Yu E, Mrus JM, Carnie J, Heeren T, et al. Influence of human immunodeficiency virus infection on the course of hepatitis C virus infection: a meta-analysis. Clin Infect Dis. 2001;33(4):562–9.
87. Graham CS, Wells A, Liu T, Sherman KE, Peters M, Chung RT, et al. Antigen-specific immune responses and liver histology in HIV and hepatitis C coinfection. AIDS. 2005;19(8):767–73.
88. Dienes HP, Drebber U, von Both I. Liver biopsy in hepatitis C. J Hepatol. 1999;31 Suppl 1:43–6.
89. Munshi N, Balasubramanian A, Koziel M, Ganju RK, Groopman JE. Hepatitis C and human immunodeficiency virus envelope proteins cooperatively induce hepatocytic apoptosis via an innocent bystander mechanism. J Infect Dis. 2003;188(8):1192–204.
90. Castedo M, Perfettini JL, Andreau K, Roumier T, Piacentini M, Kroemer G. Mitochondrial apoptosis induced by the HIV-1 envelope. Ann N Y Acad Sci. 2003;1010:19–28.
91. Roumier T, Castedo M, Perfettini JL, Andreau K, Metivier D, Zamzami N, et al. Mitochondrion-dependent caspase activation by the HIV-1 envelope. Biochem Pharmacol. 2003;66(8):1321–9.
92. Balasubramanian A, Ganju RK, Groopman JE. Hepatitis C virus and HIV envelope proteins collaboratively mediate interleukin-8 secretion through activation of p38 MAP kinase and SHP2 in hepatocytes. J Biol Chem. 2003;278(37):35755–66.
93. Klatt NR, Brenchley JM. Th17 cell dynamics in HIV infection. Curr Opin HIV AIDS. 2010;5(2):135–40.
94. Hofer U, Speck RF. Disturbance of the gut-associated lymphoid tissue is associated with disease progression in chronic HIV infection. Semin Immunopathol. 2009;31(2):257–66.
95. Cecchinato V, Trindade CJ, Laurence A, Heraud JM, Brenchley JM, Ferrari MG, et al. Altered balance between Th17 and Th1 cells at mucosal sites predicts AIDS progression in simian immunodeficiency virus-infected macaques. Mucosal Immunol. 2008;1(4):279–88.
96. Balagopal A, Ray SC, De Oca RM, Sutcliffe CG, Vivekanandan P, Higgins Y, et al. Kupffer cells are depleted with HIV immunodeficiency and partially recovered with antiretroviral immune reconstitution. AIDS. 2009;23(18):2397–404.
97. Blackard JT, Komurian-Pradel F, Perret M, Sodoyer M, Smeaton L, St Clair JB, et al. Intrahepatic cytokine expression is downregulated during HCV/HIV co-infection. J Med Virol. 2006;78(2):202–7.
98. Yim HC, Li JC, Lau JS, Lau AS. HIV-1 Tat dysregulation of lipopolysaccharide-induced cytokine responses: microbial interactions in HIV infection. AIDS. 2009;23(12):1473–84.

Host Gene Polymorphisms and Disease/Treatment Outcomes in HIV and Viral Coinfections

Jacob K. Nattermann and Jürgen K. Rockstroh

Introduction

Since the early days of the current HIV type 1 (HIV-1) pandemic, it has been observed that both susceptibility to HIV-1 infection and natural course of disease are highly variable. These differences are the result of multifaceted interactions between virus, host, and environment, and these interactions may be even more complex in the case of coinfection with other viruses such as HBV or HCV. With respect to the host, it is known that genetic differences importantly contribute to this variation.

However, our current knowledge of the relevant host genetic factors is still limited for two main reasons [1, 2]. First, many studies have suffered from suboptimal study design, which is a common theme in the genetic-association literature [3]. Second, until recent years most of the discoveries were the result of single candidate gene studies in which allelic variants with a known or suspected role in HIV-associated immune responses and pathology have been analyzed. Thus, a limited number of host genes have been studied so far and most of the identified genetic markers relevant to HIV-1 infection are either implicated in HIV-1 life cycle, including viral entry, replication, and propagation or are involved in the modulation of antiviral immunity [4].

This candidate-gene approach is based on a priori knowledge of the (potential) role of a specific gene in HIV pathogenesis. Following identification/selection of a candidate gene, the corresponding genomic region can be genotyped at known polymorphic positions, or resequenced to identify unknown variants. Association analysis can address the individual contributions of any single-nucleotide polymorphism (SNP) within this region, or of a series of linked SNPs (a haplotype), to a study phenotype.

However, by using this approach, statistical analysis needs to take into account several issues. For instance, multiple testing will lead to an increasing number of false-positive tests as the number of SNPs, alleles, study end points, phenotypes, or subgroups increase. The ongoing expansion of the global HIV-1 epidemic, its impact on human health, and the limitations of the candidate-gene approach represent a strong argument for the adoption of genome-wide association studies (GWAS). This approach enables investigators to assess genetic interactions, copy number polymorphisms, enrichment of genetic sets and of functional variants in the whole genome, or in large genomic regions even in the absence of a priori knowledge of the most important genes. Indeed, a series of GWAS have been performed in the field of HIV infection during recent years and provided important information that will help to better understand the underlying mechanisms associated with disease expression in variable population groups [5–10].

Host Genetics and HIV-1 Disease

Genetic Polymorphisms Affecting HIV Life-Cycle

Chemokines and Chemokine Receptors

Chemokines, a group of *chemo*tactic cyto*kines*, exert chemotactic and immunoregulatory actions [11]. Furthermore, these molecules are involved in modulation of adhesion processes at the endothelium and thus promote the transendothelial migration of leukocytes (haptotaxis). In addition, some chemokines stimulate angiogenesis or angiostasis and thus may play a further role in the suppression of tumor growth or the establishment of an inflammatory response.

J.K. Nattermann (✉)
Department of Internal Medicine I, University of Bonn,
Sigmund-Freud Str 25, Bonn 53125, Germany
e-mail: jacob.nattermann@ukb.uni-bonn.de

Currently, about 50 human chemokines and 20 chemokine receptors have been described.

CC-chemokines bind to specific G-protein coupled receptors to trigger cell activation and migration. In particular, the CC-chemokines CCL3 (macrophagic inflammatory protein 1, MIP-1), CCL4 (macrophagic inflammatory protein 1, MIP-1), and CCL5 (regulated upon activation, normal T cell expressed and secreted, RANTES) are ligands for the CC-chemokine receptor 5 (CCR5) and attract monocytes and T lymphocytes [12]. Moreover, CCR5 represents the main coreceptor for macrophage-tropic (R5) strains of HIV-1, normally expressed on CD4-positive T lymphocytes.

The CCR5 gene is subject to several mutations which have gained major scientific and clinical interest as these represent the only allelic variants that have been consistently associated with protection against infection with HIV-1.

The most prominent CCR5 polymorphism is a 32-bp deletion in the coding region of the CCR5 gene (CCR5Δ32) which leads to a frame shift and a truncated protein which is not expressed on the cell surface [13, 14]. In a Caucasian population the CCR5Δ32 allele frequency is about 10–20% (corresponding to a 1% frequency of homozygous individuals) [13] and this frequency decreases in a southeast cline toward Mediterranean and gradually disappears in the African and Asian populations.

Of note, the CCR5-Δ 32 mutation confers protection against infection with R5-tropic viruses in individuals that are homozygous for this allele and has been shown to slow down disease progression in heterozygotes [13].

Besides CCR5Δ32 there are several other uncommon polymorphisms within the coding region of CCR5. However, the impact of these allelic variants on HIV-1 coreceptor function has not been completely established [15], except for CCR5 303T>A SNP (also referred to as C101X or m303) [15, 16]. This rare mutation inserts a premature stop codon which prevents expression of a functional coreceptor, thereby blocking entry of R5-tropic HIV-1 strains in vitro [17].

Some reports suggested an influence of CCR5 promotor variants on disease progression owing to modulated susceptibility of target cells as a result of altered CCR5 surface expression [18–21].

Of note, CCR5 and its ligands may not only interfere with viral entry of HIV into the cell but also affect antiviral responses via modulating cellular immunity [22]. The complexity of these associations was further emphasized by studies analyzing the effects of CCR5 haplotypes (defined as a set of SNPs in combination with the CCR5Δ32 mutation). Here, the authors observed that the CCR5 haplotype (HHG*2) comprising the Δ32-mutation (both homozygous or in combination with another specific haplotype (HHE)) is a predictor of a weak cell-mediated immune response and a rapid progression of HIV infection. However, the same CCR5 HHG*2 haplotype in combination with the CCR5 HHC haplotype was associated with a slower progression of infection and possibly with a stronger immune response [22].

CCR2 is a minor HIV-1 coreceptor that is not directly used for cell entry in vivo. A mutation within the first transmembrane region of the CCR2 chemokine gene (CCR2-64I; a valine to isoleucine change) has been found to delay progression to AIDS [23].

At the moment it is still controversial how the CCR2 64I variant exerts its protective. A proposed mechanism is an increased ability of CCR2 64I to downmodulate CCR5 expression [24, 25]. However, other studies could not confirm an association between CCR2A 64I and CCR5 expression levels and suggested that CCR2 64I does not act by influencing CCR5 transcription or mRNA levels [26].

CXCR1 (IL-8RA) and CXCR2 (IL-8RB) are receptors for proinflammatory cytokine IL-8. Several polymorphisms within the CXCR1 [27] and CXCR2 genes have been classified into distinct haplotypes. Two SNPs T92G (CXCR1 2300) and C1003T (CXCR1 2142) are an integral part of the CXCR1 haplotype "Ha," which has been described to be in strong association with protection against rapid progression to AIDS possibly mediated by suppressing CD4 and CXCR4 expression [28].

Moreover, genetic variants in the genes encoding for the chemokines CX3CR1 [29–36] and CXCR6 [37] have been reported to be associated with different outcomes of HIV infection. However, the exact role of these polymorphisms remains to be clarified in larger studies.

Duffy Antigen Receptor for Chemokines

Duffy antigen receptor for chemokines (DARC), a nonspecific chemokine receptor expressed on red blood cells (RBCs), represents a known receptor for *Plasmodium vivax*. Moreover DARC can aid HIV-1 attachment to RBCs and modulate its transinfection to target cells by affecting both chemokine–HIV interactions and chemokine-driven inflammation [38–40]. A SNP in the promoter region of DARC (46T-C) is widely prevalent in African populations. The homozygous 246CC genotype confers the malaria-resisting, Duffy-null phenotype. With respect to HIV-1 infection, this genotype has been shown to be associated not only with a high risk of HIV-1 infection but, on the contrary, also with slower progression in terms of death or development of dementia [40]. Interestingly, this survival advantage became increasingly pronounced in those with progressively lower WBC counts, suggesting interactions between DARC genotype and the cellular milieu defined by WBC counts may influence HIV-1 pathogenesis [41].

Chemokines represent the natural ligands for the same receptors used by HIV for cell entry and thus can interfere with HIV entry by two means: First, they compete with HIV for the same receptor, and second, they can reduce surface expression of the respective chemokine receptor by inducing its internalization upon binding [42].

A variety of polymorphisms in genes encoding for chemokine have been analyzed with respect to its potential effects on HIV disease. CCL5, a ligand for the CCR5 receptor, is a potent inhibitor of HIV entry in vitro. In vivo studies demonstrated decreased CCL5 levels to be associated with accelerated disease progression, whereas the opposite effect could be observed in patients with upregulated CCL5 expression [42].

Several polymorphisms within regulatory regions of the CCL5 gene have been grouped in haplotypes that appear to modulate CCL5 gene expression, thereby affecting HIV susceptibility as well as the course of infection [32, 43–55]. However, these data need to be confirmed in larger cohorts [56].

Studies on the CCL2-CCL7-CCL11 genes cluster revealed additional chemokine polymorphisms potentially affecting course of HIV disease, whereby again increase in chemokine expression levels has been suggested as the underlying mechanism [28, 57, 58].

Furthermore, allelic variants in the coding and noncoding regions of the CCL3 gene have been shown to be associated with both resistance and progression [59–61].

The gene encoding for CCL3L1 harbors various SNPs. Moreover, the region on chromosome 17q that encodes this gene represents a hotspot for duplication [62]. As a result individuals vary with respect to the number of CCL3L1-containing segmental duplications (copy number variations) [62]. Of note, a low CCL3L1 copy number has been associated with reduced chemokine levels and a higher proportion of CCR5-positive CD4+ cells [63].

This is important because CCL3L1 is a potent ligand for CC chemokine receptor 5 (CCR5) and has been shown to be a dominant HIV-suppressive chemokine [64].

Of note, copy number variations in CCL3L1 have been reported to be associated with susceptibility to HIV-1 infection [60, 63, 65–67] and the course of disease [63, 66, 68, 69]. However, recent studies could not confirm these findings [70, 71].

Based on the combination of genotypes for CCL3L1 copy numbers and CCR5 deletion mutation, genetic risk groups (GRKs) have been defined that are associated with the risk of acquiring HIV infection and the extent of HIV replication [22, 69, 72].

Individuals with CCL3L1 high copy numbers and CCR5 deletion point toward low risk compared with those with CCL3L1 low copy numbers and CCR5 nondeletion genotypes. Furthermore, these genotypes have been shown to influence CD4 recovery and immune reconstitution after highly active antiretroviral therapy [69] and seemed to affect cell-mediated immune response.

SDF-1 (CXCL12) is a powerful chemoattractant cytokine that regulates the maturation, trafficking, and homing of lymphocytes and represents the natural ligand for CXCR4, the main coreceptor for lymphotropic HIV-1 strains (X4 strains). Numerous studies have analyzed allelic variants with the SDF-1 gene with respect to its potential effects on HIV susceptibility and progression of disease.

In particular, a SNP located in the 3′-untranslated region, which might affect SDF-1 production, has been suggested to have various effects [73, 74]. However, in a large meta-analysis these findings could not be convincingly confirmed [75]. Thus, the exact role of CXCL12 variants remains unclear.

HIV-1 Dependency Factors (TSG101 and PPIA)

After cell entry, HIV-1 interacts with various host proteins. Some function as antiviral factors but the majority are HIV dependency factors (HDFs). These specific proteins are essential for sustaining viral replication. Therefore, HDFs would represent ideal candidate genes and thus have been studied in several host genetic studies. Until now, only two allelic variants in genes encoding for such HDFs have been shown to affect pathogenesis of HIV-1 infection und confirmed in subsequent studies, including TSG101 (encoding tumor susceptibility gene 101) and PPIA (peptidyl-prolyl cis-trans isomerase, encoding cyclophilin A).

TSG101 directly interacts with a highly conserved motif in the p6 region of the HIV-1 Gag protein, Pro-Thr/Ser-Ala-Pro (PTAP), and thus was shown to be critical for the release of HIV-1 particles from the cellular membrane [76–80]. Haplotypes constructed from SNPs located in the 5′-region (+181A>C and −183T>C) were shown to affect disease progression, the rate of CD4 T-cell depletion and viral load increase over time, and to possibly influence on HIV-1 infection [81].

The cyclophilin A protein is incorporated into the viral particle through selective interaction with viral capsid. At the moment, it is only incompletely understood how cyclophilin A enhances HIV-1 infection. However, recent studies suggest that this molecule is involved in uncoating of the viral core and may act as a cofactor for the anti-HIV protein TRIM5. Several allelic variants within the regulatory region of PPIA have been found to modulate CD4+ T cell loss in African Americans and to possibly affect susceptibility to HIV-1 infection [82–84]. Considering the important role of cyclophilin A in HIV-1 replication, manipulation of CypA activity may represent a interesting novel therapeutic approach [83].

Intrinsic Antiretroviral Factors

In addition to genes that modulate viral entry, there are others that are critically involved in HIV restriction and influence the anti-HIV immune response. Most notably, the antiviral APOBEC3G gene family and the virus restriction factor TRIM5a have been shown to exert a potent antiretroviral function.

TRIM5a (Tripartite interaction motif 5a) is a species-specific antiviral factor that protects humans and other primates against a broad range of retroviruses. It targets the capsid molecules of the incoming retrovirus in the cytosol and promotes its premature disassembly. Human TRIM5a has been shown to effectively block N-tropic murine leukemia virus (MLV) and equine anemia virus, but is much less efficient in restricting HIV-1 replication [85–87].

Several TRIM5a polymorphisms have been reported to have functional consequences with regard to the antiviral activity of Trim5α in vitro (e.g., H43Y, R136Q, G110R, and G176del) and to affect natural course of and/or susceptibility to HIV infection. However, most in vivo data suggest that common variants of human TRIM5a may only have limited effect on HIV-1 disease, and thus, the exact in vivo role of TRIM5a variants is still under discussion [85, 88, 89].

APOBEC3G (Apolipoprotein B mRNA-editing enzyme, catalytic polypeptide-like 3G), a cellular cytidine deaminase, was first identified as a host antiviral factor able to restrict replication of human immune deficiency viruses lacking the accessory protein Vif (viral infection factor) [90]. In the absence of Vif, APOBEC proteins are encapsidated by budding virus particles and either cause extensive cytidine to uridine editing of negative sense single-stranded DNA during reverse transcription or restrict virus replication through deaminase-independent mechanisms.

In African populations, an H186R coding change was reported to favor progression to AIDS. More recently, an APOBEC3H allele encoding stable APOBEC3H protein with potent activity against retroviruses including HIV has been described primarily in African populations. However, an exhaustive analysis of APOBEC3G variants in Caucasian did not reveal any association with control of HIV. Thus, further studies in larger, ethnically controlled populations are needed to exactly define the role of APOBEC3 variants in HIV infection are warranted [91–93].

Genetic Polymorphisms and Immunity

Major Histocompatibility Complex

Among the various immunogenetic determinants that are known to influence HIV/AIDS, the human leukocyte antigen (HLA) system represent the most prominent host genetic factor that has been consistently demonstrated to affect outcome of HIV disease.

Three genes (HLA-A, HLA-B, and HLA-C) encode the classical HLA class I proteins, which are critical for the development of an immune response. The major biological function of HLA class I is presentation of antigenic peptides (including viral epitopes). Thus, the genetic diversity in this locus sets the stage for effective CD8+ T cell responses against the virus. Owing to HLA driven immune selection pressure, the virus continues to evolve into new mutants, albeit with varying degrees of fitness.

Following infection with HIV, the potency of the elicited antiviral immune response critically depends on the viral epitopes that can be presented by the HLA repertoire of the infected individual. Therefore, an increased heterozygosity at HLA class I region is considered to be a selective advantage as it enables presentation of a wide range of viral antigens and thus evokes a broader T-cell response, resulting in delayed emergence of escape mutants and decelerates progression toward AIDS [94]. Moreover, the HLA status may also affect horizontal transmission of HIV infection, as it has been suggested that Major histocompatibility complex (MHC) concordance between the virus donor and the recipient facilitates the virus to passage itself to a new host [95–97].

In the case of vertical transmission from mother to child, it is generally easier for the preadapted virus to reestablish itself in the progeny (which is least HLA haploidentical) with the virus donor, even if the shared HLA allele is apparently a "protective" one like HLA-B27 [98, 99].

The HLA allele that has most consistently been associated with efficient control of HIV is B*57, with B*5701 found almost exclusively in Caucasian populations and B*5703 mostly observed in individuals of African ancestry [5, 7, 9, 100].

HLA-B*57 has been shown to exert strong selection pressure on HIV, forcing rapid viral mutation. But this comes at the cost of its replicative fitness [101]. Accordingly, a SNP (HCP5 rs2395029) that is a proxy for B*5701 showed the strongest association with viral load or long-term nonprogression in different genome-wide association studies [5, 7, 9].

Moreover, there is clear functional and epidemiological evidence indicating effective restriction of HIV by B*27. However, a recent report indicated that HIV is in the process of adaptation as a stable HLA-B27 CTL-escape strain circulating in The Netherlands has been detected. Thus, patients carrying protective HLA alleles might not be protected anymore from disease progression in the future [102].

Based on their peptide binding abilities *HLA-B*35 subtypes* can be categorized into two major groups: *B*35 "Py" and B*35Px* [28]. Of these, B*35Px (including B*3501, B*3502, B*3503, and B*3504) is associated with faster progression to AIDS [101]. However, the underlying mechanism(s) of such an association are not fully clear.

Various MHC haplotypes and several HLA-A supertypes (a group of HLA alleles with overlapping peptide-binding properties) have been reported to modulate the course of HIV infection. For instance, the B7 supertype, which encompass alleles such as *B*0702-5, *1508, *3501-3, *5101, *5301, *5401, *5501-02, *5601, *5602, *6701,* and *7801*, has been associated with high viremia and accelerated progression to AIDS in

Caucasians infected with the clade B virus, but not in Africans who are infected predominantly with clade C [94, 103].

However, most of the reported associations between HIV infection and HLA haplotypes/subtypes are likely to reflect the impact of individual alleles included in these groups and to the long-range linkage disequilibrium structure of the MHC region [2].

Moreover, there is some evidence suggesting that genetic variation in HLA-C might also affect outcome of HIV infection as a SNP (rs9264942) located in the 5' region of HLA-C has been demonstrated be in strong association with both viral set point and progression [5]. However, more work is needed to understand the precise immunological and biological function of HLA-C in the context of HIV-1 infection [104].

The nonclassical HLA class I molecules *HLA-E* and *-G* are ligands for the inhibitory NK-cell receptors CD94/NKG2A and KIR2DL4, respectively. A recent study carried out on Zimbabwean women suggested specific genetic variants of *HLA-E* (*0103*) and *HLA-G* (*0105N*) to be associated decreased risk of heterosexual HIV transmission [105]. However, due to the strong linkage disequilibrium within the HLA gene complex, the authors could not rule out the possibility that another linked gene is responsible for the observed effect. Thus, further data are warranted.

HLA and Drug Hypersensitivity

Finally, HLA gene variants play a role in terms of HAART hypersensitivity reactions which shows considerable interindividual variability among HIV-infected patients. Approximately 2–8% of HIV-positive Caucasian patients have been found to develop abacavir (NRTI) hypersensitivity syndrome (AHS) within 10–40 days after initiation of treatment. Of note, these patients show a strong association of AHS with an extended MHC Ancestral Haplotype 57.1 (AH57.1) carrying HLA-B*5701-DRB1*07 [106]. Accordingly, the presence of HLA-B*5701 is highly predictive of clinically diagnosed AHS and has been confirmed in several study cohorts [15]. Therefore, HIV treatment guidelines in the USA and Europe have recommended mandatory screening of B*5701 before prescribing abacavir therapy. Besides abacavir, a few other antiretroviral drugs have shown specific genetic associations with drug efficacy and toxicities [107]. These include associations of (1) HLA-DRB1*0101 and Cw8 with sensitivity to Nevirapine (NNRTI), (2) CYP2B6*6 with improved immunological recovery in response to NNRTIs; (3) CYP3A5*3 with faster PI (sequinavir and indinavir) oral clearance and others [107].

Killer Cell Immunoglobulin-Like Receptors

Beyond their role for the adaptive immune system, HLA molecules are also involved in the functional regulation of natural killer (NK) cells, a central part of the innate immune response against viral infections. NK cells express killer cell immunoglobulin-line receptors (KIR), which recognize HLA molecules resulting in activating or inhibitory signaling. Of note, there is increasing evidence indicating that specific HLA-KIR combinations have epistatic influences on the natural course of HIV infection [108].

KIR3DS1, an activating receptor has been associated with rapid progression to AIDS but only in the absence of HLA Bw4 molecules encoding an isoleucine at position 80 (Bw4 80I) whereas KIR3DS1 alone or in combination with Bw4-80I has a protective effect. In the absence of KIR3DS1, the HLA-Bw4-80I allele was not associated with any effect on HIV infection.

Moreover, several combinations of inhibitory KIR3DL1 alleles and HLA Bw4 molecules have been associated with lower HIV serum levels and slower progression of disease. In addition, recent reports suggest that KIR3DL1 and KIR2DS1 may also have a role in modulating susceptibility to HIV infection [108–114].

Other Molecules Involved in Immune Responses

In general, all genes related to immunity can be suspected to be involved in the pathogenesis of HIV infection. Accordingly, many of them have been analyzed in genetic studies. However, most of the reported associations have not been conclusively replicated and therefore remain controversial.

DC-SIGN (CD209) and its related protein DC-SIGNR are C-type lectins known to bind multiple pathogens including HIV-1, HIV-2, and hepatitis C virus. The extracellular portion of this molecule, which is important for pathogen binding, is composed of a tandem repeat region ("neck region") and a carbohydrate recognition domain. Of note, the number of tandem repeats may affect susceptibility to HIV infection [115]. For instance, neck regions with less than 5 repeat units have recently been demonstrated to be associated with resistance in individuals of Chinese ancestry.

Moreover, there are some reports suggesting a role of DC-SIGN promoter variants in HIV pathogenesis. The DC-SIGN 2336C allele has been associated with susceptibility to parenteral HIV-1 infection in the European Americans [116], while DC-SIGN-139C was associated with accelerated AIDS progression in HIV-1-infected Japanese hemophiliacs [117]. However, these findings could not be confirmed in other studies.

Beta-defensin-1 (DEFB1), a small molecule mainly produced by epithelial cells, plays a role against infections, in inflammatory and allergic processes. In HIV-1 infection, significant correlations between the SNPs −44 G/C and −52 A/C in the 5′-untranslated region of the DEFB1 gene and a risk of vertical transmission were reported in Italian and Brazilian populations [118–121]. Moreover, −52 G/G genotype has been associated with lower levels of HIV-1 RNA in breast milk, but not in plasma, in Mozambican women with the −52GG genotype versus women with the −52GA and −52AA genotypes [122].

Mannose-binding lectin (MBL), a major component of the innate immune response, is a circulating host-defense protein that acts as a broad-spectrum pattern-recognition molecule against a wide variety of infectious agents. MBL mediates its effects by influencing complement activation], opsonization, and phagocytosis. Of note, MBL2 contains polymorphisms in the coding and promoter region that have been associated with susceptibility to and/or progression of HIV-1 infection [123–125].

Finally, mounting evidence indicates Toll-like receptor (TLR) polymorphisms can affect susceptibility to and progression of HIV-1 infection. TLRs are innate immune sensors that are integral to resisting chronic and opportunistic infections. Toll-like receptors (TLRs) play an important role in the innate immune response to pathogens. TLR7 recognizes RNA of various viruses including HIV. A SNP in the gene encoding for TLR7 (TLR7 Gln11Leu) has been found to be associated with susceptibility to and a more severe clinical course of HIV-1 disease [126]. These results may have implications for the risk assessment of individual patients as well as for HIV-1 therapy and vaccination strategies in the future.

Moreover, TLR4 polymorphisms [1063 A/G (D299G) and 1363C/T (T399I)] have been suggested to modulate HIV-1 peak viral load [127] and polymorphisms in the gene encoding TLR9 (1635A/G and +1174G/A) have been associated with disease progression [128, 129].

Host Genetics and HCV Mono- and HCV–HIV Coinfection

Currently pegylated interferon-α in combination with ribavirin represents the backbone of HCV-specific therapy. However, in clinical studies interferon-based combination therapy sustained virologic response (SVR) is achieved in only ~40% of HCV/HIV coinfected patients [130], and SVR may be even lower in clinical practice [131].

HCV genotype [132–135] and viral load are major determinants of treatment response in HCV infection, but there is clear evidence indicating host genetic factors to also influence response to treatment. However, only a limited number of studies have been performed in HIV–HCV coinfected patients.

The Cytokine/Chemokine System

Interleukins, Interferons, and Members of the Tumor Necrosis Factor Family

Factors that have received attention as possible predictors of response to interferon therapy of hepatitis C comprise the members of the cytokine family, including the chemokines, interleukins, interferons, and members of the tumor necrosis factor (TNF) family, all which play an important role for the initiation and regulation of immune responses.

Recently, allelic variants in IL-28B have gained major scientific interest as several genome-wide association studies identified a panel of SNPs on chromosome 19q13 to be strongly associated with sustained virological response to treatment with pegylated interferon-α and ribavirin and spontaneous clearance of hepatitis C [136–141] in HCV monoinfection. These SNPs are located about 3 kb upstream of the IL28B gene, which encodes for the type III interferon IFN-3λ. Of note, IFN-λ1, another member of the type III interferons has been shown to inhibit HCV in a dose- and time-dependent fashion [138, 142, 143]. Moreover, IFN-λ1 is capable of upregulating interferon-stimulated genes (ISG) and enhances the antiviral activity of IFN-α. Whether IFN-λ3 acts in the same way remains to be clarified. However, recent in vitro data suggest that IFN-λ3 may have comparable functions as IFN-λ1 [144].

With respect to HIV–HCV coinfection two recent reports suggest that IL28B polymorphisms may also affect treatment response in HIV-positive patients with chronic HCV coinfection but do not affect treatment-induced clearance of acute hepatitis C virus.

Besides IL28B variants several other polymorphisms have been suggested to be associated with response to HCV-specific therapy in patients with HCV mono- and/or HIV–HCV coinfection, including mutations located within coding and regulatory regions of cytokine genes that are associated with either high, intermediate, or low production of the corresponding gene product [145–148].

In particular, the production of inappropriate levels of tumor necrosis factor-a (TNF-a) and interleukin-10 (IL-10) have been reported to contribute to viral persistence in HCV infection [149–152], and serum levels of IL-6 and transforming growth factor-b (TGF-b) are also reported to be elevated in chronic HCV infection compared to healthy controls [153–158].

Interleukin-6 (IL-6) is a multifunctional cytokine that has been implicated in a variety of cellular functions including stimulation of hepatocytes to produce acute-phase proteins [159], liver regeneration and protection against hepatic injury [160], and activation of STAT3 in the liver. A polymorphism within the promotor region (C>G transition at position 174) is associated with differences in the production of IL-6 [147]. Thus, individuals can be classified into high (genotypes IL-6 174 GG and 174 GC) and low (genotype IL-6 174 CC) IL-6 producers, respectively [147]. In HCV–HIV coinfection, the IL6 high producer (HP) genotype has been reported as an independent predictor of SVR [161]. This effect was seen in both HIV-positive patients with acute and chronic hepatitis C and corresponded to the in vitro observation that in HCV core-transfected HUH7 cells, IL-6 helps to overcome HCV core mediated inhibition of STAT3 activation [161]. A similar observation was made in HCV monoinfected subjects treated with standard-interferon but not in patients treated with the more potent combination of pegylated interferon plus ribavirin.

IL10 is considered to play important roles of IL10 in antiviral immune responses and several studies have examined the relevance of functional IL10 gene polymorphisms in hepatitis C. Two studies found that carriers of the −592A or −819T alleles and the corresponding extended haplotype (108-bp IL10.R microsatellite and −591A+−819T+−1082 A+−2763C+−3575T+), are more likely to achieve a sustained response to therapy with standard interferon +/− ribavirin [162, 163]. However, these data have not been confirmed in patients treated with the more potent pegylated interferon. In addition, several variants of the immunomodulatory IL10 gene have been suggested to be involved in natural clearance of HCV [164–166].

Interleukin-12 (IL-12) is a cytokine that governs the Th1-type immune response. Several studies analyzed whether the IL12B polymorphisms within the promoter region (4 bp insertion/deletion) and the 3′-UTR (1188-A/C)-loci, which have been proposed to regulate IL-12 synthesis, are associated with the natural course of hepatitis C and treatment outcome [167–170]. Houldsworth et al. [168] found chronically infected patients to be significantly more likely to be homozygous for the 3′-UTR A allele than those with resolved HCV infection. Of note, the 3′-UTR A allele has been associated with lower IL-12 production.

By contrast, in a study by Mueller et al. no association of IL12B polymorphisms and self-limited HCV infection could be demonstrated [169]. Nevertheless, these authors identified carriers of the IL12B 3′-UTR 1188-C-allele to be capable of responding more efficiently to antiviral combination therapy owing to reduced relapse rates [169]. Finally, Lee and colleagues [170] reported that interleukin-12 exerts only limited antiviral activity against certain HCV quasi-species in vivo.

Transforming growth factor (TGF)-β is involved in the control of growth, differentiation, and apoptosis of cells. In addition, TGF-β plays a major regulatory role in hepatic fibrosis and cirrhosis. Analogous to other cytokine genes, the TGF-β gene is polymorphic (codon 10 and 25), leading to differences in cytokine production. Thus, patients can be classified in TGF-β high (10T/T 25G/G; 10T/C 25G/G), intermediate (10T/C 25G/C; 10C/G 25G/G; 10T/T 25G/C), and low (10C/C 25G/C; 10C/C 25C/C; 10T/T 26C/C; 10T/C 25C/C) producers according to their TGF-β genotype.

In HIV-positive patients with acute hepatitis C genotype 1 infection the TGF-β high producer genotype has been described as independent predictor of SVR to HCV specific treatment with pegylated interferon. A comparable trend was observed in patients with chronic HCV monoinfection but failed to reach statistical significance. Moreover, a variant in the promoter of the TGF-β 1 gene (−509T/C) may affect natural course of HCV infection as the −509CC genotype and the −509C allele have been found to be significantly associated with higher HCV clearance rates [171].

Tumor necrosis factor (TNF)-α and IFN-γ are proinflammatory cytokines, that have been shown to be important pathogenic mediators in a variety of liver conditions. TNF-α has been reported to play a role in the immunopathogenesis of both acute and chronic HCV infection, in viral persistence as well as for the response to IFN-α-based therapy [150]. Genetic variants in the human TNF-α promoter region, such as the mutations at positions −308 and −238, have been shown to influence expression of TNF-α [148, 172, 173]. However, whether these polymorphisms affect the pathogenesis and progression of chronic HCV infection and/or the response to IFN-a therapy is still under discussion as conflicting data have been reported [174–177].

IFN-γ is essential for an effective host defense against a variety of intracellular pathogens. With respect to hepatitis C IFN-γ has been demonstrated to efficiently inhibit viral replication in vitro [178], and the intrahepatic IFN-γ levels appear to be associated with viral clearance in the chimpanzee model [179].

Several polymorphisms within the IFN-γ noncoding regions, such as −874A/T, CA repeat microsatellite, and −179T/G, have been implicated in several autoimmune and chronic inflammatory conditions [145, 180, 181]. Recently, Huang et al. [181] have demonstrated a SNP variant located in the proximal IFN-γ promoter region next to the binding motif of heat shock transcription factor (HSF), −764G, to be significantly associated with sustained virological response. Moreover, this polymorphism was also significantly associated with spontaneous recovery in a second study cohort. In functional studies the authors demonstrated that the G allele confers a two- to threefold higher promoter activity and stronger binding affinity to HSF1 than the C allele [179].

Whether the CCR5-Δ32 polymorphism affects susceptibility to infection with HCV is still under discussion as controversial results have been published [182–185]. By contrast, it is widely accepted that this mutation does not affect response to standard combination therapy with pegylated interferon and ribavirin [186–188].

However, certain RANTES (CCL5) haplotypes that are known to downregulate RANTES transcriptional activity in vitro, have been associated with nonresponse to antiviral therapy, which may indicate a possible role of the CCR5/RANTES axis for treatment outcome [189].

The Human Leukocyte Antigen (HLA)-System

Cell-mediated immunity is considered to be an important mechanism for resolution of primary HCV infection [190]. Thus, potential associations between the HLA system and response to interferon treatment in HCV-infected patients have been intensively studied [191]. However, the reported data are conflicting and suggest major influences from other factors unrelated to HLA alleles [192–198], although a recent large-scale study in liver transplant recipients provided some evidence for human leukocyte antigen DRB1 heterozygote advantage against hepatitis C virus infection [199].

Killer Cell Immunoglobulin-Like Receptors

Similar to data obtained in HIV-infected patients, there is increasing evidence indicating a role of specific HLA-KIR combinations for treatment-induced and spontaneous clearance of HCV infection.

Khakoo and colleagues [200] first described that genes encoding the inhibitory NK cell receptor KIR2DL3 and its ligand HLA-C1 directly influence resolution of hepatitis C virus (HCV) infection in Caucasians and African Americans with expected low infectious doses of HCV but not in those with high-dose exposure. These findings have been confirmed in several subsequent studies [201–210]. Thus, it is widely accepted that KIR and HLA-C genes are consistently beneficial determinants in the outcome of HCV infection [191, 211]. This advantage extends to the allelic level for both gene families.

Other Host Genetic Factors

In patients with HCV genotype 1 monoinfection, a polymorphism of the GNB3 gene (GNB3 C825T) has been demonstrated to be associated with response to standard interferon-α treatment [169, 189, 212, 213]. GNB3 encodes the β3 subunit of heterotrimeric G proteins. The GNB3 825T allele is associated with the generation of a truncated albeit functionally active splice variants of the human G protein β3 subunit [214] with enhanced signal transduction via G proteins [215]. The GNB3 825 CC genotype has been reported to be associated with nonresponse to HCV therapy with standard interferon-α in monoinfected patients. However, this effect could not be confirmed in patients treated with the more potent PEG-IFN [216]. This in contrast to data in HCV–HIV coinfection, where the GNB3 genotype was significantly associated with response to treatment with pegylated interferon [216].

CTLA4 is a costimulatory molecule that attenuates T-lymphocyte responses. Two studies examined potential associations of CTLA4 SNPs at promoter site −318 (C→T) and exon-1 site 49 (A→G) with clearance of hepatitis C virus (HCV) after treatment with combination interferon-α plus ribavirin therapy [217, 218]. In these studies, CTLA4 49G in exon 1 alone and as a haplotype in combination with the −318C mutation in the CTLA4 promoter region was found to be associated with SVR in Caucasian patients with HCV genotype 1 infection.

The interferon-inducible MxA protein is known to play a role in the antiviral host defense and has been suggested as specific surrogate parameter for IFN action. Studies on a SNP within promoter region of the MxA gene reported the G/T polymorphism at position nt −88 to correlate with the response of hepatitis C patients in interferon monotherapy [219–221]. However, these data could not be confirmed by Naito et al. who did not find any relationship between the efficacy of IFN-based therapy and the MxA SNP [222].

In addition, polymorphisms in the mannose binding-lectin (MBL) and LMP7 have been reported to affect treatment outcome. However, a more recent study found no association between SNPs in the MBL and LMP7 gene and response to IFN monotherapies [222].

Moreover, a SNP (rs760370A>G) in gene encoding the equilibrative nucleoside transporter type 1 (ENT1), which is considered the primary protein involved in ribavirin cellular uptake, has been shown to influences the chances of rapid virological response to pegIFN plus RBV in HIV–HCV coinfected patients.

Host Genetics and HBV Mono- and HIV–HBV Coinfection

Only a limited number of association studies have been performed in patients with hepatitis B virus infection and most of the results have not been confirmed. Thus, only little is known regarding the potential role of allelic variants and susceptibility to natural course and treatment response in HBV infection. However, some genetic factors have been identified, including variants in CTLA4, CD24, various genes encoding for cytokines as well as specific KIR-HLA combinations.

Summary

Host genetic polymorphisms are key modulators of immune response, natural history, and treatment outcomes of chronic viral infections including HIV, HCV, and HBV. Identification and characterization of these polymorphisms has the potential to significantly impact not only our understanding but also the management of patients with HIV and coinfections.

References

1. Telenti A, Goldstein DB. Genomics meets HIV-1. Nat Rev Microbiol. 2006;4:865–73.
2. Fellay J, Ge D, Shianna KV, et al. Common genetic variation and the control of HIV in humans. PLoS Genet. 2009;5:e1000791.
3. Ioannidis JP. Commentary: grading the credibility of molecular evidence for complex diseases. Int J Epidemiol. 2006;35:572–8. discussion 593–6.
4. O'Brien SJ, Nelson GW. Human genes that limit AIDS. Nat Genet. 2004;36:565–74.
5. Fellay J, Shianna KV, Ge D, et al. A whole-genome association study of major determinants for host control of HIV-1. Science. 2007;317:944–7.

6. Le Clerc S, Limou S, Coulonges C, et al. Genomewide association study of a rapid progression cohort identifies new susceptibility alleles for AIDS (ANRS Genomewide Association Study 03). J Infect Dis. 2009;200:1194–201.
7. Limou S, Le Clerc S, Coulonges C, et al. Genomewide association study of an AIDS-nonprogression cohort emphasizes the role played by HLA genes (ANRS Genomewide Association Study 02). J Infect Dis. 2009;199:419–26.
8. Herbeck JT, Gottlieb GS, Winkler CA, et al. Multistage genomewide association study identifies a locus at 1q41 associated with rate of HIV-1 disease progression to clinical AIDS. J Infect Dis. 2010;201:618–26.
9. Dalmasso C, Carpentier W, Meyer L, et al. Distinct genetic loci control plasma HIV-RNA and cellular HIV-DNA levels in HIV-1 infection: the ANRS Genome Wide Association 01 study. PLoS One. 2008;3:e3907.
10. Catano G, Kulkarni H, He W, et al. HIV-1 disease-influencing effects associated with ZNRD1, HCP5 and HLA-C alleles are attributable mainly to either HLA-A10 or HLA-B*57 alleles. PLoS One. 2008;3:e3636.
11. Mackay CR. Chemokines: immunology's high impact factors. Nat Immunol. 2001;2:95–101.
12. Loetscher P, Uguccioni M, Bordoli L, et al. CCR5 is characteristic of Th1 lymphocytes. Nature. 1998;391:344–5.
13. Dean M, Carrington M, Winkler C, et al. Genetic restriction of HIV-1 infection and progression to AIDS by a deletion allele of the CKR5 structural gene. Hemophilia Growth and Development Study, Multicenter AIDS Cohort Study, Multicenter Hemophilia Cohort Study, San Francisco City Cohort, ALIVE Study. Science. 1996;273:1856–62.
14. Liu R, Paxton WA, Choe S, et al. Homozygous defect in HIV-1 coreceptor accounts for resistance of some multiply-exposed individuals to HIV-1 infection. Cell. 1996;86:367–77.
15. Blanpain C, Libert F, Vassart G, Parmentier M. CCR5 and HIV infection. Receptors Channels. 2002;8:19–31.
16. Blanpain C, Lee B, Tackoen M, et al. Multiple nonfunctional alleles of CCR5 are frequent in various human populations. Blood. 2000;96:1638–45.
17. Quillent C, Oberlin E, Braun J, et al. HIV-1-resistance phenotype conferred by combination of two separate inherited mutations of CCR5 gene. Lancet. 1998;351:14–8.
18. Wu L, Paxton WA, Kassam N, et al. CCR5 levels and expression pattern correlate with infectability by macrophage-tropic HIV-1, in vitro. J Exp Med. 1997;185:1681–91.
19. Martin MP, Dean M, Smith MW, et al. Genetic acceleration of AIDS progression by a promoter variant of CCR5. Science. 1998;282:1907–11.
20. Gonzalez E, Bamshad M, Sato N, et al. Race-specific HIV-1 disease-modifying effects associated with CCR5 haplotypes. Proc Natl Acad Sci U S A. 1999;96:12004–9.
21. Mummidi S, Ahuja SS, Gonzalez E, et al. Genealogy of the CCR5 locus and chemokine system gene variants associated with altered rates of HIV-1 disease progression. Nat Med. 1998;4:786–93.
22. Dolan MJ, Kulkarni H, Camargo JF, et al. CCL3L1 and CCR5 influence cell-mediated immunity and affect HIV-AIDS pathogenesis via viral entry-independent mechanisms. Nat Immunol. 2007;8:1324–36.
23. Smith MW, Dean M, Carrington M, et al. Contrasting genetic influence of CCR2 and CCR5 variants on HIV-1 infection and disease progression. Hemophilia Growth and Development Study (HGDS), Multicenter AIDS Cohort Study (MACS), Multicenter Hemophilia Cohort Study (MHCS), San Francisco City Cohort (SFCC), ALIVE Study. Science. 1997;277:959–65.
24. Nakayama EE, Tanaka Y, Nagai Y, Iwamoto A, Shioda T. A CCR2-V64I polymorphism affects stability of CCR2A isoform. AIDS. 2004;18:729–38.
25. Lee B, Doranz BJ, Rana S, et al. Influence of the CCR2-V64I polymorphism on human immunodeficiency virus type 1 coreceptor activity and on chemokine receptor function of CCR2b, CCR3, CCR5, and CXCR4. J Virol. 1998;72:7450–8.
26. Mariani R, Wong S, Mulder LC, et al. CCR2-64I polymorphism is not associated with altered CCR5 expression or coreceptor function. J Virol. 1999;73:2450–9.
27. Vasilescu A, Terashima Y, Enomoto M, et al. A haplotype of the human CXCR1 gene protective against rapid disease progression in HIV-1+ patients. Proc Natl Acad Sci U S A. 2007;104:3354–9.
28. Gonzalez E, Rovin BH, Sen L, et al. HIV-1 infection and AIDS dementia are influenced by a mutant MCP-1 allele linked to increased monocyte infiltration of tissues and MCP-1 levels. Proc Natl Acad Sci U S A. 2002;99:13795–800.
29. Faure S, Meyer L, Genin E, et al. Deleterious genetic influence of CX3CR1 genotypes on HIV-1 disease progression. J Acquir Immune Defic Syndr. 2003;32:335–7.
30. McDermott DH, Colla JS, Kleeberger CA, et al. Genetic polymorphism in CX3CR1 and risk of HIV disease. Science. 2000;290:2031.
31. Kwa D, Boeser-Nunnink B, Schuitemaker H. Lack of evidence for an association between a polymorphism in CX3CR1 and the clinical course of HIV infection or virus phenotype evolution. AIDS. 2003;17:759–61.
32. Puissant B, Abbal M, Blancher A. Polymorphism of human and primate RANTES, CX3CR1, CCR2 and CXCR4 genes with regard to HIV/SIV infection. Immunogenetics. 2003;55:275–83.
33. Singh KK, Hughes MD, Chen J, Spector SA. Genetic polymorphisms in CX3CR1 predict HIV-1 disease progression in children independently of CD4+ lymphocyte count and HIV-1 RNA load. J Infect Dis. 2005;191:1971–80.
34. Suresh P, Wanchu A, Sachdeva RK, Bhatnagar A. Gene polymorphisms in CCR5, CCR2, CX3CR1, SDF-1 and RANTES in exposed but uninfected partners of HIV-1 infected individuals in North India. J Clin Immunol. 2006;26:476–84.
35. Puissant B, Roubinet F, Massip P, et al. Analysis of CCR5, CCR2, CX3CR1, and SDF1 polymorphisms in HIV-positive treated patients: impact on response to HAART and on peripheral T lymphocyte counts. AIDS Res Hum Retroviruses. 2006;22:153–62.
36. Vidal F, Vilades C, Domingo P, et al. Spanish HIV-1-infected long-term nonprogressors of more than 15 years have an increased frequency of the CX3CR1 249I variant allele. J Acquir Immune Defic Syndr. 2005;40:527–31.
37. Passam AM, Sourvinos G, Krambovitis E, et al. Polymorphisms of Cx(3)CR1 and CXCR6 receptors in relation to HAART therapy of HIV type 1 patients. AIDS Res Hum Retroviruses. 2007;23:1026–32.
38. Walton RT, Rowland-Jones SL. HIV and chemokine binding to red blood cells – DARC matters. Cell Host Microbe. 2008;4:3–5.
39. Lachgar A, Jaureguiberry G, Le Buenac H, et al. Binding of HIV-1 to RBCs involves the Duffy antigen receptors for chemokines (DARC). Biomed Pharmacother. 1998;52:436–9.
40. He W, Neil S, Kulkarni H, et al. Duffy antigen receptor for chemokines mediates trans-infection of HIV-1 from red blood cells to target cells and affects HIV-AIDS susceptibility. Cell Host Microbe. 2008;4:52–62.
41. Kulkarni H, Marconi VC, He W, et al. The Duffy-null state is associated with a survival advantage in leukopenic HIV-infected persons of African ancestry. Blood. 2009;114:2783–92.
42. Cocchi F, DeVico AL, Garzino-Demo A, Arya SK, Gallo RC, Lusso P. Identification of RANTES, MIP-1 alpha, and MIP-1 beta as the major HIV-suppressive factors produced by CD8+ T cells. Science. 1995;270:1811–5.
43. Dong HF, Wigmore K, Carrington MN, Dean M, Turpin JA, Howard OM. Variants of CCR5, which are permissive for HIV-1 infection, show distinct functional responses to CCL3, CCL4 and CCL5. Genes Immun. 2005;6:609–19.

44. Liu H, Hwangbo Y, Holte S, et al. Analysis of genetic polymorphisms in CCR5, CCR2, stromal cell-derived factor-1, RANTES, and dendritic cell-specific intercellular adhesion molecule-3-grabbing nonintegrin in seronegative individuals repeatedly exposed to HIV-1. J Infect Dis. 2004;190:1055–8.
45. Liu XL, Wang FS, Jin L, Liu MX, Xu DZ. Preliminary study on the association of chemokine RANTES gene polymorphisms with HIV-1 infection in Chinese Han population. Zhonghua Liu Xing Bing Xue Za Zhi. 2003;24:971–5.
46. Zhao XY, Lee SS, Wong KH, et al. Effects of single nucleotide polymorphisms in the RANTES promoter region in healthy and HIV-infected indigenous Chinese. Eur J Immunogenet. 2004;31:179–83.
47. An P, Nelson GW, Wang L, et al. Modulating influence on HIV/AIDS by interacting RANTES gene variants. Proc Natl Acad Sci U S A. 2002;99:10002–7.
48. Gonzalez E, Dhanda R, Bamshad M, et al. Global survey of genetic variation in CCR5, RANTES, and MIP-1alpha: impact on the epidemiology of the HIV-1 pandemic. Proc Natl Acad Sci U S A. 2001;98:5199–204.
49. McDermott DH, Beecroft MJ, Kleeberger CA, et al. Chemokine RANTES promoter polymorphism affects risk of both HIV infection and disease progression in the Multicenter AIDS Cohort Study. AIDS. 2000;14:2671–8.
50. Duggal P, Winkler CA, An P, et al. The effect of RANTES chemokine genetic variants on early HIV-1 plasma RNA among African American injection drug users. J Acquir Immune Defic Syndr. 2005;38:584–9.
51. Boulassel MR, Smith GH, Edwardes MD, et al. Influence of RANTES, SDF-1 and TGF-beta levels on the value of interleukin-7 as a predictor of virological response in HIV-1-infected patients receiving double boosted protease inhibitor-based therapy. HIV Med. 2005;6:268–77.
52. Ahlenstiel G, Iwan A, Nattermann J, et al. Distribution and effects of polymorphic RANTES gene alleles in HIV/HCV coinfection – a prospective cross-sectional study. World J Gastroenterol. 2005;11:7631–8.
53. Cooke GS, Tosh K, Ramaley PA, et al. A polymorphism that reduces RANTES expression is associated with protection from death in HIV-seropositive Ugandans with advanced disease. J Infect Dis. 2006;194:666–9.
54. Guerini FR, Delbue S, Zanzottera M, et al. Analysis of CCR5, CCR2, SDF1 and RANTES gene polymorphisms in subjects with HIV-related PML and not determined leukoencephalopathy. Biomed Pharmacother. 2008;62:26–30.
55. Rathore A, Chatterjee A, Sivarama P, Yamamoto N, Singhal PK, Dhole TN. Association of RANTES −403G/A, −28C/G and In1.1T/C polymorphism with HIV-1 transmission and progression among North Indians. J Med Virol. 2008;80:1133–41.
56. Vidal F, Peraire J, Domingo P, et al. Polymorphism of RANTES chemokine gene promoter is not associated with long-term nonprogressive HIV-1 infection of more than 16 years. J Acquir Immune Defic Syndr. 2006;41:17–22.
57. Modi WS, Goedert JJ, Strathdee S, et al. MCP-1-MCP-3-Eotaxin gene cluster influences HIV-1 transmission. AIDS. 2003;17:2357–65.
58. Singh KK, Hughes MD, Chen J, Spector SA. Impact of MCP-1-2518-G allele on the HIV-1 disease of children in the United States. AIDS. 2006;20:475–8.
59. Modi WS, Lautenberger J, An P, et al. Genetic variation in the CCL18-CCL3-CCL4 chemokine gene cluster influences HIV Type 1 transmission and AIDS disease progression. Am J Hum Genet. 2006;79:120–8.
60. Kuhn L, Schramm DB, Donninger S, et al. African infants' CCL3 gene copies influence perinatal HIV transmission in the absence of maternal nevirapine. AIDS. 2007;21:1753–61.
61. Paximadis M, Mohanlal N, Gray GE, Kuhn L, Tiemessen CT. Identification of new variants within the two functional genes CCL3 and CCL3L encoding the CCL3 (MIP-1alpha) chemokine: implications for HIV-1 infection. Int J Immunogenet. 2009;36:21–32.
62. Modi WS. CCL3L1 and CCL4L1 chemokine genes are located in a segmental duplication at chromosome 17q12. Genomics. 2004;83:735–8.
63. Gonzalez E, Kulkarni H, Bolivar H, et al. The influence of CCL3L1 gene-containing segmental duplications on HIV-1/AIDS susceptibility. Science. 2005;307:1434–40.
64. Menten P, Wuyts A, Van Damme J. Macrophage inflammatory protein-1. Cytokine Growth Factor Rev. 2002;13:455–81.
65. Huik K, Sadam M, Karki T, et al. CCL3L1 copy number is a strong genetic determinant of HIV seropositivity in Caucasian intravenous drug users. J Infect Dis. 2010;201:730–9.
66. Nakajima T, Ohtani H, Naruse T, et al. Copy number variations of CCL3L1 and long-term prognosis of HIV-1 infection in asymptomatic HIV-infected Japanese with hemophilia. Immunogenetics. 2007;59:793–8.
67. Nakajima T, Kaur G, Mehra N, Kimura A. HIV-1/AIDS susceptibility and copy number variation in CCL3L1, a gene encoding a natural ligand for HIV-1 co-receptor CCR5. Cytogenet Genome Res. 2008;123:156–60.
68. Shalekoff S, Meddows-Taylor S, Schramm DB, et al. Host CCL3L1 gene copy number in relation to HIV-1-specific CD4+ and CD8+ T-cell responses and viral load in South African women. J Acquir Immune Defic Syndr. 2008;48:245–54.
69. Ahuja SK, Kulkarni H, Catano G, et al. CCL3L1-CCR5 genotype influences durability of immune recovery during antiretroviral therapy of HIV-1-infected individuals. Nat Med. 2008;14:413–20.
70. Bhattacharya T, Stanton J, Kim EY, et al. CCL3L1 and HIV/AIDS susceptibility. Nat Med. 2009;15:1112–5.
71. Urban TJ, Weintrob AC, Fellay J, et al. CCL3L1 and HIV/AIDS susceptibility. Nat Med. 2009;15:1110–2.
72. Kulkarni H, Marconi VC, Agan BK, et al. Role of CCL3L1-CCR5 genotypes in the epidemic spread of HIV-1 and evaluation of vaccine efficacy. PLoS One. 2008;3:e3671.
73. Winkler C, Modi W, Smith MW, et al. Genetic restriction of AIDS pathogenesis by an SDF-1 chemokine gene variant. ALIVE Study, Hemophilia Growth and Development Study (HGDS), Multicenter AIDS Cohort Study (MACS), Multicenter Hemophilia Cohort Study (MHCS), San Francisco City Cohort (SFCC). Science. 1998;279:389–93.
74. van Rij RP, Broersen S, Goudsmit J, Coutinho RA, Schuitemaker H. The role of a stromal cell-derived factor-1 chemokine gene variant in the clinical course of HIV-1 infection. AIDS. 1998;12:F85–90.
75. Ioannidis JP, Rosenberg PS, Goedert JJ, et al. Effects of CCR5-Delta32, CCR2-64I, and SDF-1 3′A alleles on HIV-1 disease progression: an international meta-analysis of individual-patient data. Ann Intern Med. 2001;135:782–95.
76. VerPlank L, Bouamr F, LaGrassa TJ, et al. Tsg101, a homologue of ubiquitin-conjugating (E2) enzymes, binds the L domain in HIV type 1 Pr55(Gag). Proc Natl Acad Sci U S A. 2001;98:7724–9.
77. Garrus JE, von Schwedler UK, Pornillos OW, et al. Tsg101 and the vacuolar protein sorting pathway are essential for HIV-1 budding. Cell. 2001;107:55–65.
78. Demirov DG, Ono A, Orenstein JM, Freed EO. Overexpression of the N-terminal domain of TSG101 inhibits HIV-1 budding by blocking late domain function. Proc Natl Acad Sci U S A. 2002;99:955–60.
79. Medina G, Zhang Y, Tang Y, et al. The functionally exchangeable L domains in RSV and HIV-1 Gag direct particle release through pathways linked by Tsg101. Traffic. 2005;6:880–94.
80. Martin-Serrano J, Zang T, Bieniasz PD. HIV-1 and Ebola virus encode small peptide motifs that recruit Tsg101 to sites of particle assembly to facilitate egress. Nat Med. 2001;7:1313–9.

81. Bleiber G, May M, Martinez R, et al. Use of a combined ex vivo/in vivo population approach for screening of human genes involved in the human immunodeficiency virus type 1 life cycle for variants influencing disease progression. J Virol. 2005;79: 12674–80.
82. Berthoux L, Sebastian S, Sokolskaja E, Luban J. Cyclophilin A is required for TRIM5{alpha}-mediated resistance to HIV-1 in Old World monkey cells. Proc Natl Acad Sci U S A. 2005;102: 14849–53.
83. Rits MA, van Dort KA, Kootstra NA. Polymorphisms in the regulatory region of the cyclophilin A gene influence the susceptibility for HIV-1 infection. PLoS One. 2008;3:e3975.
84. Abdurahman S, Hoglund S, Hoglund A, Vahlne A. Mutation in the loop C-terminal to the cyclophilin A binding site of HIV-1 capsid protein disrupts proper virus assembly and infectivity. Retrovirology. 2007;4:19.
85. van Manen D, Rits MA, Beugeling C, van Dort K, Schuitemaker H, Kootstra NA. The effect of Trim5 polymorphisms on the clinical course of HIV-1 infection. PLoS Pathog. 2008;4:e18.
86. Lin TY, Emerman M. Determinants of cyclophilin A-dependent TRIM5 alpha restriction against HIV-1. Virology. 2008;379: 335–41.
87. Sokolskaja E, Luban J. Cyclophilin, TRIM5, and innate immunity to HIV-1. Curr Opin Microbiol. 2006;9:404–8.
88. Goldschmidt V, Bleiber G, May M, Martinez R, Ortiz M, Telenti A. Role of common human TRIM5alpha variants in HIV-1 disease progression. Retrovirology. 2006;3:54.
89. Speelmon EC, Livingston-Rosanoff D, Li SS, et al. Genetic association of the antiviral restriction factor TRIM5alpha with human immunodeficiency virus type 1 infection. J Virol. 2006;80:2463–71.
90. Sheehy AM, Gaddis NC, Choi JD, Malim MH. Isolation of a human gene that inhibits HIV-1 infection and is suppressed by the viral Vif protein. Nature. 2002;418:646–50.
91. An P, Bleiber G, Duggal P, et al. APOBEC3G genetic variants and their influence on the progression to AIDS. J Virol. 2004;78: 11070–6.
92. Do H, Vasilescu A, Diop G, et al. Exhaustive genotyping of the CEM15 (APOBEC3G) gene and absence of association with AIDS progression in a French cohort. J Infect Dis. 2005;191: 159–63.
93. OhAinle M, Kerns JA, Li MM, Malik HS, Emerman M. Antiretroelement activity of APOBEC3H was lost twice in recent human evolution. Cell Host Microbe. 2008;4:249–59.
94. Carrington M, Nelson GW, Martin MP, et al. HLA and HIV-1: heterozygote advantage and B*35-Cw*04 disadvantage. Science. 1999;283:1748–52.
95. Dalmau J, Puertas MC, Azuara M, et al. Contribution of immunological and virological factors to extremely severe primary HIV type 1 infection. Clin Infect Dis. 2009;48:229–38.
96. Dorak MT, Tang J, Penman-Aguilar A, et al. Transmission of HIV-1 and HLA-B allele-sharing within serodiscordant heterosexual Zambian couples. Lancet. 2004;363:2137–9.
97. Tang J, Shao W, Yoo YJ, et al. Human leukocyte antigen class I genotypes in relation to heterosexual HIV type 1 transmission within discordant couples. J Immunol. 2008;181:2626–35.
98. Goulder PJ, Pasquier C, Holmes EC, et al. Mother-to-child transmission of HIV infection and CTL escape through HLA-A2-SLYNTVATL epitope sequence variation. Immunol Lett. 2001;79: 109–16.
99. Goulder PJ, Brander C, Tang Y, et al. Evolution and transmission of stable CTL escape mutations in HIV infection. Nature. 2001;412:334–8.
100. Migueles SA, Sabbaghian MS, Shupert WL, et al. HLA B*5701 is highly associated with restriction of virus replication in a subgroup of HIV-infected long term nonprogressors. Proc Natl Acad Sci U S A. 2000;97:2709–14.
101. Gao X, Bashirova A, Iversen AK, et al. AIDS restriction HLA allotypes target distinct intervals of HIV-1 pathogenesis. Nat Med. 2005;11:1290–2.
102. Cornelissen M, Hoogland FM, Back NK, et al. Multiple transmissions of a stable human leucocyte antigen-B27 cytotoxic T-cell-escape strain of HIV-1 in The Netherlands. AIDS. 2009;23:1495–500.
103. Flores-Villanueva PO, Hendel H, Caillat-Zucman S, et al. Associations of MHC ancestral haplotypes with resistance/susceptibility to AIDS disease development. J Immunol. 2003;170: 1925–9.
104. Goulder PJ, Bunce M, Luzzi G, Phillips RE, McMichael AJ. Potential underestimation of HLA-C-restricted cytotoxic T-lymphocyte responses. AIDS. 1997;11:1884–6.
105. Lajoie J, Hargrove J, Zijenah LS, Humphrey JH, Ward BJ, Roger M. Genetic variants in nonclassical major histocompatibility complex class I human leukocyte antigen (HLA)-E and HLA-G molecules are associated with susceptibility to heterosexual acquisition of HIV-1. J Infect Dis. 2006;193:298–301.
106. Mallal S, Nolan D, Witt C, et al. Association between presence of HLA-B*5701, HLA-DR7, and HLA-DQ3 and hypersensitivity to HIV-1 reverse-transcriptase inhibitor abacavir. Lancet. 2002;359: 727–32.
107. Mahungu TW, Johnson MA, Owen A, Back DJ. The impact of pharmacogenetics on HIV therapy. Int J STD AIDS. 2009;20: 145–51.
108. Martin MP, Gao X, Lee JH, et al. Epistatic interaction between KIR3DS1 and HLA-B delays the progression to AIDS. Nat Genet. 2002;31:429–34.
109. Boulet S, Sharafi S, Simic N, et al. Increased proportion of KIR3DS1 homozygotes in HIV-exposed uninfected individuals. AIDS. 2008;22:595–9.
110. Pascal V, Yamada E, Martin MP, et al. Detection of KIR3DS1 on the cell surface of peripheral blood NK cells facilitates identification of a novel null allele and assessment of KIR3DS1 expression during HIV-1 infection. J Immunol. 2007;179:1625–33.
111. Carrington M, Martin MP, van Bergen J. KIR-HLA intercourse in HIV disease. Trends Microbiol. 2008;16:620–7.
112. O'Connell KA, Han Y, Williams TM, Siliciano RF, Blankson JN. Role of natural killer cells in a cohort of elite suppressors: low frequency of the protective KIR3DS1 allele and limited inhibition of human immunodeficiency virus type 1 replication in vitro. J Virol. 2009;83:5028–34.
113. Long BR, Erickson AE, Chapman JM, et al. Increased number and function of natural killer cells in human immunodeficiency virus 1-positive subjects co-infected with herpes simplex virus 2. Immunology. 2010;129(2):186–96.
114. Li H, Cui Y, Fu QX, et al. Kinetics of interaction of HLA-B2705 with natural killer cell immunoglobulin-like receptor 3DS1. Protein Pept Lett. 2010;17(5):547–54.
115. Wichukchinda N, Kitamura Y, Rojanawiwat A, et al. The polymorphisms in DC-SIGNR affect susceptibility to HIV type 1 infection. AIDS Res Hum Retroviruses. 2007;23:686–92.
116. Martin MP, Lederman MM, Hutcheson HB, et al. Association of DC-SIGN promoter polymorphism with increased risk for parenteral, but not mucosal, acquisition of human immunodeficiency virus type 1 infection. J Virol. 2004;78:14053–6.
117. Koizumi Y, Kageyama S, Fujiyama Y, et al. RANTES −28G delays and DC-SIGN −139C enhances AIDS progression in HIV type 1-infected Japanese hemophiliacs. AIDS Res Hum Retroviruses. 2007;23:713–9.
118. Milanese M, Segat L, Pontillo A, Arraes LC, de Lima Filho JL, Crovella S. DEFB1 gene polymorphisms and increased risk of HIV-1 infection in Brazilian children. AIDS. 2006;20:1673–5.
119. Segat L, Milanese M, Boniotto M, et al. DEFB-1 genetic polymorphism screening in HIV-1 positive pregnant women and their children. J Matern Fetal Neonatal Med. 2006;19:13–6.

120. Ricci E, Malacrida S, Zanchetta M, Montagna M, Giaquinto C, De Rossi A. Role of beta-defensin-1 polymorphisms in mother-to-child transmission of HIV-1. J Acquir Immune Defic Syndr. 2009;51:13–9.
121. Braida L, Boniotto M, Pontillo A, Tovo PA, Amoroso A, Crovella S. A single-nucleotide polymorphism in the human beta-defensin 1 gene is associated with HIV-1 infection in Italian children. AIDS. 2004;18:1598–600.
122. Baroncelli S, Ricci E, Andreotti M, et al. Single-nucleotide polymorphisms in human beta-defensin-1 gene in Mozambican HIV-1-infected women and correlation with virologic parameters. AIDS. 2008;22:1515–7.
123. Boniotto M, Crovella S, Pirulli D, et al. Polymorphisms in the MBL2 promoter correlated with risk of HIV-1 vertical transmission and AIDS progression. Genes Immun. 2000;1:346–8.
124. Boniotto M, Braida L, Pirulli D, Arraes L, Amoroso A, Crovella S. MBL2 polymorphisms are involved in HIV-1 infection in Brazilian perinatally infected children. AIDS. 2003;17:779–80.
125. Crovella S, Bernardon M, Braida L, et al. Italian multicentric pilot study on MBL2 genetic polymorphisms in HIV positive pregnant women and their children. J Matern Fetal Neonatal Med. 2005;17:253–6.
126. Oh DY, Baumann K, Hamouda O, et al. A frequent functional toll-like receptor 7 polymorphism is associated with accelerated HIV-1 disease progression. AIDS. 2009;23:297–307.
127. Pine SO, McElrath MJ, Bochud PY. Polymorphisms in toll-like receptor 4 and toll-like receptor 9 influence viral load in a seroincident cohort of HIV-1-infected individuals. AIDS. 2009;23: 2387–95.
128. Bochud PY, Hersberger M, Taffe P, et al. Polymorphisms in Toll-like receptor 9 influence the clinical course of HIV-1 infection. AIDS. 2007;21:441–6.
129. Soriano-Sarabia N, Vallejo A, Ramirez-Lorca R, et al. Influence of the Toll-like receptor 9 1635A/G polymorphism on the CD4 count, HIV viral load, and clinical progression. J Acquir Immune Defic Syndr. 2008;49:128–35.
130. Rockstroh JK, Spengler U. HIV and hepatitis C virus co-infection. Lancet Infect Dis. 2004;4:437–44.
131. Falck-Ytter Y, Kale H, Mullen KD, Sarbah SA, Sorescu L, McCullough AJ. Surprisingly small effect of antiviral treatment in patients with hepatitis C. Ann Intern Med. 2002;136:288–92.
132. Fried MW, Shiffman ML, Reddy KR, et al. Peginterferon alfa-2a plus ribavirin for chronic hepatitis C virus infection. N Engl J Med. 2002;347:975–82.
133. Manns MP, McHutchison JG, Gordon SC, et al. Peginterferon alfa-2b plus ribavirin compared with interferon alfa-2b plus ribavirin for initial treatment of chronic hepatitis C: a randomised trial. Lancet. 2001;358:958–65.
134. Hagemann T, Wilson J, Kulbe H, et al. Macrophages induce invasiveness of epithelial cancer cells via NF-kappa B and JNK. J Immunol. 2005;175:1197–205.
135. Hadziyannis SJ, Sette Jr H, Morgan TR, et al. Peginterferon-alpha2a and ribavirin combination therapy in chronic hepatitis C: a randomized study of treatment duration and ribavirin dose. Ann Intern Med. 2004;140:346–55.
136. Suppiah V, Moldovan M, Ahlenstiel G, et al. IL28B is associated with response to chronic hepatitis C interferon-alpha and ribavirin therapy. Nat Genet. 2009;41:1100–4.
137. Tanaka Y, Nishida N, Sugiyama M, et al. Genome-wide association of IL28B with response to pegylated interferon-alpha and ribavirin therapy for chronic hepatitis C. Nat Genet. 2009;41:1105–9.
138. Ge D, Fellay J, Thompson AJ, et al. Genetic variation in IL28B predicts hepatitis C treatment-induced viral clearance. Nature. 2009;461:399–401.
139. Thomas DL, Thio CL, Martin MP, et al. Genetic variation in IL28B and spontaneous clearance of hepatitis C virus. Nature. 2009;461:798–801.
140. McCarthy JJ, Li JH, Thompson A, et al. Replicated association between an IL28B gene variant and a sustained response to pegylated interferon and ribavirin. Gastroenterology. 2010;138: 2307–14.
141. Rauch A, Kutalik Z, Descombes P, et al. Genetic variation in IL28B is associated with chronic hepatitis C and treatment failure: a genome-wide association study. Gastroenterology. 2010;138: 1338–45.
142. Sheppard P, Kindsvogel W, Xu W, et al. IL-28, IL-29 and their class II cytokine receptor IL-28R. Nat Immunol. 2003;4:63–8. Epub 2002 Dec 2.
143. Kotenko SV, Gallagher G, Baurin VV, et al. IFN-lambdas mediate antiviral protection through a distinct class II cytokine receptor complex. Nat Immunol. 2003;4:69–77.
144. Marcello T, Grakoui A, Barba-Spaeth G, et al. Interferons alpha and lambda inhibit hepatitis C virus replication with distinct signal transduction and gene regulation kinetics. Gastroenterology. 2006;131:1887–98.
145. Pravica V, Asderakis A, Perrey C, Hajeer A, Sinnott PJ, Hutchinson IV. In vitro production of IFN-gamma correlates with CA repeat polymorphism in the human IFN-gamma gene. Eur J Immunogenet. 1999;26:1–3.
146. Turner DM, Williams DM, Sankaran D, Lazarus M, Sinnott PJ, Hutchinson IV. An investigation of polymorphism in the interleukin-10 gene promoter. Eur J Immunogenet. 1997;24:1–8.
147. Fishman D, Faulds G, Jeffery R, et al. The effect of novel polymorphisms in the interleukin-6 (IL-6) gene on IL-6 transcription and plasma IL-6 levels, and an association with systemic-onset juvenile chronic arthritis. J Clin Invest. 1998;102:1369–76.
148. Wilson AG, Symons JA, McDowell TL, McDevitt HO, Duff GW. Effects of a polymorphism in the human tumor necrosis factor alpha promoter on transcriptional activation. Proc Natl Acad Sci U S A. 1997;94:3195–9.
149. Tilg H, Wilmer A, Vogel W, et al. Serum levels of cytokines in chronic liver diseases. Gastroenterology. 1992;103:264–74.
150. Larrea E, Garcia N, Qian C, Civeira MP, Prieto J. Tumor necrosis factor alpha gene expression and the response to interferon in chronic hepatitis C. Hepatology. 1996;23:210–7.
151. Fukuda R, Ishimura N, Ishihara S, et al. Intrahepatic expression of pro-inflammatory cytokine mRNAs and interferon efficacy in chronic hepatitis C. Liver. 1996;16:390–9.
152. Nelson DR, Lim HL, Marousis CG, et al. Activation of tumor necrosis factor-alpha system in chronic hepatitis C virus infection. Dig Dis Sci. 1997;42:2487–94.
153. Malaguarnera M, Di Fazio I, Romeo MA, et al. Elevation of interleukin 6 levels in patients with chronic hepatitis due to hepatitis C virus Serum interleukin 6 concentrations in chronic hepatitis C patients before and after interferon-alpha treatment. J Gastroenterol. 1997;32:211–5.
154. Oyanagi Y, Takahashi T, Matsui S, et al. Enhanced expression of interleukin-6 in chronic hepatitis C. Liver. 1999;19:464–72.
155. Tsushima H, Kawata S, Tamura S, et al. Reduced plasma transforming growth factor-beta1 levels in patients with chronic hepatitis C after interferon-alpha therapy: association with regression of hepatic fibrosis. J Hepatol. 1999;30:1–7.
156. Cotler SJ, Reddy KR, McCone J, et al. An analysis of acute changes in interleukin-6 levels after treatment of hepatitis C with consensus interferon. J Interferon Cytokine Res. 2001;21: 1011–9.
157. Lapinski TW. The levels of IL-1beta, IL-4 and IL-6 in the serum and the liver tissue of chronic HCV-infected patients. Arch Immunol Ther Exp (Warsz). 2001;49:311–6.

158. Malaguarnera M, Di Fazio I, Romeo MA, Restuccia S, Laurino A, Trovato BA. Elevation of interleukin 6 levels in patients with chronic hepatitis due to hepatitis C virus. J Gastroenterol. 1997;32:211–5.
159. Ramadori G, Christ B. Cytokines and the hepatic acute-phase response. Semin Liver Dis. 1999;19:141–55.
160. Gao B. Cytokines, STATs and liver disease. Cell Mol Immunol. 2005;2:92–100.
161. Nattermann J, Vogel M, Berg T, et al. Effect of the interleukin-6 C174G gene polymorphism on treatment of acute and chronic hepatitis C in human immunodeficiency virus coinfected patients. Hepatology. 2007;1:1.
162. Yee LJ, Tang J, Gibson AW, Kimberly R, Van Leeuwen DJ, Kaslow RA. Interleukin 10 polymorphisms as predictors of sustained response in antiviral therapy for chronic hepatitis C infection. Hepatology. 2001;33:708–12.
163. Edwards-Smith CJ, Jonsson JR, Purdie DM, Bansal A, Shorthouse C, Powell EE. Interleukin-10 promoter polymorphism predicts initial response of chronic hepatitis C to interferon alfa. Hepatology. 1999;30:526–30.
164. Oleksyk TK, Thio CL, Truelove AL, et al. Single nucleotide polymorphisms and haplotypes in the IL10 region associated with HCV clearance. Genes Immun. 2005;6:347–57.
165. Mangia A, Santoro R, Piattelli M, et al. IL-10 haplotypes as possible predictors of spontaneous clearance of HCV infection. Cytokine. 2004;25:103–9.
166. Lio D, Caruso C, Di Stefano R, et al. IL-10 and TNF-alpha polymorphisms and the recovery from HCV infection. Hum Immunol. 2003;64:674–80.
167. Yin LM, Zhu WF, Wei L, et al. Association of interleukin-12 p40 gene 3′-untranslated region polymorphism and outcome of HCV infection. World J Gastroenterol. 2004;10:2330–3.
168. Houldsworth A, Metzner M, Rossol S, et al. Polymorphisms in the IL-12B gene and outcome of HCV infection. J Interferon Cytokine Res. 2005;25:271–6.
169. Mueller T, Mas-Marques A, Sarrazin C, et al. Influence of interleukin 12B (IL12B) polymorphisms on spontaneous and treatment-induced recovery from hepatitis C virus infection. J Hepatol. 2004;41:652–8.
170. Lee JH, Teuber G, von Wagner M, Roth WK, Zeuzem S. Antiviral effect of human recombinant interleukin-12 in patients infected with hepatitis C virus. J Med Virol. 2000;60:264–8.
171. Kimura T, Saito T, Yoshimura M, et al. Association of transforming growth factor-beta 1 functional polymorphisms with natural clearance of hepatitis C virus. J Infect Dis. 2006;193:1371–4.
172. D'Alfonso S, Richiardi PM. A polymorphic variation in a putative regulation box of the TNFA promoter region. Immunogenetics. 1994;39:150–4.
173. Wilson AG, de Vries N, Pociot F, di Giovine FS, van der Putte LB, Duff GW. An allelic polymorphism within the human tumor necrosis factor alpha promoter region is strongly associated with HLA A1, B8, and DR3 alleles. J Exp Med. 1993;177:557–60.
174. Hohler T, Kruger A, Gerken G, Schneider PM, Meyer zum Buschenfelde KH, Rittner C. Tumor necrosis factor alpha promoter polymorphism at position −238 is associated with chronic active hepatitis C infection. J Med Virol. 1998;54:173–7.
175. Dai CY, Chuang WL, Chang WY, et al. Tumor necrosis factor-alpha promoter polymorphism at position −308 predicts response to combination therapy in hepatitis C virus infection. J Infect Dis. 2006;193:98–101. Epub 2005 Nov 16.
176. Yee LJ, Tang J, Herrera J, Kaslow RA, van Leeuwen DJ. Tumor necrosis factor gene polymorphisms in patients with cirrhosis from chronic hepatitis C virus infection. Genes Immun. 2000;1:386–90.
177. Schiemann U, Glas J, Torok P, et al. Response to combination therapy with interferon alfa-2a and ribavirin in chronic hepatitis C according to a TNF-alpha promoter polymorphism. Digestion. 2003;68:1–4. Epub 2003 Aug 29.
178. Frese M, Schwarzle V, Barth K, et al. Interferon-gamma inhibits replication of subgenomic and genomic hepatitis C virus RNAs. Hepatology. 2002;35:694–703.
179. Woollard DJ, Grakoui A, Shoukry NH, Murthy KK, Campbell KJ, Walker CM. Characterization of HCV-specific Patr class II restricted CD4+ T cell responses in an acutely infected chimpanzee. Hepatology. 2003;38:1297–306.
180. Bream JH, Carrington M, O'Toole S, et al. Polymorphisms of the human IFNG gene noncoding regions. Immunogenetics. 2000;51:50–8.
181. Huang Y, Yang H, Borg BB, et al. A functional SNP of interferon-gamma gene is important for interferon-alpha-induced and spontaneous recovery from hepatitis C virus infection. Proc Natl Acad Sci U S A. 2007;104:985–90. Epub 2007 Jan 10.
182. Woitas RP, Ahlenstiel G, Iwan A, et al. Frequency of the HIV-protective CC chemokine receptor 5-Delta32/Delta32 genotype is increased in hepatitis C. Gastroenterology. 2002;122:1721–8.
183. Promrat K, McDermott DH, Gonzalez CM, et al. Associations of chemokine system polymorphisms with clinical outcomes and treatment responses of chronic hepatitis C. Gastroenterology. 2003;124:352–60.
184. Hellier S, Frodsham AJ, Hennig BJ, et al. Association of genetic variants of the chemokine receptor CCR5 and its ligands, RANTES and MCP-2, with outcome of HCV infection. Hepatology. 2003;38:1468–76.
185. Goulding C, McManus R, Murphy A, et al. The CCR5-delta32 mutation: impact on disease outcome in individuals with hepatitis C infection from a single source. Gut. 2005;54:1157–61. Epub 2005 Apr 29.
186. Ahlenstiel G, Berg T, Woitas RP, et al. Effects of the CCR5-Delta 32 mutation on antiviral treatment in chronic hepatitis C. J Hepatol. 2003;39:245–52.
187. Goyal A, Suneetha PV, Kumar GT, Shukla DK, Arora N, Sarin SK. CCR5Delta32 mutation does not influence the susceptibility to HCV infection, severity of liver disease and response to therapy in patients with chronic hepatitis C. World J Gastroenterol. 2006;12:4721–6.
188. Glas J, Torok HP, Simperl C, et al. The Delta 32 mutation of the chemokine-receptor 5 gene neither is correlated with chronic hepatitis C nor does it predict response to therapy with interferon-alpha and ribavirin. Clin Immunol. 2003;108:46–50.
189. Wasmuth HE, Werth A, Mueller T, et al. Haplotype-tagging RANTES gene variants influence response to antiviral therapy in chronic hepatitis C. Hepatology. 2004;40:327–34.
190. Neumann-Haefelin C, Blum HE, Chisari FV, Thimme R. T cell response in hepatitis C virus infection. J Clin Virol. 2005;32:75–85.
191. Singh R, Kaul R, Kaul A, Khan K. A comparative review of HLA associations with hepatitis B and C viral infections across global populations. World J Gastroenterol. 2007;13:1770–87.
192. Thursz M, Yallop R, Goldin R, Trepo C, Thomas HC. Influence of MHC class II genotype on outcome of infection with hepatitis C virus. The HENCORE group. Hepatitis C European Network for Cooperative Research. Lancet. 1999;354:2119–24.
193. Jiao J, Wang JB. Hepatitis C virus genotypes, HLA-DRB alleles and their response to interferon-alpha and ribavirin in patients with chronic hepatitis C. Hepatobiliary Pancreat Dis Int. 2005;4:80–3.
194. Sim H, Wojcik J, Margulies M, Wade JA, Heathcote J. Response to interferon therapy: influence of human leucocyte antigen alleles in patients with chronic hepatitis C. J Viral Hepat. 1998;5:249–53.

195. Piekarska A, Woszczek G, Sidorkiewicz M, Kuydowicz J. HLA class II alleles and response to hepatitis C treatment with interferon alpha2b. Przegl Epidemiol. 2002;56:123–8.
196. Alric L, Fort M, Izopet J, et al. Study of host- and virus-related factors associated with spontaneous hepatitis C virus clearance. Tissue Antigens. 2000;56:154–8.
197. Romero-Gomez M, Gonzalez-Escribano MF, Torres B, et al. HLA class I B44 is associated with sustained response to interferon+ribavirin therapy in patients with chronic hepatitis C. Am J Gastroenterol. 2003;98:1621–6.
198. Kikuchi I, Ueda A, Mihara K, et al. The effect of HLA alleles on response to interferon therapy in patients with chronic hepatitis C. Eur J Gastroenterol Hepatol. 1998;10:859–63.
199. Hraber P, Kuiken C, Yusim K. Evidence for human leukocyte antigen heterozygote advantage against hepatitis C virus infection. Hepatology. 2007;46:1713–21.
200. Khakoo SI, Thio CL, Martin MP, et al. HLA and NK cell inhibitory receptor genes in resolving hepatitis C virus infection. Science. 2004;305:872–4.
201. Zuniga J, Romero V, Azocar J, et al. Protective KIR-HLA interactions for HCV infection in intravenous drug users. Mol Immunol. 2009;46:2723–7.
202. Rauch A, Gaudieri S, Thio C, Bochud PY. Host genetic determinants of spontaneous hepatitis C clearance. Pharmacogenomics. 2009;10:1819–37.
203. Askar M, Avery R, Corey R, et al. Lack of killer immunoglobulin-like receptor 2DS2 (KIR2DS2) and KIR2DL2 is associated with poor responses to therapy of recurrent hepatitis C virus in liver transplant recipients. Liver Transpl. 2009;15:1557–63.
204. de Arias AE, Haworth SE, Belli LS, et al. Killer cell immunoglobulin-like receptor genotype and killer cell immunoglobulin-like receptor-human leukocyte antigen C ligand compatibility affect the severity of hepatitis C virus recurrence after liver transplantation. Liver Transpl. 2009;15:390–9.
205. Lu Z, Zhang B, Chen S, et al. Association of KIR genotypes and haplotypes with susceptibility to chronic hepatitis B virus infection in Chinese Han population. Cell Mol Immunol. 2008;5:457–63.
206. Rauch A, Laird R, McKinnon E, et al. Influence of inhibitory killer immunoglobulin-like receptors and their HLA-C ligands on resolving hepatitis C virus infection. Tissue Antigens. 2007;69 Suppl 1:237–40.
207. Paladino N, Flores AC, Marcos CY, et al. Increased frequencies of activating natural killer receptors are associated with liver injury in individuals who do not eliminate hepatitis C virus. Tissue Antigens. 2007;69 Suppl 1:109–11.
208. Lopez-Vazquez A, Rodrigo L, Martinez-Borra J, et al. Protective effect of the HLA-Bw4I80 epitope and the killer cell immunoglobulin-like receptor 3DS1 gene against the development of hepatocellular carcinoma in patients with hepatitis C virus infection. J Infect Dis. 2005;192:162–5.
209. Thio CL, Gao X, Goedert JJ, et al. HLA-Cw*04 and hepatitis C virus persistence. J Virol. 2002;76:4792–7.
210. Knapp S, Warshow U, Hegazy D, et al. Consistent beneficial effects of killer cell immunoglobulin-like receptor 2DL3 and group 1 human leukocyte antigen-C following exposure to hepatitis C virus. Hepatology. 2010;51(4):1168–75.
211. Gardiner CM. Killer cell immunoglobulin-like receptors on NK cells: the how, where and why. Int J Immunogenet. 2008;35:1–8.
212. Siffert W, Rosskopf D, Siffert G, et al. Association of a human G-protein beta3 subunit variant with hypertension. Nat Genet. 1998;18:45–8.
213. Sarrazin C, Berg T, Weich V, et al. GNB3 C825T polymorphism and response to interferon-alfa/ribavirin treatment in patients with hepatitis C virus genotype 1 (HCV-1) infection. J Hepatol. 2005;43:388–93.
214. Rosskopf D, Koch K, Habich C, et al. Interaction of Gbeta3s, a splice variant of the G-protein Gbeta3, with Ggamma- and Galpha-proteins. Cell Signal. 2003;15:479–88.
215. Rosskopf D, Manthey I, Siffert W. Identification and ethnic distribution of major haplotypes in the gene GNB3 encoding the G-protein beta3 subunit. Pharmacogenetics. 2002;12:209–20.
216. Ahlenstiel G, Nischalke HD, Bueren K, et al. The GNB3 C825T polymorphism affects response to HCV therapy with pegylated interferon in HCV/HIV co-infected but not in HCV mono-infected patients. J Hepatol. 2007;47:348–55. Epub 2007 May 24.
217. Yee LJ, Perez KA, Tang J, van Leeuwen DJ, Kaslow RA. Association of CTLA4 polymorphisms with sustained response to interferon and ribavirin therapy for chronic hepatitis C virus infection. J Infect Dis. 2003;187:1264–71. Epub 2003 Apr 2.
218. Schott E, Witt H, Hinrichsen H, et al. Gender-dependent association of CTLA4 polymorphisms with resolution of hepatitis C virus infection. J Hepatol. 2007;46:372–80. Epub 2006 Nov 2.
219. Hijikata M, Ohta Y, Mishiro S. Identification of a single nucleotide polymorphism in the MxA gene promoter (G/T at nt −88) correlated with the response of hepatitis C patients to interferon. Intervirology. 2000;43:124–7.
220. Hijikata M, Mishiro S, Miyamoto C, Furuichi Y, Hashimoto M, Ohta Y. Genetic polymorphism of the MxA gene promoter and interferon responsiveness of hepatitis C patients: revisited by analyzing two SNP sites (−123 and −88) in vivo and in vitro. Intervirology. 2001;44:379–82.
221. Suzuki F, Arase Y, Suzuki Y, et al. Single nucleotide polymorphism of the MxA gene promoter influences the response to interferon monotherapy in patients with hepatitis C viral infection. J Viral Hepat. 2004;11:271–6.
222. Naito M, Matsui A, Inao M, et al. SNPs in the promoter region of the osteopontin gene as a marker predicting the efficacy of interferon-based therapies in patients with chronic hepatitis C. J Gastroenterol. 2005;40:381–8.

Effects of HIV on Liver Cell Populations

Meena B. Bansal and Jason T. Blackard

Introduction

Approximately one third of the body's blood supply passes through the liver each minute [1], and the majority of the blood flow is derived from the portal circulation. As blood enters the liver, it is distributed through the hepatic sinusoids, which are lined by a uniquely fenestrated endothelium interspersed with resident hepatic macrophages, also known as Kupffer cells. Additionally, hepatic stellate cells (HSCs) reside in the Space of Disse between the fenestrated endothelial cells and hepatocytes. Consequently, the low pressure flow combined with the uniquely fenestrated endothelium within the hepatic sinusoids create an environment that is primed for interactions between gut-derived pathogens, intrahepatic cell populations, and circulating cells of the immune system. While HIV clearly affects the immune system in patients with chronic liver injury, the focus of this chapter is to detail what is currently known about the effects of HIV on both parenchymal and nonparenchymal cells of the liver in isolation and during coinfection with other hepatotropic pathogens such as hepatitis B virus (HBV) and hepatitis C virus (HCV). Potential mechanisms by which infectious HIV, as well as its viral antigens, effects hepatocyte apoptosis, stellate cell activation, and stimulation of profibrogenic and proinflammatory cytokines by both parenchymal and nonparenchymal cells of the liver are discussed.

When considering interactions between HIV and liver cell populations, several possibilities exist. First, viral antigens may engage liver cell populations without the need for viral infection per se. Importantly, these viral antigens may be part of infectious virions – even if the virions themselves cannot infect the particular cell type being engaged – or defective virions that are unable to productively infect any cell type. Such viral antigens may also represent antigens that have been shed from virions and are freely circulating. In the case of HIV, these soluble antigens consist largely of the envelope glycoprotein (gp120), although the transactivator protein Tat may also be present. Low concentrations of other HIV proteins may result from lysis of HIV-infected cells but are diluted in the systemic circulation and, therefore, unlikely to have any appreciable effect in vivo. Separate from interactions between viral antigens and liver cells, there is evidence to suggest that several distinct liver cell populations also support productive HIV infection. This chapter provides a comprehensive review of the interactions of HIV proteins with and HIV infection of liver cell populations, including hepatocytes, hepatic stellate cells, and Kupffer cells, as well as several other minor liver cell types when data are available.

Shortly after the discovery of HIV, it was recognized that there were a variety of hepatobiliary disorders, as well as nonspecific hepatic changes, associated with HIV infection [2–5]. Moreover, liver enzyme elevations are relatively frequent in persons with HIV infection. Nonetheless, due to frequent coinfection with HBV or HCV, which also lead to characteristic elevations in liver enzymes, the effects of HIV itself on the liver was inadequately explored for a number of years. Similarly, the inability to detect the primary HIV receptor – CD4 – on hepatocyte-derived cells lines in an early study [6], as well as conflicting reports on the ability of HIV to productively infect hepatocyte cell lines [6, 7], has lead to the assumption that HIV is nonhepatotropic.

It has been well established that HIV gains entry into most target cells by forming a complex consisting of its outer envelope glycoprotein (trimeric gp120), CD4 receptor, and members of the chemokine coreceptor family [8]. A variety of chemokine receptors may serve as HIV entry cofactors, with CCR5 (R5) and CXCR4 (X4) being the most common. Binding of HIV virions or soluble gp120 to their receptors

M.B. Bansal (✉)
Department of Medicine, Mount Sinai School of Medicine, 1425 Madison Ave, Box 1123, New York, NY 10029 USA
e-mail: meena.bansal@mssm.edu

J.T. Blackard (✉)
Division of Digestive Diseases, University of Cincinnati College of Medicine, ML 0595, 231 Albert Sabin Way, Cincinnati, OH 45267, USA
e-mail: jason.blackard@uc.edu

triggers a broad spectrum of signaling pathways that modulates the activation state of target cells (reviewed in [9–11]). Interestingly, HIV is also capable of infecting several CD4-negative cell types, including fibroblasts, neural cells, trophoblasts, cervical epithelial cells, and renal tubular cells [12–16]. Astrocytes are also susceptible to HIV in a CD4-independent manner, although the infection is not productive; entry is dependent upon mannose receptor and endocytic trafficking [17]. Moreover, CD4-independent HIV variants that interact directly with chemokine coreceptors have been identified in vivo (reviewed in [18]), and minor viral mutations can significantly alter the requirement for particular entry receptors and dramatically alter tropism. In addition, gp120 is capable of binding C-type lectin receptors, such as the mannose receptor or dendritic cell-specific intercellular adhesion molecule-3-grabbing nonintegrin (DC-SIGN) found on antigen-presenting cells (APCs) such as macrophages and dendritic cells [19–21]. This pathway of viral entry appears to be relevant for transinfection, wherein input virus is transferred via virologic synapses to susceptible CD4+ cells [22]. While the role of gp120 was initially thought to be primarily that of viral fusion, more recent studies demonstrate that gp120 can activate cells in the absence of viral infection. Additionally, gp120 can activate a variety of signaling pathways in lymphocytes, including phosphatidylinositol-3 kinase (PI3K), the protein tyrosine kinases pyk2 and lck, focal adhesion kinase, the serine/threonine kinase Raf-1, and MAPK p42/44 (reviewed in [23]). Furthermore, using envelope-truncated or envelope-deleted HIVs, gp120-independent infection has also been reported [24–26]. While these findings suggest that viral proteins can significantly impact cell function separate from actual infection of the cell type(s), similar studies on the effects of gp120 on both parenchymal and nonparenchymal cells of the liver are quite limited as outlined below. One critical issue is whether concentrations of gp120 used to elicit biologic effects in vitro are present in vivo. Because of the presence of anti-gp120 antibodies, the effective amount of gp120 available for binding to receptors in the plasma of HIV-infected patients is very low [27]. However, tissue concentrations are disproportionately higher than plasma levels, persist even when patients are on effective ART, and may be underestimated by current techniques used to measure them [28–30]. The hepatic concentration of gp120 in HIV patients is not known and would be helpful to clarify the physiologic relevance of in vitro effects of gp120 on hepatic cell types.

As mentioned, there are limited studies on the identification and characterization of the possible cellular targets of HIV in the liver. However, several lines of evidence highlight the potential for HIV to interact directly with multiple liver cell populations (reviewed in [31]). For example, HIV proviral DNA was detected in liver biopsies from patients with AIDS [32], while HIV proteins and viral RNA have been detected in hepatocytes, Kupffer cells, inflammatory mononuclear cells, and sinusoidal cells using liver samples from HIV-infected patients [32, 33]. Similarly, Jiang et al. [34] detected intracellular expression of p24 antigen in Kupffer cells, endothelial cells, and hepatocytes. As well, there were more HIV-positive liver cells in patients with more severe liver damage compared to those with milder liver damage. While Hoda et al. [35] also detected p24 and/or gp41 in Kupffer cells and other lymphoid cells by immunostaining, these findings were not related to the degree of histological abnormality [35]. Lang et al. [36] also used immunostaining for HIV proteins to demonstrate HIV infection of Kupffer cells and some intrahepatic lymphocytes, although hepatocytes were HIV negative in this study. Collectively, such findings would suggest that HIV is present within the liver, although the consequences of HIV's interactions with specific hepatic cell types are largely unknown.

HIV's Interactions with Hepatocytes

Hepatocytes represent the major hepatic cell type and thus a logical cell type in which to examine HIV infection and/or the pathways altered by viral proteins. Expression of HIV entry receptors has been explored in hepatocytes, albeit with ambiguous results. Cao et al. found that two distinct hepatocyte-derived cell lines – Huh7 and HepG2 – were CD4 negative [6], while others have reported that HepG2 cells were CD4 positive [37, 38]. Recent data suggest that HepG2 cells also express the chemokine coreceptors CXCR4, CCR3, and CCR5 [38, 39]. Vlahakis et al. [7] reported that the Huh7, HepG2, and Hep3B cell lines, as well as primary hepatocytes, express CXCR4, although data on CD4 and other chemokine receptors were not provided. Iser et al. [40] were unable to detect CXCR4 or CCR5 on HepG2 cells via flow cytometry, although HIV infection of these cells could be blocked using CXCR4 or CCR5 antagonists. Thus, low-level expression of CXCR4 and CCR5 receptors on hepatocytes seems likely, although flow cytometry may not be sufficiently sensitive for their detection. Divergent findings among these studies may also reflect the conditions under which the cells are maintained, the length of time cells have been in culture, the method used to prepare cells for analysis, the sensitivity of the detection method employed, and/or clonal variation in the cell types analyzed. Moreover, there are extremely limited data on expression of nonconventional HIV entry receptors that may also be pertinent to HIV's interactions with hepatocytes. Similarly, data on HIV entry receptor expression in primary hepatocytes are not available for the most part, and it is not known how levels of these receptors may be different in distinct individuals based on common comorbid conditions such as HBV, HCV, and/or chronic alcohol consumption.

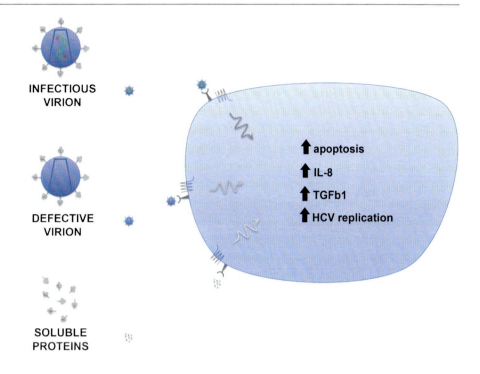

Fig. 9.1 The effects of HIV may occur either as a result of direct viral infection or from the activation of cells, in part, by soluble viral proteins

HIV Proteins

As outlined above, the effects of HIV may occur either as a result of direct viral infection or from the activation of cells, in part, by soluble viral proteins (Fig. 9.1). Utilizing an "innocent bystander" in which only viral proteins and uninfected hepatocytes are present, it was found that the HCV E2 and HIV gp120 envelope proteins cooperatively induce apoptosis in hepatocytes through the CXCR4 chemokine coreceptor [7, 38]. Downstream signaling events were also characterized and included upregulation of Fas ligand and degradation of the antiapoptotic molecule AKT and enhanced caspase expression [38, 41]. Subsequent studies further demonstrated that HIV glycoproteins stimulate hepatocyte expression of the TNF-related apoptosis inducing ligand (TRAIL) and induce TRAIL-mediated apoptosis in a JNK II-dependent manner [42], as well as enhance signal transducer and activator of transcription 1 (STAT1)-mediated apoptosis in uninfected hepatocytes [43]. This is an intriguing finding give that STATs are key components of the Jak-Stat signaling pathway and play critical roles in antiviral defense, hepatic injury, and hepatic inflammation [44].

Moreover, gp120 can also activate hepatic expression of interleukin 8 (IL-8), a proinflammatory chemokine that represents an important mediator of hepatic inflammation and is known to antagonize the antiviral effects of interferon (IFN) [39, 45–47]. Thus, induction of IL-8 expression may represent an important pathogenic link between HIV and increased replication of hepatitis viruses by abrogating the innate antiviral effects of IFN. Furthermore, as both hepatocyte apoptosis and inflammation are important stimuli for stellate cell activation and the fibrogenic response [48], HIV infection and/or its envelope proteins may accelerate fibrosis progression by both promoting hepatocyte apoptosis and hepatic inflammation. Other HIV proteins may also be important in the pathogenesis of liver disease. For example, transgenic mice expressing HIV Tat – a regulatory protein necessary for viral replication and secreted by HIV-infected cells – have an increased incidence of hepatocellular carcinoma [49]. Despite these intriguing findings, it should be noted that the majority of in vitro studies were performed in the HepG2 cell line; confirmation in additional hepatocyte-derived cell lines, as well as in primary hepatocytes, has not been reported to date. Moreover, the effects of viral proteins on important hepatocyte functions, such as drug and alcohol metabolism, remain largely unexplored.

HIV Infection

Despite several published studies assessing the effects of HIV proteins on hepatocytes in vitro, the contradictory reports related to HIV entry receptor expression may have dampened enthusiasm for investigating whether HIV can actually infect and productively replicate within hepatocytes. Nonetheless, in 1990, Cao et al. [6] utilized infectious HIV molecular clones to achieve productive viral infection of several distinct hepatocyte-derived cell lines. Expression of viral p24 antigen lasted for at least 3 months, and HIV antigens were observed in cells by immunohistochemical staining and radioimmunoprecipitation assay. Viral RNA and HIV-like particles were also detected via in situ hybridization and electron microscopy, respectively. Nonetheless, hepatocyte-derived cell lines were negative for CD4 by immunofluorescence and for CD4 mRNA by slot-blot hybridization. Moreover, HIV infection was not blocked by anti-CD4 monoclonal antibody or soluble CD4 suggesting a CD4-independent mechanism of infection. Vlahakis et al. [7] also evaluated HIV infection of hepatocytes by assessing HIV infection of the Huh7 cell line via detection of intracellular p24 levels at 48 h post infection. However, the authors found no HIV infection of hepatocytes. The conflicting findings in these studies may reflect inadequate time to achieve sufficient viral replication for detection and/or heterogeneity in the cell lines or maintenance conditions utilized.

More recently, several reports have provided additional evidence that HIV can productively infect hepatocytes. For example, Xiao et al. [50] isolated a CD4-independent strain of HIV from a patient with advanced HIV disease that was able to infect hepatocytes. Interestingly, preexposure of the Huh7 cell line to the CCR5 antagonist TAK-779 failed to block HIV infection, whereas the CXCR4 antagonist AMD3100 suppressed infection. Primary human hepatocytes were also susceptible to HIV infection, although CD4 and CCR5 receptors were not detected via flow cytometry or real-time PCR. Fromentin et al. [51] demonstrated that Huh7.5 cells bind to and internalize HIV particles. Furthermore, HIV infection of CD4+ T cells was enhanced after interactions with virus-loaded hepatocytes compared to cell-free virus. Finally, the absence of CD4 expression, as well as the low expression levels of both CXCR4 and CCR5 led the authors to suggest that HIV infection of hepatocytes may occur in a gp120-independent manner. Finally, Iser et al. [40] observed increased HIV reverse transcriptase activity following HIV infection of hepatocyte cell lines with X4 or R5 HIV. Despite no detection of surface CD4, CCR5, or CXCR4 by flow cytometry in the AD38 hepatocyte cell line, infection of R5 or X4 HIV was inhibited by maraviroc or AMD3100, respectively, suggesting CCR5- or CXCR4-dependent entry. These findings are further supported by studies demonstrating efficient activation of the HIV long terminal repeat (LTR) activation in hepatocyte-derived cell lines, as well as the presence of hepatocyte-specific factors that regulate LTR activity [52–54]. However, this intriguing avenue of research has remained unexplored in vivo; thus, it is currently unknown if signature mutations within the LTR may permit more robust expression of HIV in hepatocytes compared to other susceptible cell types.

HIV's Interactions with Hepatic Stellate Cells

Few studies have examined the effects of direct HIV infection and/or the indirect effects of HIV proteins on nonparenchymal cells of the liver in vivo. In vitro, primary cultures of Kupffer cells [55], liver sinusoidal endothelial cells (LSECs) [56], and activated HSCs [57] are permissive to HIV entry and replication.

HIV Proteins

Activated HSCs – the main effector cell in liver fibrosis – express both CXCR4 [58] and CCR5 coreceptors [59]. Interactions between HSCs and gp120 (CCR5-utilizing) promote the secretion of proinflammatory cytokines/chemokines such as IL-6 and MCP-1, promote the chemotaxis of HSCs, and to a lesser extent exert profibrogenic effects by stimulating secretion of collagen I and increasing expression of tissue inhibitor of metalloproteinases-1 (TIMP-1), which inhibits degradation of the scar matrix. Gp120 mediates its chemotactic effects through the PI3K/Akt pathway, while it proinflammatory effects are mediated through nuclear factor kappa B (NF-kB) and p38^{MAPK} (Fig. 9.2) [60]. Similarly, X4 gp120 promotes HSC activation, collagen I expression, and proliferation [61]. Together, these findings suggest that HIV envelope proteins elicit both proinflammatory and profibrogenic effects through direct interaction with stellate cells. In the case of CXCR4, it has been shown that expression of CXCR4 increases with culture-induced activation of HSCs [58], suggesting that the effects of X4 gp120 could be accentuated during chronic liver disease in which an initial injury activates HSCs and thus increases cell-surface expression of CXCR4. It has not been reported whether HSC expression of the CCR5 receptor also increases with HSC activation.

HIV Infection

Activated HSCs have recently been shown to be permissive to HIV entry and gene expression [57]. HIV infects culture-activated HSCs predominantly in a CD4/CXCR4/CCR5-independent manner and causes increased expression of collagen I, the collagen characteristic of the cirrhotic liver, and of monocyte chemotactic protein-1 (MCP-1), a potent proinflammatory cytokine. Interestingly, much like what has been reported for dendritic cells or other APCs, HSCs can transfer infectious HIV to susceptible CD4+ cells *in trans* [57]. Therefore, direct interaction between HIV and HSCs may be an important mechanism for enhancing hepatic inflammation and fibrosis in patients with underlying chronic liver injury.

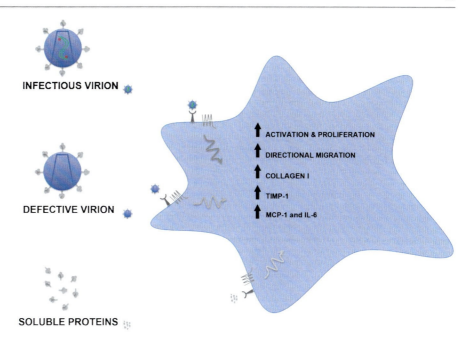

Fig. 9.2 Gp120 mediates its chemotactic effects on hepatic stellate cells through the PI3K/Akt pathway, while it proinflammatory effects are mediated through nuclear factor kappa B (NF-kB) and p38^{MAPK}

HIV's Interactions with Liver Sinusoidal Endothelial Cells

Only a limited number of studies have addressed HIV's interactions with LSECs, although the description of hepatic sinusoidal lesions in a significant number of AIDS patients prompted Scoazec et al. [62] to examine sinusoidal barrier abnormalities in a series of 29 individuals with HIV and liver abnormalities. The authors observed ultrastructural lesions of the sinusoidal barrier in all cases. Numerous hyperplastic sinusoidal macrophages were also common, suggesting that HIV may directly or indirectly injure hepatic endothelial cells. The same group subsequently demonstrated that LSECs were CD4 positive, suggesting that they may serve as putative targets of HIV infection in the liver [63]. Finally, Steffan et al. [56] reported that primary LSECs were permissive to HIV infection in vitro in a CD4-dependent manner. Once infected, LSECs are capable of producing infectious virus in culture supernatant that can infect susceptible CD4$^+$ cells. In addition, the synthesis of von Willebrand's factor and excretion of endothelin-1 were decreased in HIV-infected LSECs, while other functions such as phagocytosis and pinocytosis were preserved [64]. These findings suggest that while some secretory functions that may promote liver pathology are disrupted by HIV infection, the overall actin cytoskeleton is preserved [65]. Interestingly, LSECs express liver/lymph node-specific ICAM-3-grabbing nonintegrin (L-SIGN), which behaves similarly to DC-SIGN on dendritic cells in that it has high affinity for intercellular adhesion molecule 3 (ICAM-3), captures HIV through gp120 binding, and enhances HIV infection of T cells *in trans* [66]. Whether LSECs are able to infect CD4$^+$ cells *in trans* through a similar mechanism has not yet been demonstrated but would be in keeping with their ability to act as APCs and their position within the hepatic sinusoid.

HIV's Interactions with Kupffer Cells

While blood monocytes/macrophages support HIV replication, there are limited data on HIV infection of liver resident macrophages such as Kupffer cells. Using Kupffer cells purified from liver tissues from AIDS patients, Hufert et al. [67] analyzed HIV proviral DNA and found that Kupffer cells were indeed infected in three of seven patients. Interestingly, Kupffer cells harbored HIV proviral DNA only if matched peripheral blood monocytes were also infected. Schmitt et al. [55] subsequently demonstrated that primary cultures of Kupffer cells support HIV replication in vitro. Moreover, Kupffer cell infection was increased in the presence of morphine [68], a substance commonly used among persons with HIV infection transmitted via intravenous injection. It has also been reported that Kupffer cell density is correlated with the degree of HIV-related immunosuppression and may increase upon initiation of antiretroviral therapy [69]. The authors suggest that since Kupffer cells play a critical role in controlling microbial translocation, this reduction may be important for systemic immune activation and profibrogenic effects of LPS on HSCs (discussed further below). Finally, Kupffer cells can be infected *in trans* with virus from lymphocytes resulting in robust HIV replication [70]. While these reports are intriguing, no studies have examined the direct impact of HIV infection on the biology of Kupffer cells. HIV gp120 has been shown to induce the release of cytokines and chemokines in human mononuclear cells and rat Kupffer cells likely through the release of reactive oxygen species (ROS) [71]. Mannose-specific receptors are thought to be the putative binding sites for gp120 in rat cells [72]. Nonetheless, these studies have not been performed using human cells but clearly warrant further investigation.

Alteration of the Cytokine Milieu by HIV and Its Relevance to Liver Pathogenesis

Cytokines are immunologic signaling molecules that play a central role in generating immune responses to viral infections by regulation of the host response, as well as direct inhibition of viral replication. For example, a T-helper type 1 (Th1) cytokine response may result in a self-limited, acute response to HCV [73]. By contrast, Th2 cytokines inhibit the effects of Th1 cytokines and are decreased during chronic HCV infection [74]. Several studies have reported that proinflammatory cytokines, such as IL-8 and tumor necrosis factor a (TNFα), are associated with severe hepatitis activity, inflammation, steatosis, and/or decreased interferon sensitivity [45, 46, 75–78]. The fibrogenic cytokine transforming growth factor β_1 (TGFβ_1) is also a key regulator of liver fibrosis [79] and is increased in patients with HIV infection [80, 81]. Recently, the intrahepatic expression of TGFβ_1 was shown to be significantly increased in HIV–HCV coinfected patients compared to HCV-monoinfected patients [82]. Furthermore, HCV-induced TGFβ_1 secretion by hepatocytes is enhanced by receptor-mediated binding of the HIV envelope protein gp120 to hepatocytes [83]. TGFβ_1 may then promote fibrosis via direct effects on stellate cells [84]. However, fibrogenic cytokines may be offset, in part, by antifibrotic cytokines, such as the interferons. Clearly, any perturbation of this balance could profoundly impact liver disease, as well as treatment sensitivity [75, 78, 85] as summarized in Fig. 9.3.

Cytokine dysregulation is a hallmark of HIV infection [86]; thus, HIV coinfection may contribute to liver disease by altering the cytokine milieu and/or by providing inappropriate immunologic signals. By contrast, antiretroviral therapy (ART) utilization in HIV–HCV coinfected persons may have beneficial effects with respect to liver disease progression [87, 88]. We have previously reported that hepatic mRNA levels of IFN, TNFα, IL-2, IL-8, and IL-10 were lower in HIV–HCV coinfected persons compared to HCV monoinfected persons, although hepatic expression of TGFβ_1 was higher in the HIV–HCV coinfected group [82]. Similarly, Kuntzen et al. [89] reported that intrahepatic mRNA levels of several proinflammatory cytokines/chemokines were significantly higher in HIV-positive compared to HIV-negative persons, whereas mRNA levels of profibrogenic cytokines did not differ between the two groups. These differences were less pronounced among individuals receiving HAART compared to treatment naïve individuals. Therefore, an

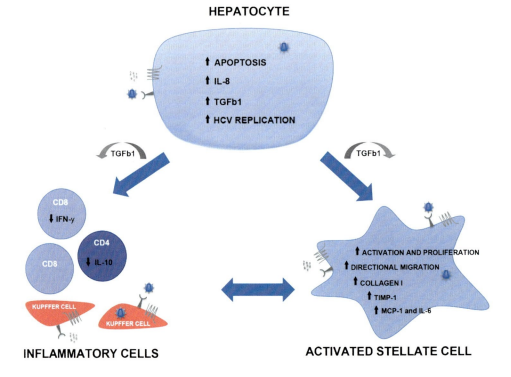

Fig. 9.3 TGFb$_1$ may then promote fibrosis via direct effects on stellate cells. HIV and/or its envelope protein gp120 elicit pro-inflammatory and pro-fibrogenic effects on both parenchymal and non-parenchymal cells of the liver. Impact on one cell has clear implications for eliciting effects on neighboring cells within the liver. The net result is a pro-inflammatory and pro-fibrogenic milieu

enhanced inflammatory response may also contribute to accelerated liver disease and HCV persistence, particularly during HIV–HCV coinfection. Despite these intriguing findings, characterization of cytokine expression among the various intrahepatic cell types outlined here has not been fully explored in vivo.

HIV-Related Microbial Translocation Is Associated with Liver Pathogenesis

HIV infection causes $CD4^+$ lymphocyte depletion in the gut within the first months of infection [90]. This HIV-related mucosal depletion of $CD4^+$ lymphocytes has been linked to the disruption of gut epithelial integrity and increased microbial translocation as evidenced by increased plasma lipopolysaccharide (LPS) levels, the inflammatory component of gram-negative bacteria cell wall [91]. Interestingly, even though mucosal $CD4^+$ T cell depletion occurs during the acute phase of HIV infection, plasma LPS does not increase until the chronic phase of infection. This suggests that the consequences of depletion and mucosal damage are counteracted by transient mobilization of factors that neutralize circulating LPS and likely the ability of healthy Kupffer cells to clear increased LPS levels [91]. Furthermore, in a cohort of HCV-infected persons at different stages of liver disease, microbial translocation in HIV coinfected patients was strongly associated with liver disease progression [92]. Additionally, HIV–HCV coinfection is associated with Kupffer cell depletion which is only partially recovered upon initiation of antiretroviral therapy [69]. Whether increased systemic LPS during chronic liver disease is due to increased shunting in the setting of portal hypertension and/or the inability of impaired Kupffer cells to clear LPS or is actually the cause of liver disease progression is not clear. However, potential effects of LPS on intrahepatic cell types include the following: (1) TLR4-mediated increased responsiveness of HSCs to $TGF\beta_1$ [93] and (2) increased cytokine/chemokine secretion by both Kupffer and activated HSCs creating a proinflammatory milieu [94]. In addition, LPS stimulation enhances replication of R5 HIV but has minimal effect on replication of X4 HIV [95]. Thus, examining whether a similar situation exists for Kupffer cells would be an interesting area for future research.

Interactions of HIV with Hepatitis B Virus and Hepatitis C Virus

Since the widespread utilization of highly active antiretroviral therapy (HAART), the survival of persons with HIV infection has improved dramatically. Unfortunately, liver disease has now surpassed AIDS-defining illnesses as a major cause of morbidity and mortality in several cohorts [96–98]. Hepatitis C virus is a significant public health threat with over 170 million infected persons. Moreover, 350 million people are chronically infected with hepatitis B virus – the world's leading cause of cirrhosis and hepatocellular carcinoma [99, 100]. Owing to shared routes of transmission, coinfection with HBV and/or HCV is a major cause of morbidity and mortality among HIV positive persons [97].

In HIV–HBV coinfected individuals, increased HBV DNA levels are frequently observed [101, 102]. Similarly, HCV RNA levels are significantly elevated during HIV–HCV coinfection compared to HCV monoinfection [96, 103]. While diminished immune responses in persons with HIV partially explain these observations, immune-mediated mechanisms are not the sole interactions between HIV and HBV or HCV. For instance, in vivo HCV RNA levels are more strongly associated with HIV RNA levels than with $CD4^+$ cell counts [104], further supporting the hypothesis that direct virus–virus interactions contribute to the pathogenesis of HIV–HBV or HIV–HCV coinfection.

By contrast, the presence of viral hepatitis may also impact HIV expression and/or disease progression. For instance, Daar et al. reported that increased HCV RNA levels were associated with accelerated progression to AIDS even after controlling for $CD4^+$ cell count and HIV RNA level [105]. Similarly, others have reported that HCV seropositivity was associated with progression to a new AIDS-defining illness or death, slower $CD4^+$ cell rebound during antiretroviral therapy, and decreased adherence to anti-HIV therapy [106–112]. In vitro studies have demonstrated that the HCV NS3/4A protein activates HIV transcription through its LTR, while the HCV core protein suppresses the HIV LTR [113–115]. Furthermore, the HBV X protein acts as a nuclear coactivator that induces transcriptional activation of the HIV long terminal repeat [116, 117], resulting in increased HIV replication and further impairment of the host immune function. Nonetheless, the precise pathways by which hepatitis viruses may interact with HIV in vivo remain to be fully elucidated.

HIV proteins may also have a more direct effect on replication of hepatotropic viruses. For example, a recent study by Lin et al. [83] showed that recombinant, monomeric gp120 protein increased HCV replication and enhanced HCV regulated $TGF\beta_1$ expression in vitro. This enhancement of HCV expression by gp120 could also be blocked using antibodies against CXCR4 or CCR5. These provocative data suggest a novel mechanism by which HIV regulates HCV replication and may accelerate liver fibrosis. Nonetheless, other mediators of liver fibrosis, as well as $TGF\beta_1$ signal transducers, have not been well characterized in hepatocytes in the presence of HIV proteins in vitro or during HIV–HCV coinfection in vivo.

While Iser et al. [40] demonstrated HIV infection of the HBV-expressing AD38 cell line, perhaps the most interesting finding was that coinfection of this cell line with HIV resulted in increased levels of intracellular HBV surface antigen. These data would suggest that HIV could dramatically impact

HBV pathogenesis and accelerate liver disease in HIV–HBV coinfected individuals. Similarly, preliminary studies within our group have shown increased HCV protein expression and RNA synthesis in an HCV-expressing cell line after HIV coinfection [118]. Unfortunately, to date, there are no published reports on HIV regulation of HCV entry receptors gene expression. However, engagement of the CD81 receptor – a putative receptor for HCV – results in increased HIV LTR activation and HIV replication in lymphocytes [119, 120]. Thus, it is conceivable that HCV–CD81 interactions in hepatocytes and/or lymphocytes could impact HIV gene expression, although this has not been evaluated to date.

Summary

Given the immense public health burdens of the overlapping HIV and viral hepatitis epidemics, more effective strategies to combat viral replication, as well as complementary therapies to ameliorate the complications of liver disease, are urgently required. A number of clinical studies have clearly demonstrated that HIV coinfection is associated with increased HBV or HCV replication and decreased treatment response rates, as well as progressive liver disease. While these observations have led many to conclude that HIV suppression may be the most critical factor in controlling liver disease if the underlying liver disease is not treated, this must be supported by understanding the mechanisms by which HIV accelerates inflammation and fibrosis through effects on individual cell populations. However, the influence of HIV on distinct liver cell populations has only recently begun to be examined in detail. Moreover, characterization of the intracellular pathways by which HIV infection and/or viral proteins impact liver cell function will significantly improve our understanding of HIV pathogenesis and virus–virus interactions and may ultimately improve treatment modalities for HIV-mediated liver disease.

References

1. Sheth K, Bankey P. The liver as an immune organ. Curr Opin Crit Care. 2001;7:99–104.
2. Kahn J, Walker B. Acute human immunodeficiency virus type 1 infection. N Engl J Med. 1998;339(1):33–9.
3. Keaveny AP, Karasik M. Hepatobiliary and pancreatic infections in AIDS: Part one. AIDS Patient Care STDS. 1998;12(5):347–57.
4. Bonacini M. Hepatobiliary complications in patients with human immunodeficiency virus infection. Am J Med. 1992;92:404–11.
5. Lefkowitch J. Pathology of AIDS-related liver disease. Dig Dis. 1994;12:321–30.
6. Cao Y et al. CD4-independent, productive human immunodeficiency virus type 1 infection of hepatoma cell lines in vitro. J Virol. 1990;64(6):2553–9.
7. Vlahakis S et al. Human immunodeficiency virus-induced apoptosis of human hepatocytes via CXCR4. J Infect Dis. 2003;188:1455–60.
8. Littman D. Chemokine receptors: keys to AIDS pathogenesis? Cell Death Differ. 1998;93(5):677–80.
9. Popik W, Pitha P. Exploitation of cellular signaling by HIV-1: unwelcome guests with master keys that signal their entry. Virology. 2000;276(1):1–6.
10. Zlotnik A, Yoshie O. Chemokines: a new classification system and their role in immunity. Immunity. 2000;12:121–7.
11. Mellado M et al. Chemokine signaling and functional responses: the role of receptor dimerization and TK pathway activation. Annu Rev Immunol. 2001;19:397–421.
12. Pearce-Pratt R, Malamud D, Phillips D. Role of the cytoskeleton in cell-to-cell transmission of human immunodeficiency virus. J Virol. 1994;68(5):2898–905.
13. Douglas GC et al. Cell-mediated infection of human placental trophoblast with HIV in vitro. AIDS Res Hum Retroviruses. 1991;7(9):735–40.
14. Hatsukari I et al. DEC-205-mediated internalization of HIV-1 results in the establishment of silent infection in renal tubular cells. J Am Soc Nephrol. 2007;18(3):780–7.
15. Lusso P, Lori F, Gallo R. CD4-independent infection by human immunodeficiency virus type 1 after phenotypic mixing with human T-cell leukemia viruses. J Virol. 1990;64(12):6341–4.
16. Harouse JM et al. CD4-independent infection of human neural cells by human immunodeficiency virus type 1. J Virol. 1989;63(6):2527–33.
17. Liu Y et al. CD4-independent infection of astrocytes by human immunodeficiency virus type 1: requirement for the human mannose receptor. J Virol. 2004;78(8):4120–33.
18. Bhattacharya J, Peters PJ, Clapham P. CD4-independent infection of HIV and SIV: implications for envelope conformation and cell tropism in vivo. AIDS. 2003;17 Suppl 4:S3–43.
19. Cameron P et al. Dendritic cells exposed to human immunodeficiency virus type-1 transmit a vigorous cytopathic infection to CD4+ T cells. Science. 1992;257:383–7.
20. Geijtenbeek T et al. DC-SIGN, a dendritic cell-specific HIV-1 binding protein that enhances trans-infection of T cells. Cell. 2000;100:587–97.
21. Nguyen DG, Hildreth J. Involvement of macrophage mannose receptor in the binding and transmission of HIV by macrophages. Eur J Immunol. 2003;33(2):483–93.
22. Chen P et al. Predominant mode of human immunodeficiency virus transfer between T cells is mediated by sustained Env-dependent neutralization-resistant virological synapses. J Virol. 2007;81:12582–95.
23. Popik W, Pitha P. Exploitation of cellular signaling by HIV-1: unwelcome guests with master keys that signal their entry. Virology. 2000;2000:1–6.
24. Zheng J et al. gp120-independent HIV infection of cells derived from the female reproductive tract, brain, and colon. J Acquir Immune Defic Syndr. 2006;43(2):137–6.
25. Vidricaire G, Gauthier S, Tremblay M. HIV-1 infection of trophoblasts is independent of gp120/CD4 interactions but relies on heparan sulfate proteoglycans. J Infect Dis. 2007;195(10):1461–71.
26. Chow YH et al. gp120-Independent infection of CD4(−) epithelial cells and CD4(+) T-cells by HIV-1. J Acquir Immune Defic Syndr. 2002;30(1):1–8.
27. Klasse P, Moore J. Is there enough gp120 in the body fluids of HIV-1 infected individuals to have biologically significant effects. Virology. 2004;323:1–8.
28. Popovic M et al. Persistence of HIV-1 structural proteins and glycoproteins in lymph nodes of patients under highly active antiretroviral therapy. Proc Natl Acad Sci U S A. 2005;102:14807–12.
29. Santosuosso M et al. HIV-1 envelope protein gp120 is present at high concentrations in secondary lymphoid organs of individuals with chronic HIV-1 infection. J Infect Dis. 2009;200(7):1050–3.

30. Cummins NW, Rizza SA, Badley AD. How much gp120 is there? J Infect Dis. 2010;201(8):1273–4. author reply 1274–5.
31. Blackard JT, Sherman K. HCV/HIV co-infection: time to re-evaluate the role of HIV in the liver? J Viral Hepat. 2008;15(5):323–30.
32. Cao Y et al. Identification and quantitation of HIV-1 in the liver of patients with AIDS. AIDS. 1992;6(1):65–70.
33. Housset C, Lamas E, Brechot C. Detection of HIV1 RNA and p24 antigen in HIV-1-infected human liver. Res Virol. 1990;141:153–9.
34. Jiang TJ et al. Immunohistochemical evidence for HIV-1 infection in the liver of HIV-infected patients. Zhonghua Shi Yan He Lin Chuang Bing Du Xue Za Zhi. 2005;19(2):152–4.
35. Hoda SA, White JE, Gerber M. Immunohistochemical studies of human immunodeficiency virus-1 in liver tissues of patients with AIDS. Mod Pathol. 1991;4(5):578–81.
36. Lang ZW et al. A pathological study on liver tissues of patients with HIV infection. Zhonghua Gan Zang Bing Za Zhi. 2005;13(12):930–2.
37. Banerjee R et al. Inhibition of HIV-1 productive infection in hepatoblastoma HepG2 cells by recombinant tumor necrosis factor-a. AIDS. 1992;6(10):1127–31.
38. Munshi N et al. Hepatitis C and human immunodeficiency virus envelope proteins cooperatively induce hepatocytic apoptosis via an innocent bystander mechanism. J Infect Dis. 2003;188:1192–204.
39. Balasubramanian A, Ganju R, Groopman J. HCV and HIV envelope proteins collaboratively mediate IL-8 secretion through activation of p38 MAP kinase and SHP2 in hepatocytes. J Biol Chem. 2003;278(37):35755–66.
40. Iser DM et al. Coinfection of hepatic cell lines with human immunodeficiency virus and hepatitis B virus leads to an increase in intracellular hepatitis B surface antigen. J Virol. 2010;84(12):5860–7.
41. Balasubramanian A et al. Molecular mechanism of hepatic injury in coinfection with hepatitis C virus and HIV. Clin Infect Dis. 2005;41 Suppl 1:S32–7.
42. Babu CK et al. HIV induces TRAIL sensitivity in hepatocytes. PLoS One. 2009;4(2):e4623.
43. Balasubramanian A, Ganju RK, Groopman JE. Signal transducer and activator of transcription factor 1 mediates apoptosis induced by hepatitis C virus and HIV envelope proteins in hepatocytes. J Infect Dis. 2006;194(5):670–81.
44. Gao B. Cytokines, STATs and liver disease. Cell Mol Immunol. 2005;2(2):92–100.
45. Polyak S et al. Elevated levels of interleukin-8 in serum are associated with hepatitis C infection and resistance to interferon therapy. J Virol. 2001;75(13):6209–11.
46. Polyak S et al. Hepatitis C virus nonstructural 5A protein induces interleukin-8, leading to partial inhibition of the interferon-induced antiviral response. J Virol. 2001;75(13):6095–106.
47. Khabar K et al. The alpha chemokine, interleukin 8, inhibits the antiviral action of interferon a. J Exp Med. 1997;186(7):1077–85.
48. Canbay A, Friedman S, Gores G. Apoptosis: the nexus of liver injury and fibrosis. Hepatology. 2004;39:273–8.
49. Altavilla G et al. Enhancement of chemical carcinogenesis by the HIV-1 tat gene. Am J Pathol. 2000;157(4):1081–9.
50. Xiao P et al. Characterization of a CD4-independent clinical HIV-1 that can efficiently infect human hepatocytes through chemokine (C-X-C motif) receptor 4. AIDS. 2008;22(14):1749–57.
51. Fromentin R, MR T, Tremblay M. Human hepatoma cells transmit surface bound HIV-1 to CD4+ T cells through an ICAM-1/LFA-1-dependent mechanism. Virology. 2010;398:168–75.
52. Zhu M, Duan L, Pomerantz R. TAR- and Tat-independent replication of human immunodeficiency virus type 1 in human hepatoma cells. AIDS Res Hum Retroviruses. 1996;12(12):1093–101.
53. Pizzella T, Banerjee R. Identification of a human immunodeficiency virus type 1 TAR binding protein in human hepatoblastoma HepG2 cells that trans-activates HIV-1 LTR-directed gene expression. DNA Cell Biol. 1994;13(1):67–74.
54. Hsu ML et al. Cytokine regulation of HIV-1 LTR transactivation in human hepatocellular carcinoma cell lines. Cancer Lett. 1995;94(1):41–8.
55. Schmitt MP et al. Multiplication of human immunodeficiency virus in primary cultures of human kupffer cells – possible role of liver macrophage infection in the physiopathology of AIDS. Res Virol. 1990;141:143–52.
56. Steffan A et al. Primary cultures of endothelial cells from the human liver sinusoid are permissive for human immunodeficiency virus type 1. Proc Natl Acad Sci U S A. 1992;89:1582–6.
57. Ana C, Tuyama A, Hong F, Saiman Y, Wang C, Mosoian A, et al. HIV infects human hepatic stellate cells and promotes collagen I and MCP-1 expression: implications for hepatic fibrosis in HIV/HCV coinfection. Hepatology. 2010;52:612–21.
58. Hong F et al. Hepatic stellate cells express functional CXCR4: role in stromal cell-derived factor-1alpha-mediated stellate cell activation. Hepatology. 2009;49(6):2055–67.
59. Schwabe R, Bataller R, Brenner D. Human hepatic stellate cells express CCR5 and RANTES to induce proliferation and migration. Am J Physiol Gastrointest Liver Physiol. 2003;285:G949–58.
60. Bruno R et al. gp120 modulates the biology of human hepatic stellate cells: a link between HIV infection and liver fibrogenesis. Gut. 2010;59(4):513–20.
61. Hong F, Bansal M. HIV gp120(X4) promotes hepatic stellate cell activation, fibrogenesis, and proliferation: a potential mechanism for rapid fibrosis progression in HIV/HCV coinfected patients. Hepatology. 2009;50(4) Suppl:128A.
62. Scoazec JY et al. Peliosis hepatis and sinusoidal dilation during infection by the human immunodeficiency virus (HIV): an ultrastructural study. Am J Pathol. 1988;131(1):38–47.
63. Scoazec JY, Feldmann G. Both macrophages and endothelial cells of the human hepatic sinusoid express the CD4 molecule, a receptor for the human immunodeficiency virus. Hepatology. 1990;12(1):505–10.
64. Lafon ME et al. HIV-1 infection induces functional alterations in human liver endothelial cells in primary culture. AIDS. 1994;8(6):747–52.
65. Lafon ME et al. Interaction of human immunodeficiency virus with human macrovascular endothelial cells in vitro. AIDS Res Hum Retroviruses. 1992;8(9):1567–70.
66. Bashirova AA et al. A dendritic cell-specific intercellular adhesion molecule 3-grabbing nonintegrin (DC-SIGN)-related protein is highly expressed on human liver sinusoidal endothelial cells and promotes HIV-1 infection. J Exp Med. 2001;193(6):671–8.
67. Hufert FT et al. Human Kupffer cels infected with HIV-1 in vivo. J Acquir Immune Defic Syndr. 1993;6(7):772–7.
68. Schweitzer C et al. Morphine stimulates HIV replication in primary cultures of human Kupffer cells. Res Virol. 1991;142(2–3):189–95.
69. Balagopal A et al. Kupffer cells are depleted with HIV immunodeficiency and partially recovered with antiretroviral immune reconstitution. AIDS. 2009;23(18):2397–404.
70. Gendrault JL et al. Interaction of cultured human Kupffer cells with HIV-infected CEM cells: an electron microscopic study. Pathobiology. 1991;59(4):223–6.
71. Bautista AP. Impact of alcohol on the ability of Kupffer cells to produce chemokines and its role in alcoholic liver disease. J Gastroenterol Hepatol. 2000;15(4):349–56.
72. Bautista AP. Chronic alcohol intoxication induces hepatic injury through enhanced macrophage inflammatory protein-2 production and intercellular adhesion molecule-1 expression in the liver. Hepatology. 1997;25(2):335–42.
73. Jacobson-Brown P, Neuman M. Immunopathogenesis of hepatitis C viral infection: Th1/Th2 responses and the role of cytokines. Clin Biochem. 2001;34:167–71.
74. Spanakis N et al. Cytokine serum levels in patients with chronic HCV infection. J Clin Lab Anal. 2002;16:40–6.
75. Fukuda R et al. Intrahepatic expression of pro-inflammatory cytokine mRNAs and interferon efficacy in chronic hepatitis C. Liver. 1996;16:390–9.

76. Shimoda K et al. Interleukin-8 and hIRH (SDF1-a/PBSF) mRNA expression and histological activity index in patients with chronic hepatitis C. Hepatology. 1998;28(1):108–15.
77. Neuman M et al. Serum tumour necrosis factor-a and transforming growth factor-b levels in chronic hepatitis C patients are immunomodulated by therapy. Cytokine. 2002;17(2):108–17.
78. Gochee P et al. Steatosis in chronic hepatitis C: association with increased messenger RNA expression of collagen I, tumor necrosis factor-a and cytochrome P4502E1. J Gastroenterol Hepatol. 2003;18:386–92.
79. Schuppan D et al. Hepatitis C and liver fibrosis. Cell Death Differ. 2002;10 Suppl 1:S59–67.
80. Pal S, Schnapp L. HIV-infected lymphocytes regulate fibronectin synthesis by TGFb1 secretion. J Immunol. 2004;172:3189–95.
81. Navikas V et al. Increased levels of interferon-gamma(IFN-gamma), IL-4 and tranforming growth factor-beta (TGF-beta) mRNA expressing blood mononuclear cells in human HIV infection. Clin Exp Immunol. 1994;96:59–63.
82. Blackard J et al. Intrahepatic cytokine expression is downregulated during HCV/HIV co-infection. J Med Virol. 2006;78:202–7.
83. Lin W et al. HIV increases HCV replication in a TGF-beta1-dependent manner. Gastroenterology. 2008;164(3):803–11.
84. Friedman S. Cytokines and fibrogenesis. Semin Liver Dis. 1999;19(2):129–40.
85. Masaki N, Fukushima S, Hayashi S. Lower Th-1/Th-2 ratio before interferon therapy may favor long-term virological responses in patients with chronic hepatitis C. Dig Dis Sci. 2002;47(10):2163–9.
86. Breen E. Pro- and anti-inflammatory cytokines in human immunodeficiency virus infection and acquired immunodeficiency syndrome. Pharmacol Ther. 2002;95(3):295–304.
87. Mehta S et al. The effect of antiretroviral therapy on liver disease among adults with HIV and hepatitis C coinfection. Hepatology. 2005;41(1):123–31.
88. Qurishi N et al. Effect of antiretroviral therapy on liver-related mortality in patients with HIV and hepatitis C virus coinfection. Lancet. 2003;362:1708–13.
89. Kuntzen T et al. Intrahepatic mRNA expression in hepatitis C virus and HIV/hepatitis C virus co-infection: infiltrating cells, cytokines, and influence of HAART. AIDS. 2008;22(2):203–10.
90. Mehandru S et al. Mechanisms of gastrointestinal CD4+ T-cell depletion during acute and early human immunodeficiency virus type 1 infection. J Virol. 2007;81(2):599–612.
91. Brenchley J et al. Microbial translocation is a cause of systemic immune activation in chronic HIV infection. Nat Med. 2006;12:1365–71.
92. Balagopal A et al. Human immunodeficiency virus-related microbial translocation and progression of hepatitis C. Gastroenterology. 2008;135(1):226–33.
93. Seki E et al. TLR4 enhances TGF-beta signaling and hepatic fibrosis. Nat Med. 2007;13(11):1324–32.
94. Paik YH et al. Toll-like receptor 4 mediates inflammatory signaling by bacterial lipopolysaccharide in human hepatic stellate cells. Hepatology. 2003;37(5):1043–55.
95. Moriuchi M et al. Exposure to bacterial products renders macrophages highly susceptible to T-tropic HIV-1. J Clin Invest. 1998;102(8):1540–50.
96. Tedaldi E et al. Influence of coinfection with hepatitis C virus on morbidity and mortality due to human immunodeficiency virus infection in the era of highly active antiretroviral therapy. Clin Infect Dis. 2003;36:363–7.
97. Bica I et al. Increasing mortality due to end-stage liver disease in patients with human immunodeficiency virus infection. Clin Infect Dis. 2001;32:492–7.
98. Salmon-Ceron D et al. Liver disease as a major cause of death among HIV infected patients: role of hepatitis C and B viruses and alcohol. J Hepatol. 2005;42(6):799–805.
99. Shi J et al. A meta-analysis of case-control studies on the combined effect of hepatitis B and C virus infections in causing hepatocellular carcinoma in China. Br J Cancer. 2005;92(3):607–12.
100. World Health Organization. Fact Sheet, Hepatitis B. 2000. 10 Apr 2003. Available from: http://www.who.int/inf-fs/en/fact204.html.
101. Colin JF et al. Influence of human immunodeficiency virus infection on chronic hepatitis B in homosexual men. Hepatology. 1999;29(4):1306–10.
102. Gilson RJ et al. Interactions between HIV and hepatitis B virus in homosexual men: effects on the natural history of infection. AIDS. 1997;11(5):597–606.
103. Yokozaki S et al. Immunological dynamics in hemophiliac patients infected with hepatitis C and human immunodeficiency virus: influence of antiretroviral therapy. Blood. 2000;96(13):4293–9.
104. Thomas D et al. Multicenter evaluation of hepatitis C RNA levels among female injection drug users. J Infect Dis. 2001;183:973–6.
105. Daar E et al. Hepatitis C viral load is associated with human immunodeficiency virus type 1 disease progression in hemophiliacs. J Infect Dis. 2001;193:589–95.
106. Greub G et al. Clinical progression, survival, and immune recovery during antiretroviral therapy in patients with HIV-1 and hepatitis C virus coinfection: the Swiss HIV Cohort Study. Lancet. 2000;356:1800–5.
107. Braitstein P et al. Hepatitis C coinfection is independently associated with decreased adherence to antiretroviral therapy in a population-based HIV cohort. AIDS. 2006;20(3):323–31.
108. Piroth L et al. Hepatitis C virus co-infection is a negative prognostic factor for clinical evolution in human immunodeficiency virus-positive patients. J Viral Hepat. 2000;7(4):302–8.
109. Piroth L et al. Does hepatitis C virus co-infection accelerate clinical and immunological evolution of HIV-infected patients? AIDS. 1998;12(4):381–8.
110. Macias J et al. Impaired recovery of CD4+ cell counts following highly active antiretroviral therapy in drug-naive patients coinfected with human immunodeficiency virus and hepatitis C virus. Eur J Clin Microbiol Infect Dis. 2003;22:675–80.
111. Ruys T, et al. Impaired recovery of CD4 cells in HIV-1 HCV co-infected patients using highly active antiretroviral therapy. In XV International AIDS Conference. Bangkok, Thailand. 2004.
112. Anderson K, Guest J, Rimland D. Hepatitis C virus coinfection increases mortality in HIV-infected patients in the highly active antiretroviral therapy era: data from the HIV Atlanta Cohort Study. Clin Infect Dis. 2004;39:1507–13.
113. Wu X et al. HCV NS3/4A protein activates HIV-1 transcription from its long terminal repeat. Virus Res. 2008;135(1):155–60.
114. Srinivas R et al. Hepatitis C virus core protein inhibits human immunodeficiency virus type 1 replication. Virus Res. 1996;45(2):87–92.
115. Ray RB et al. Transcriptional regulation of cellular and viral promoters by the hepatitis C virus core protein. Virus Res. 1995;37(3):209–20.
116. Balsano C et al. The hepatitis B virus X gene product transactivates the HIV-LTR in vivo. Arch Virol. 1993;8:63–71.
117. Gomez-Gonzalo M et al. The hepatitis B virus X protein induces HIV-1 replication and transcription in synergy with T-cell activation signals: functional roles of NF-kappaB/NF-AT and SP1-binding sites in the HIV-1 long terminal repeat promoter. J Biol Chem. 2001;276(38):35435–43.
118. Ma G, et al. HIV infection of an HCV-producing hepatocyte cell line – a model system for exploring HIV-HCV co-infection in vitro. In 13th International Symposium on Viral Hepatitis and Liver Disease. Washington, DC. 2009.
119. Tardif MR, Tremblay M. Tetraspanin CD81 provides a costimulatory signal resulting in increased human immunodeficiency virus type 1 gene expression in primary CD4+ T lymphocytes through NF-kappaB, NFAT, and AP-1 transduction pathways. J Virol. 2005;79(7):4316–28.
120. Gordón-Alonso M et al. Tetraspanins CD9 and CD81 modulate HIV-1-induced membrane fusion. J Immunol. 2006;177(8):5129–37.

HIV Replication

Vladimir A. Novitsky and Max Essex

Introduction

Knowledge of HIV replication is critical for understanding AIDS pathogenesis and the proper design of therapeutic interventions. HIV-1 replication is a complex, multistep process of virus–host interaction, dependent on both viral and host cell factors. HIV-1 utilizes host cell machinery extensively at each step of viral replication. Transient events that occur during HIV-1 replication include viral fusion, trafficking of the viral nucleoprotein complex in the cytoplasm, reverse transcription, relocation of proviral DNA into the nucleus, integration, transcription, and export of mRNA to the cytoplasm, assembly of new virions at the host cell membrane, budding, and maturation of viral particles (see Fig. 10.1). The proteolytically cleaved HIV proteins are essential for forming infectious virus particles able to start the next round of viral infection.

The HIV-1 virion contains two copies of a single-stranded RNA genome. The HIV-1 RNA genome consists of nine genes flanked by long terminal repeats (LTRs) and encodes structural and nonstructural proteins (see Table 10.1). Three structural HIV-1 proteins are encoded by the *gag*, *pol*, and *env* genes. The *gag* gene encodes the structural proteins of the viral core, *pol* encodes the enzymes responsible for viral replication and integration, and *env* encodes the viral envelope glycoproteins.

The *gag* gene encodes a polyprotein precursor, $Pr55^{Gag}$, that is cleaved by the viral protease (PR) to the mature Gag proteins matrix (MA) p17, capsid (CA) p24, nucleocapsid (NC) p7, p6, and two spacer peptides, p2 and p1, upon release of the viral particle.

The *pol* gene encodes a large polyprotein precursor, $Pr160^{GagPol}$, as a result of the −1 (minus one) frameshift during $Pr55^{Gag}$ translation. In HIV-1, the −1 ribosomal frameshift occurs at a frequency of 5–10% during Gag synthesis [1]. The ratio of Gag to Gag-Pol molecules is maintained strictly at the level of 20:1, which is critical for RNA dimerization, viral assembly, replication, and infectivity [2]. The −1 frameshift is promoted by two *cis*-acting RNA elements, the "slippery" sequence represented by a UUUUUUA heptamer and a stem-loop. Both the slippery sequence and the stem-loop are located in the overlapping region of the *gag* and *pol* genes directly following the coding region for NC.

The *env* encodes the surface Env glycoprotein gp120 and the transmembrane glycoprotein gp41. Env proteins are synthesized as a single polypeptide precursor, gp160, which is cleaved by the viral PR during transit to the cellular membrane. gp120 contains the determinants that interact with the CD4 receptor and coreceptor. gp41 anchors the gp120/gp41 complex in the membrane and contains domains critical for catalyzing the membrane fusion between viral and host lipid bilayers during virus entry. gp120 is organized into five conserved regions (C1–C5) and five highly variable domains (V1–V5). The variable loops, along with multiple glycosylation sites, provide evolving epitopes interacting with the host immune response. The gp41 protein contains a large extracellular ectodomain, a transmembrane spanning anchor, and a large cytoplasmic domain inside the virion membrane. The ectodomain contains a hydrophobic, N′-terminal fusion peptide and two heptad-repeat domains, HR1 and HR2, which are critical for fusion. The native Env spikes on the surface of HIV-1 are assembled as trimers.

HIV-1 encodes two regulatory gene products – Tat and Rev. Tat transactivates viral transcription from the LTR by binding to the transactivation response region (TAR) at the 5′ end of viral mRNA. Rev is an essential HIV-1 regulatory protein that binds to the Rev-responsive element (RRE) RNA and is responsible for transport of unspliced and singly spliced viral transcripts from the cell nucleus to the cytoplasm.

V.A. Novitsky (✉)
Department of Immunology and Infectious Diseases,
Harvard School of Public Health, FXB 402 651 Huntington Avenue,
Boston, MA 02115, USA
e-mail: vnovi@hsph.harvard.edu

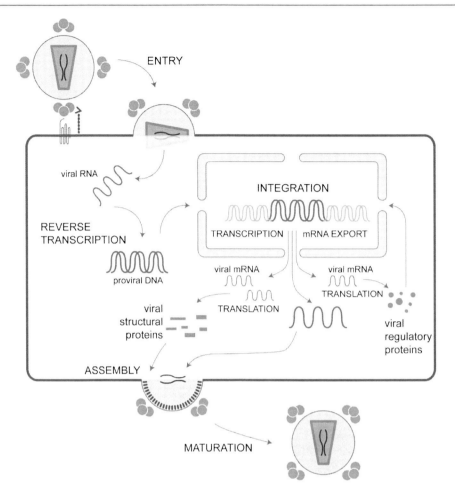

Fig. 10.1 Replication of HIV-1. The replication of HIV-1 begins with viral entry into the target cell by fusion of the viral envelope and plasma membrane of the cell. Binding of gp120 to the cellular receptor CD4 and interaction with the coreceptor triggers a series of conformation changes in both gp120 and gp41 that mediate membrane fusion and delivery of the viral core to the cytoplasm. The viral core is composed of a capsid protein that encapsidates the single-stranded, dimeric viral RNA genome in complex with the viral nucleocapsid protein and the viral enzymes RT and IN. After the core uncoats, RT copies the RNA genome into a double-stranded viral DNA, which is transported into the nucleus and integrates into the host cell genome by IN. The integrated proviral DNA is transcribed to full-length viral RNA and to a number of spliced mRNA transcripts that are translated in the cytoplasm. Cellular machinery is employed for transcription and translation of major structural proteins, Gag polyprotein precursor and Env glycoprotein precursor, which are transported to the site of virus particle assembly together with viral genomic RNA. Viral assembly is coordinated by Gag, and is followed by budding of the nascent virion from the plasma membrane. Viral PR cleaves the Gag and Gag-Pol precursors, which leads to virion maturation with a condensed conical core

HIV-1 also encodes four accessory proteins: viral infectivity factor (Vif), viral protein U (Vpu), negative factor (Nef), and viral protein R (Vpr). Vif is essential for enhancing viral infectivity. Vif induces degradation of the cytidine deaminases APOBEC-3G and APOBEC-3F. This counteraction of the innate antiviral defense results in reduction or prevention of viral hypermutation caused by APOBEC-3G and APOBEC-3F. Vpu is responsible for CD4 receptor degradation, induction of apoptosis, and enhancement of viral particle release. Nef is involved in T-cell receptor activation, downregulating surface expression of CD4 and major histocompatibility complex I (MHC-I), modulating cell activation pathways, enhancing particle infectivity, and acting as an auxiliary factor of HIV-1 reverse transcription. Vpr contributes to the nuclear import of the preintegration complex and induces arrest of cell cycle, stimulates transcription from some cellular promoters, and influences virus-induced apoptosis in activated peripheral blood mononuclear cells (PBMCs) and Jurkat T cells. Vpr can contribute to the depletion of CD4+ lymphocytes either directly by activating caspases 3/7, 8 and 9, or by enhancing Fas-mediated apoptosis [3]. In experiments on mice, Vpr expressed in adipose tissues and liver was able to alter lipid and fatty acid metabolism [4].

Two classes of HIV-1 genes can be distinguished: the early genes and the late genes [5]. The completely spliced messages that are exported to cytoplasm by the normal mRNA export pathway are Rev-independent and are early genes. During the early stage of HIV-1 infection, the completely

Table 10.1 HIV-1 genes and gene products

Gene symbol	Gene name	Major function	Gene product(s)	Function
gag	Group-specific antigen	Structural	Matrix protein, p17	Coats the inner leaflet of the viral membrane. Stabilizes viral particle. Facilitates nuclear transport of viral DNA
			Core protein, p24	Forms a cone-shaped core
			p2	Spacer protein
			Nucleocapsid (NC)	A highly basic protein with two zinc fingers; associated with viral RNA. Responsible for recognition of packaging signal and encapsidation of genomic viral RNA
			p1	Spacer protein
			p6	Mediates interactions between p55 and Vpr and initiates incorporation of Vpr
pol	Polymerase	Structural	Protease, PR	Cleaves newly synthesized polyproteins during viral replication, which leads to virion maturation
			Reverse transcriptase (RT)	Transcribes single-stranded viral RNA into double-stranded DNA
			Integrase (IN)	Exonuclease activity (trims 3′-end of linear DNA), endonuclease activity (cleaves the host DNA), and ligase activity (links ends of viral DNA)
env	Envelope	Structural	Surface glycoprotein, gp120	Binds to CD4+ cells and chemokine coreceptor
			Transmembrane glycoprotein, gp41	Viral fusion and internalization
tat	Transactivator	Regulatory	Tat	Transactivates viral transcription from LTR by binding to TAR
rev	Regulator of viral expression	Regulatory	Rev	Promotes export of unspliced and partially spliced mRNAs from the nucleus; binds to RRE
vif	Viral infectivity protein	Accessory	Vif	Enhances viral infectivity; counteracts APOBEC-3G and APOBEC-3F, preventing viral hypermutation
vpr	R protein	Accessory	Vpr	Enhances nuclear import of the preintegration complex; induces cell arrest in G2 phase; stimulates transcription; and influences apoptosis
vpu	U protein	Accessory	Vpu	Responsible for CD4 receptor degradation; and enhances viral particle release
nef	Negative regulation factor	Accessory	Nef	Activates T-cell receptor; downregulates surface expression of CD4 and MHC-I; modulates cell activation pathways; and enhances viral particle infectivity

spliced 1.8-kb mRNAs encode the viral regulatory proteins Tat, Rev, and Nef and are transported for translation to the cytoplasm. Transport of spliced and unspliced RNA from the nucleus to the cytoplasm is facilitated by the viral regulatory protein Rev which interacts with the RRE RNA in the *env* gene. Later, at the time of HIV-1 infection, Rev becomes available, and the intron-containing mRNA that are incompletely spliced or unspliced viral mRNA use Rev as an adapter. These are late genes. HIV-1 uses spliced mRNAs for viral protein synthesis and unspliced viral RNA for genome RNA and mRNA. Regulation of HIV-1 splicing is essential for efficient virus replication. Based on the size and extent of processing, there are three types of mRNAs: the 9-kb unspliced RNA that encode Gag and Pol, the 4-kb singly spliced RNA forming Vif, Vpr, Vpu, and Env, and the 2-kb completely spliced RNA that codes Tat, Rev, and Nef [6, 7]. HIV-1 Rev is a mediator of HIV-1 RNA transport from the nucleus to the cytoplasm, and acts as a traffic signal in the nucleus, directing the viral mRNA from spliced to unspliced and singly spliced viral mRNA [8]. Rev decreases the amount of viral spliced messages by generating a negative feedback loop. The expression levels of Rev are strictly regulated, which is important for balancing the products of viral gene expression and increasing levels of virion production [5].

Entry

HIV-1 infection begins with the interaction between viral Env proteins and host cell proteins. HIV-1 entry into cells is mediated by a trimeric complex consisting of noncovalently associated surface gp120 and transmembrane gp41 Env glycoproteins. The initial steps of viral entry are facilitated by nonspecific interactions between positively charged domains on the gp120 and negatively charged proteoglycans on the cellular membrane, or by specific interactions with cell surface lectin-binding proteins such as DC-SIGN that can enhance the efficiency of HIV infection. The primary HIV-1 receptor is CD4, a member of the immunoglobulin superfamily that is expressed on monocytes, macrophages, and subsets of T cells and dendritic cells. CD4 binding is a prerequisite to the formation and exposure of the coreceptor binding site of gp120. The CD4-binding site in gp120 is represented by highly conserved residues. Attachment of viral gp120 to CD4 triggers a conformational change in the glycoprotein spike. Specifically, two sets of β (beta)-sheets that are spatially separated in unbound gp120 are brought together by CD4, binding into a four-stranded β (beta)-sheet, the bridging sheet. CD4 binding results in exposure of the V1/V2 and V3 loops of gp120. Binding of CD4 changes the orientation of gp120, and the bridging sheet and the V3 loop become directed toward the host cell membrane. Such a series of conformational changes in gp120 makes the coreceptor binding site accessible and allows high-affinity interaction with the coreceptor.

In HIV-1 infection, the primary coreceptor on the surface of T-cells and macrophages is CCR5, although under certain circumstances CXCR4 can also be utilized as a coreceptor for virus entry. Utilization of coreceptors for virus entry, including a few alternative coreceptors, is associated with HIV-1 subtype. For example, HIV-1 subtype B shows robust entry via alternative coreceptor CCR3, and HIV-1 subtypes A and C are able to use the alternative coreceptor FPRL1 more efficiently than CCR3, while subtype D viruses are unable to use either CCR3 or FPRL1 efficiently [9]. Both coreceptors are members of the seven-transmembrane G protein-coupled receptor family. Spatially separated domains of CCR5 interact with distinct regions of gp120 including the N' terminus with the bridging sheet, the base, and the tip of the V3 loop. Engagement of the N' terminus by gp120 requires the formation of a conserved sulfotyrosine binding pocket and converts the V3 stem from a flexible structure into a rigid β (beta)-hairpin [10]. Binding of the coreceptor results in further glycoprotein spike rearrangement and internalization of the viral gp41 protein, leading to a fusion of viral and cellular membranes. Following insertion of the fusion peptide, the heptad repeat regions HR1 and HR2 of gp41 undergo a highly energetically favorable rearrangement in which they fold back on each other. In a functional trimer spike, this forms a six-helix bundle structure where the three HR1 domains form a central coiled-coil, and the three HR2 domains wrap in an antiparallel direction around the central coil [10]. This structural rearrangement brings the transmembrane region of gp41, which is embedded in the viral membrane, into close proximity with the fusion peptide, which is inserted into the host cell membrane. This results in the formation of the fusion pore, allowing the viral capsid to enter the cell [10].

After the fusion and delivery of the viral core into the cytoplasm of the target host cell, the viral core releases the RNA genome. Uncoating is the specific dissociation of the capsid shell from the viral core in the host cell cytoplasm, and is an essential step in the HIV-1 life cycle. Cyclophilin A incorporates into the HIV-1 virion through interaction with the Gag capsid antigen, and facilitates uncoating of the virus. While the Gag capsid antigen appears to be lost during this process, some other HIV-1 proteins, such as MA, NC, RT, IN, and Vpr, which entered the host cell with the viral RNA genome, remain associated with the functional reverse transcription complex.

Reverse Transcription

HIV-1 reverse transcription is catalyzed by RT, which is a multifunctional enzyme, reviewed by Sarafianos et al. [11]. Two enzymatic activities of RT include a DNA polymerase and ribonuclease hybrid (RNase H) activity. The DNA polymerase can copy either a DNA or an RNA template. The RNase H cleaves RNA in the RNA–DNA duplex. These enzymatic functions of RT convert the viral RNA into a double-stranded linear DNA in the cytoplasm of the infected cell.

The HIV-1 reverse transcription is a multistep process (see Fig. 10.2). HIV-1 RT requires both a primer and a template. DNA synthesis is initiated from a host tRNA primer, which hybridizes to the primer binding site (PBS) on the viral RNA genome. The PBS is located near the 5' end of the viral RNA genome and has a sequence complementary to the site at the 3' end of the host tRNA primer. The viral RNA genome is plus-strand. First minus-strand DNA synthesis is initiated from the tRNA primer toward the 5' end of the viral RNA genome. The synthesized stretch is represented by the RNA/DNA hybrid between the viral RNA and newly generated minus-strand DNA. The RNase H degrades the plus-strand RNA (see faded stretch in Fig. 10.2), and the minus-strand DNA becomes single stranded. Owing to identical sequences at the 5' and 3' ends of the viral RNA genome, minus-strand DNA relocates and hybridizes at the 3' end of the viral RNA. This is the first jump, or the minus-strand transfer. The first jump is followed by the minus-strand extension, which results in a long minus-strand DNA synthesized along the viral RNA. During or shortly after the DNA synthesis, RNase H degrades the RNA strand (see faded stretch in Fig. 10.2) except the polypurine tract (PPT) near the 3' end of the viral RNA. The PPT is resistant to RNase H degradation and is used as the primer for second-strand DNA synthesis, plus-strand DNA. The synthesis of plus-strand DNA toward the 3' end continues until RT copies almost the entire tRNA primer. After this, the RNase H cleaves the 3' end of the viral minus-strand DNA, which prepares the second jump, or plus-strand transfer. The second jump is required for synthesis of the second DNA strand. Removal of the tRNA primer exposes a portion of the plus-strand DNA that has the sequence complementary to the PBS.

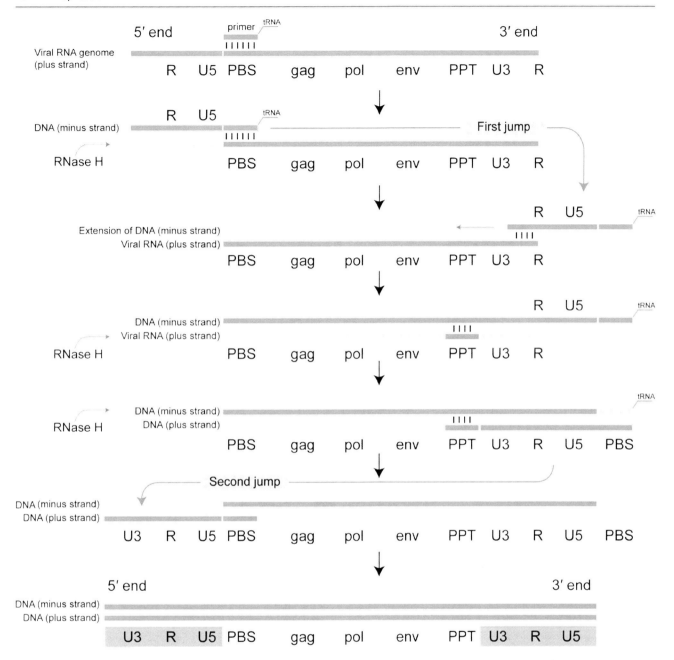

Fig. 10.2 HIV-1 Reverse Transcription. A host tRNA functions as a primer and hybridizes to the PBS near the 5′ end of the viral RNA genome. The synthesized short stretch of single-stranded DNA relocates and hybridizes to the 3′ end of the viral genome. After the first jump, synthesis of the first DNA minus-strand occurs. Owing to RNase H cleavage, a unique plus-strand RNA primer is formed at the PPT region that uses minus-strand DNA as a template for synthesis of a portion of DNA plus-strand toward the 3′ end of the viral genome. RNase H removes tRNA, which stops the synthesis and facilitates the second jump. After the second jump, elongation of the plus- and minus-strands continues. The DNA copy of the viral genome is completed when RT copies the plus and minus strands entirely. The final product is a blunt-ended linear duplex DNA with LTR at both ends. Degraded strands by RNase H are shown fainted

Exposure of the 3′ end of the plus-strand DNA allows the 5′ end of the minus-strand to be transferred to the plus-strand. After the second transfer, both the minus- and plus-strands are elongated until the entire DNA is double stranded. The two strands of DNA generated have similar LTR sequences at both ends (shaded in Fig. 10.2). The generated DNA is longer than the RNA genome from which it was derived. This allows the integrated proviral DNA to be used as the template from which new copies of the viral genome and the viral mRNAs are copied by the host enzyme DNA-dependent RNA polymerase.

The final product of the reverse transcription is the substrate for viral IN. Linear double-stranded viral DNA is translocated to the nucleus where the viral DNA is inserted into the host genome by IN.

If RT makes a double-stranded viral DNA by copying from two different RNA genomes, the resulting DNA may contain sequences that are derived from both of the parental genomes, resulting in a recombined HIV-1 genome. Recombination during the process of reverse transcription is very common in HIV-1.

Integration

HIV-1 integrase (IN) is an essential viral enzyme that binds to and mediates integration of the double-stranded viral DNA into the genomic DNA of the infected host cell. HIV-1 IN mediates two critical reactions during viral replication: 3'-end processing of the double-stranded viral DNA ends and strand transfer. The result of IN activity is a functional integrated proviral DNA within the host chromosomal DNA. During the 3'-processing reaction IN removes few nucleotides from the ends of viral DNA. After import of the viral DNA into the nucleus, IN inserts both 3' ends of the viral DNA into opposing strands of cellular genomic DNA.

In cytoplasm, after completion of the reverse transcription step, IN binds the newly synthesized double-stranded viral DNA and initiates 3'-end processing. IN binds to the LTR of the viral DNA and cleaves GT nucleotides at both 3'-ends of viral DNA. IN bounded to both LTR ends forms the preintegration complex that also includes viral matrix protein, p7/nucleocapsid, Vpr, and RT, as well as some host cellular proteins [12]. The preintegration complex is transported through the nuclear membrane to the nucleus. The host cell cofactor lens epithelium-derived growth factor/transcriptional coactivator 75 (LEDGF/p75) plays an important role in the integration process by tethering IN to chromatin [13].

Integration of HIV-1 into the human genome is not random but favors regions containing transcriptionally active genes [14]. In the nucleus, the preintegration complex is targeted to the host genomic DNA, which results in the strand transfer reaction. IN within the preintegration complex binds to host genomic DNA and performs nucleophilic attack on the phosphodiester bonds of the host genomic DNA. The 3'-OH ends of the viral DNA ligate to the 5'-phosphate ends of the host genomic DNA. The two nucleotides at the 5'-end of the viral DNA form a "flap" and are trimmed [12]. Gap filling from the 3'-end of the host genomic DNA completes the process of integration. The resulting integrated proviral DNA represents the template for transcription of new viral RNAs for translation of viral proteins and transcription of viral RNAs for packaging new virions.

Transcription

The transcription of HIV-1 provirus is regulated by viral proteins and host cellular factors by the binding of both host and viral proteins to the viral LTR, which serves as the viral promoter, reviewed by Knipe and Howley [15]. Host transcription factors such as the Sp family, nuclear factor kappa B (NF-κB) family, activator protein 1 (AP-1) proteins, nuclear factor of activated T cells (NFAT), and CCAAT enhancer binding protein (C/EBP) family members play critical roles in the regulation of HIV-1 transcription. This interaction becomes possible through the presence of multiple binding sites for host transcription factors across the viral LTR [16]. In addition, viral regulatory protein Tat binds to the viral LTR and interacts with host cellular factors. HIV-1 exhibits extraordinary plasticity and capacity to adapt its transcriptional strategy to different cellular environments during infection in lymphocytes, thymocytes, monocytes, macrophages, and microglial cells.

The transcription of HIV-1 is initiated in the 5'-LTR, from the first nucleotide position of the R region. The HIV-1 LTR includes functional regions such as TAR, core, enhancer, and modulatory elements. The LTR sequence contains a wide range of *cis*-acting elements for cellular transcription factors. The enhancer region has two consensus NF-κB sites which are considered the key host transcription factor in HIV-1 transcription [17]. However, two HIV-1 subtypes break the rule: the majority of circulating HIV-1 subtype C viruses has three NF-κB sites, while HIV-1 subtype E viruses have only one NF-κB binding site. HIV-1 uses the NF-κB sites to enhance its replication in host cells. Activation of CD4+ cells induces the host NFκB, which binds to promoters in both the host DNA and viral LTR, initiating the transcription of viral RNA by the cellular RNA polymerase. The major role in activating the HIV-1 LTR is played by the p50–RelA heterodimer. Two other host factors, NFAT1 and NFAT5, also participate in activation of HIV-1 transcription [18–20]. The activity of NF-κB is inhibited by IκB α, [21–23] which is degraded by signals that activate NF-κB [24–26]. In turn, the synthesis of IκB α is upregulated by NF-κB [23]. The two p50–RelA dimers bind the adjacent NF-κB sites and interact through a protein contact. The two dimers clamp DNA from opposite faces of the double helix and form a topological trap of the bound DNA [27]. The modulatory region of HIV-1 LTR harbors numerous target sequences for a variety of cellular transcription factors such as NF–interleukin (IL)-6, cyclic AMP (cAMP) response element binding protein (CREB), Ets, and nuclear hormone receptors.

HIV-1 transcription is activated by viral Tat protein, which is a major viral transactivator required for HIV-1 replication. Tat plays a central role in the regulation of HIV-1 gene expression both at the level of mRNA and protein synthesis.

In the nucleus, Tat stimulates transcriptional elongation and the synthesis of full-length transcripts from the HIV-1 promoter. Tat binds to the bulge of HIV-1 viral RNA in the 5'-nontranslated region, TAR-RNA. In the cytoplasm, Tat acts as a translational activator of HIV-1 mRNAs. HIV-1 Tat also interacts with different cellular transcription factors. For example, to activate viral transcription, Tat binds to positive transcription elongation factor b (P-TEFb), which contains the kinase CDK9, [28, 29], interacts with cyclin T1 [30], and recruits histone acetyl transferases [31, 32].

Three other HIV-1 proteins – Vpr, Rev, and Nef – also affect viral transcription. Vpr functions as a positive regulator of HIV-1 transcription by arresting the cell cycle of infected cells in the G2 phase, which results in optimizing LTR-directed gene transcription and cooperating with Tat to enhance viral transcription [33, 34]. Rev shuttles between nucleus and cytoplasm and facilitates export of unspliced and singly spliced viral transcripts containing RRE RNA [5]. Although not participating in HIV-1 transcription directly, Nef enhances viral expression by upregulating the expression of factors that positively regulate LTR-driven transcription such as NF-AT [35, 36], NF-κB, AP-1, [37], signal transducers and activators of transcription STAT1 [38] and STAT3 [39], and CDK9 [40].

Assembly

Gag is the major driving force of HIV-1 assembly which occurs with assistance from host factors and cellular machinery at the host cell plasma membrane. HIV-1 assembly is a multistep process that includes (1) Gag targeting to the site of virus assembly, (2) binding of Gag to the lipid membrane bilayer, (3) Gag multimerization, and (4) budding and release of nascent virus particles (reviewed in Dupont et al. [41]). Gag and Gag-Pol are synthesized in the host cell cytoplasm and then transported to the plasma membrane where the evolving viral particle obtains its envelope and buds from the host cell. During assembly, viral genomic RNA, the Env glycoprotein complex, and the Gag-Pol precursor protein Pr160^{GagPol} are incorporated into the assembling particle.

The HIV-1 MA domain of Gag encodes a nuclear export signal, [42] and is responsible for targeting and binding to the plasma membrane. The N-terminal myristate moiety and highly basic region in MA interact with the negatively charged inner leaflet of the plasma membrane, resulting in stable binding. Interaction between the CA regions of Gag and Gag-Pol are critical for proper packaging of the Gag-Pol precursor. Gag polyproteins form small multimers in the cytoplasm and assemble into larger complexes at the cell membrane.

The membrane binding of Gag is regulated by the myristoyl switch, a conformation change during which the exposure and sequestration of the myristate moiety is affected by the degree of Gag multimerization [43]. When Gag multimerizes, the N-terminal myristate becomes exposed from the MA globular domain, resulting in higher affinity for the membrane [41]. The viral RNA facilitates Gag multimerization, and is critical for the formation of stable Gag/Gag-Pol complexes. The HIV-1 RNA acts as a scaffold for the multimerization of Gag and Gag-Pol, and stabilizes the viral core, preventing the collapse of the particle during processing of the Gag and Gag-Pol precursor proteins.

The packaging signal is the *cis*-acting sequence that directs viral RNA encapsidation. The HIV-1 packaging signal is represented by the four stem-loop structures. The secondary structure of the packaging signal and interaction between the packaging signal and the NC domain of Gag are critical for efficient encapsidation of viral RNA. NC contains two zinc-finger motifs flanked by highly basic sequences. RNA-mediated bridging by NC also plays an important role in Gag multimerization.

Nef plays a supporting role in Gag-Pol packaging by allowing a Gag/Gag-Pol/Nef complex to be more efficiently transported to the cell membrane. The HIV-1 accessory proteins Vpr and Vif are packaged into virions. Vpr incorporates into the virus particles via interaction with Gag p6. Association of HIV-1 Vif with the viral core at the time of viral RNA packaging is important for core stability. Efficient viral budding is closely related to HIV-1 PR activity. The regulation of PR function and timing is critical for proper viral assembly. During the later steps of the HIV-1 replication cycle, the interaction between Env and Gag (Pr55^{Gag}) proteins is critical for Env incorporation into infectious HIV-1 virions. Assembly is completed by budding of the immature particle from the cell.

Budding of virus particles from cellular membranes is driven by cellular endosomal sorting machinery including ESCRT-1 complex (endosomal sorting complexes required for transport) and associated factors, which are recruited by p6 to the site of virus assembly [44–46].

Maturation

Following budding, HIV maturation is initiated by proteolytic processing of Gag and Gag-Pol polyproteins, which induces conformational changes in the CA domain and results in the assembly of the distinctive conical capsid. The processing of the Gag and Gag-Pol precursors generates a critical transformation of virion morphology resulting in a remarkable transition from noninfectious viral particles to infectious virus with cone-shaped cores. The HIV-1 capsid is organized following the principles of fullerene cones, and the hexagonal CA lattice is stabilized by distinct interfaces [47].

Sequential processing of the Gag protein is critical for the maturation of HIV-1 from immature particles with a spherical capsid shell to mature particles with an electron-dense cone-shaped capsid core, reviewed in Morikawa [48]. HIV-1 PR recognizes the asymmetric shape of the peptide substrates as a target for cleavage. The first cleavage of the Gag-Pol polyprotein occurs between p2 and NC to release MA-CA-p2 and NC-PR-RT-IN. The second cleavage releases p6Pol-PR-RT-IN. The subsequent cleavages separate MA from CA-p2 and NC-p1 from p6, leading to capsid condensation and the formation of a spherical shell. Separation of the spacer proteins p2 and p1 is the final cleavage, which generates the mature conical core.

HIV-1 maturation converts the immature, donut-shaped particle to the mature virion, which contains a condensed conical core composed of a CA shell surrounding the viral RNA genome in a complex with NC and the viral enzymes RT and IN. In the mature HIV-1 envelope glycoprotein trimer, the three gp120 subunits are noncovalently bound to three membrane-anchored gp41 subunits.

Summary

This overview of HIV replication covers the most basic aspects of this complex and multistep process. For more detailed descriptions of HIV replication, the following reviews are recommended: Freed and Martin [49], Knipe and Howley [15], Sarafianos et al. [11], Mougel et al. [50], Neckhai et al. [51], Brady and Kashanchi [52], Ganser-Pornillos et al. [47], Morikawa [48], and Ono [41].

References

1. Jacks T, Power MD, Masiarz FR, Luciw PA, Barr PJ, Varmus HE. Characterization of ribosomal frameshifting in HIV-1 gag-pol expression. Nature. 1988;331:280–3.
2. Hill M, Tachedjian G, Mak J. The packaging and maturation of the HIV-1 Pol proteins. Curr HIV Res. 2005;3:73–85.
3. Arokium H, Kamata M, Chen I. Virion-associated Vpr of human immunodeficiency virus type 1 triggers activation of apoptotic events and enhances fas-induced apoptosis in human T cells. J Virol. 2009;83:11283–97.
4. Balasubramanyam A, Mersmann H, Jahoor F, Phillips TM, Sekhar RV, Schubert U, et al. Effects of transgenic expression of HIV-1 Vpr on lipid and energy metabolism in mice. Am J Physiol Endocrinol Metab. 2007;292:E40–48.
5. Cao Y, Liu X, De Clercq E. Cessation of HIV-1 transcription by inhibiting regulatory protein Rev-mediated RNA transport. Curr HIV Res. 2009;7:101–8.
6. Favaro JP, Borg KT, Arrigo SJ, Schmidt MG. Effect of Rev on the intranuclear localization of HIV-1 unspliced RNA. Virology. 1998;249:286–96.
7. Perales C, Carrasco L, Gonzalez ME. Regulation of HIV-1 env mRNA translation by Rev protein. Biochim Biophys Acta. 2005;1743:169–75.
8. Arnold M, Nath A, Hauber J, Kehlenbach RH. Multiple importins function as nuclear transport receptors for the Rev protein of human immunodeficiency virus type 1. J Biol Chem. 2006;281:20883–90.
9. Nedellec R, Coetzer M, Shimizu N, Hoshino H, Polonis VR, Morris L, et al. Virus entry via the alternative coreceptors CCR3 and FPRL1 differs by human immunodeficiency virus type 1 subtype. J Virol. 2009;83:8353–63.
10. Tilton JC, Doms RW. Entry inhibitors in the treatment of HIV-1 infection. Antiviral Res. 2010;85:91–100.
11. Sarafianos SG, Marchand B, Das K, et al. Structure and function of HIV-1 reverse transcriptase: molecular mechanisms of polymerization and inhibition. J Mol Biol. 2009;385:693–713.
12. McColl DJ, Chen X. Strand transfer inhibitors of HIV-1 integrase: bringing IN a new era of antiretroviral therapy. Antiviral Res. 2010;85:101–18.
13. Poeschla EM. Integrase, LEDGF/p75 and HIV replication. Cell Mol Life Sci. 2008;65:1403–24.
14. Schroder AR, Shinn P, Chen H, Berry C, Ecker JR, Bushman F. HIV-1 integration in the human genome favors active genes and local hotspots. Cell. 2002;110:521–9.
15. Knipe DM, Howley PM, editors. Fields virology. 5th ed. Philadelphia: Wolters Kluwer Health/Lippincott Williams & Wilkins; 2007.
16. Brass AL, Dykxhoorn DM, Benita Y, et al. Identification of host proteins required for HIV infection through a functional genomic screen. Science. 2008;319:921–6.
17. Nabel G, Baltimore D. An inducible transcription factor activates expression of human immunodeficiency virus in T cells [published erratum appears in Nature 1990 Mar 8;344(6262):178]. Nature. 1987;326:711–3.
18. Cron RQ, Bartz SR, Clausell A, Bort SJ, Klebanoff SJ, Lewis DB. NFAT1 enhances HIV-1 gene expression in primary human CD4 T cells. Clin Immunol. 2000;94:179–91.
19. Ranjbar S, Tsytsykova AV, Lee SK, et al. NFAT5 regulates HIV-1 in primary monocytes via a highly conserved long terminal repeat site. PLoS Pathog. 2006;2:e130.
20. Bates DL, Barthel KK, Wu Y, et al. Crystal structure of NFAT bound to the HIV-1 LTR tandem kappaB enhancer element. Structure. 2008;16:684–94.
21. Davis N, Ghosh S, Simmons DL, et al. Rel-associated pp 40: an inhibitor of the rel family of transcription factors. Science. 1991;253:1268–71.
22. Ganchi PA, Sun SC, Greene WC, Ballard DW. I kappa B/MAD-3 masks the nuclear localization signal of NF-kappa B p65 and requires the transactivation domain to inhibit NF-kappa B p65 DNA binding. Mol Biol Cell. 1992;3:1339–52.
23. Sun SC, Ganchi PA, Ballard DW, Greene WC. NF-kappa B controls expression of inhibitor I kappa B alpha: evidence for an inducible autoregulatory pathway. Science. 1993;259:1912–5.
24. DiDonato JA, Hayakawa M, Rothwarf DM, Zandi E, Karin M. A cytokine-responsive IkappaB kinase that activates the transcription factor NF-kappaB. Nature. 1997;388:548–54.
25. Mercurio F, Murray BW, Shevchenko A, et al. IkappaB kinase (IKK)-associated protein 1, a common component of the heterogeneous IKK complex. Mol Cell Biol. 1999;19:1526–38.
26. Mercurio F, Zhu H, Murray BW, et al. IKK-1 and IKK-2: cytokine-activated IkappaB kinases essential for NF-kappaB activation. Science. 1997;278:860–6.
27. Stroud JC, Oltman A, Han A, Bates DL, Chen L. Structural basis of HIV-1 activation by NF-kappaB–a higher-order complex of p50:RelA bound to the HIV-1 LTR. J Mol Biol. 2009;393:98–112.
28. Mancebo HS, Lee G, Flygare J, et al. P-TEFb kinase is required for HIV Tat transcriptional activation in vivo and in vitro. Genes Dev. 1997;11:2633–44.
29. Yang X, Gold MO, Tang DN, et al. TAK, an HIV Tat-associated kinase, is a member of the cyclin-dependent family of protein kinases and is induced by activation of peripheral blood lymphocytes and differentiation of promonocytic cell lines. Proc Natl Acad Sci U S A. 1997;94:12331–6.

30. Garber ME, Wei P, Jones KA. HIV-1 Tat interacts with cyclin T1 to direct the P-TEFb CTD kinase complex to TAR RNA. Cold Spring Harb Symp Quant Biol. 1998;63:371–80.
31. Deng L, de la Fuente C, Fu P, et al. Acetylation of HIV-1 Tat by CBP/P300 increases transcription of integrated HIV-1 genome and enhances binding to core histones. Virology. 2000;277:278–95.
32. Kiernan RE, Vanhulle C, Schiltz L, et al. HIV-1 tat transcriptional activity is regulated by acetylation. EMBO J. 1999;18:6106–18.
33. Jowett JB, Planelles V, Poon B, Shah NP, Chen ML, Chen IS. The human immunodeficiency virus type 1 vpr gene arrests infected T cells in the G2+M phase of the cell cycle. J Virol. 1995;69: 6304–13.
34. Planelles V, Jowett JB, Li QX, Xie Y, Hahn B, Chen IS. Vpr-induced cell cycle arrest is conserved among primate lentiviruses. J Virol. 1996;70:2516–24.
35. Manninen A, Huotari P, Hiipakka M, Renkema GH, Saksela K. Activation of NFAT-dependent gene expression by Nef: conservation among divergent Nef alleles, dependence on SH3 binding and membrane association, and cooperation with protein kinase C-theta. J Virol. 2001;75:3034–7.
36. Manninen A, Renkema GH, Saksela K. Synergistic activation of NFAT by HIV-1 nef and the Ras/MAPK pathway. J Biol Chem. 2000;275:16513–7.
37. Varin A, Manna SK, Quivy V, et al. Exogenous Nef protein activates NF-kappa B, AP-1, and c-Jun N-terminal kinase and stimulates HIV transcription in promonocytic cells. Role in AIDS pathogenesis. J Biol Chem. 2003;278:2219–27.
38. Federico M, Percario Z, Olivetta E, et al. HIV-1 Nef activates STAT1 in human monocytes/macrophages through the release of soluble factors. Blood. 2001;98:2752–61.
39. Percario Z, Olivetta E, Fiorucci G, et al. Human immunodeficiency virus type 1 (HIV-1) Nef activates STAT3 in primary human monocyte/macrophages through the release of soluble factors: involvement of Nef domains interacting with the cell endocytotic machinery. J Leukoc Biol. 2003;74:821–32.
40. Simmons A, Aluvihare V, McMichael A. Nef triggers a transcriptional program in T cells imitating single-signal T cell activation and inducing HIV virulence mediators. Immunity. 2001;14: 763–77.
41. Ono A. HIV-1 assembly at the plasma membrane: Gag trafficking and localization. Future Virol. 2009;4:241–57.
42. Dupont S, Sharova N, DeHoratius C, et al. A novel nuclear export activity in HIV-1 matrix protein required for viral replication. Nature. 1999;402:681–5.
43. Tang C, Loeliger E, Luncsford P, Kinde I, Beckett D, Summers MF. Entropic switch regulates myristate exposure in the HIV-1 matrix protein. Proc Natl Acad Sci U S A. 2004;101:517–22.
44. Bieniasz PD. Late budding domains and host proteins in enveloped virus release. Virology. 2006;344:55–63.
45. Demirov DG, Freed EO. Retrovirus budding. Virus Res. 2004;106:87–102.
46. Morita E, Sundquist WI. Retrovirus budding. Annu Rev Cell Dev Biol. 2004;20:395–425.
47. Ganser-Pornillos BK, Yeager M, Sundquist WI. The structural biology of HIV assembly. Curr Opin Struct Biol. 2008;18:203–17.
48. Morikawa Y. HIV capsid assembly. Curr HIV Res. 2003;1:1–14.
49. Freed EO, Martin MA. HIVs and their replication. In: Howley PM, Knipe DM, editors. Fields virology. Philadelphia: Lippincott, Williams and Wilkins; 2007. p. 2107–85.
50. Mougel M, Houzet L, Darlix JL. When is it time for reverse transcription to start and go? Retrovirology. 2009;6:24.
51. Nekhai S, Jerebtsova M, Jackson A, Southerland W. Regulation of HIV-1 transcription by protein phosphatase 1. Curr HIV Res. 2007;5:3–9.
52. Brady J, Kashanchi F. Tat gets the "green" light on transcription initiation. Retrovirology. 2005;2:69.

Hepatitis C: Natural History

Mark S. Sulkowski

Introduction

Overall, HIV infection has a detrimental effect on the natural history of HCV disease; HIV-infected patients are less likely to clear hepatitis C viremia following acute infection, have higher HCV RNA loads, and experience more rapid progression of HCV-related liver disease than those without HIV infection [1–4].

Acute HCV Infection

Following acute HCV infection, HIV-infected persons are more likely to progress to chronic infection compared to those who are HIV seronegative. In the era before effective ART was available, Thomas et al. [1] reported that HCV clearance occurred more frequently in nonblacks and those not infected with HIV (adjusted OR, 2.19; 95% CI, 1.26–3.47). More recently, clearance of acute HCV infection has been linked to a single-nucleotide polymorphism (rs12979860) located ~3 kilobases upstream of the IL28B gene, which encodes the type III interferon (lambda interferon) [5–7]. In one study, HIV-infected and uninfected persons C/C genotype were significantly more likely to resolve their infection. Interestingly, among persons with the C/C genotype, the rate of HCV resolution was 52.2 and 53.1% in those with and without HIV infection, respectively; by contrast, HIV-infected persons with the unfavorable genotype (C/T or T/T) were less likely to clear hepatitis C viremia (20.6%) compared to those not infected with HIV (30%) (Fig. 11.1) [6]. Interestingly, HIV infection and IL28B genotype does not seem to affect adversely the likelihood of HCV clearance following the treatment of acute HCV infection with interferon-based therapy [8, 9].

Chronic HCV Infection

As early as 1993, Eyster and colleagues [3] reported that HCV RNA levels were higher in people with hemophilia who became HIV infected than in those who remained HIV negative, and liver failure occurred exclusively in coinfected patients. Among HCV-positive patients with hemophilia who were prospectively monitored, Goedert and colleagues estimated the 16-year cumulative incidence of end-stage liver disease (ESLD) among men with and without HIV to be 14.0 and 2.6%, respectively [4]. Among those men with coinfection, the ESLD risk increased 8.1-fold with HBV surface antigenemia, 2.1-fold with CD4 cell counts below 200 cells/mm^3, and 1.04-fold per additional year of age. The impact of HIV on HCV disease in the time era prior to effective HIV therapy was summarized in a meta-analysis of multiple studies that assessed the correlation between HIV coinfection and the progression of HCV-related liver disease. HIV coinfection was associated with a relative risk of ESLD of 6.14 and a relative risk of cirrhosis of 2.07 when compared with HCV monoinfection [10]. Thus, in the absence of effective antiretroviral therapy, HCV disease is clearly worsened by coinfection with HIV.

Since the availability of effective HIV therapy [highly active antiretroviral therapy (HAART)] in 1996, there has been more uncertainty regarding the impact of HIV on the natural history of hepatitis C. While some studies have been contradictory, the treatment of HIV disease has generally been associated with decreased risk of liver disease progression, particularly with the use of antiretroviral agents with minimal hepatotoxicity risk. For example, Qurishi et al. [11] reported a lower risk of liver mortality in persons who lived long enough to receive effective ART. Brau and colleagues [12] estimated the liver fibrosis progression rate in 274 HIV-infected and 382 HIV-uninfected patients. Among persons

M.S. Sulkowski (✉)
Department of Medicine, Johns Hopkins University
School of Medicine, Room 445, 600 N. Wolfe Street,
1830 Bldg, Baltimore, MD 21212, USA
e-mail: msulkowski@jhmi.edu

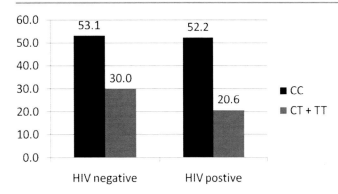

Fig. 11.1 Frequency of hepatitis C clearance according to HIV serostatus and IL28B genotype (rs1299860) adapted from Thomas DL, Thio CL, Martin MP, Qi Y, Ge D, O'Huigin C et al. Genetic variation in IL28B and spontaneous clearance of hepatitis C virus. Nature 2009; 461(7265):798–801 [6]

with effectively controlled HIV-infection, defined as an HIV RNA level <400 c/mL and/or CD4 cell count >500/mm^3, the fibrosis progression rate was similar in persons with and without HIV infection. By contrast, those with inadequately treated HIV disease had accelerated liver disease progression compared to those without HIV coinfection. Similarly, Verma and coworkers [13] found that persons treated initially with effective ART had a risk of developing cirrhosis which was similar to HCV monoinfected control patients. More recently, two studies failed to detect evidence of significant fibrosis progression in HCV coinfected who underwent paired liver biopsies. The first study was a prospective study designed to assess the effect of long-term interferon therapy on HCV disease progression. In this trial, Sherman et al. [14] observed no or minimal fibrosis in the control subjects, leading the study to stopped early due to the lack of observed progression in the cohort of coinfected patients. In a second study, Schuppan and colleagues [15] observed similar fibrosis progression rate in HCV-infected patients with and without HIV disease. Together, these and other studies have led some expert panels to recommend that all HIV-infected patients receive antiretroviral therapy independent of other factors such as CD4 cell count due to the benefit of delaying liver disease progression [16, 17].

However, other studies have found that while ART may be beneficial, HIV/HCV coinfected patients remain at greater risk for liver disease progression than those with HCV monoinfection. For example, in the Amsterdam Cohort study, the coinfected drug users had an increased risk of dying of HCV disease compared to those without HIV infection; this risk did not decrease in the era of effective antiretroviral therapy [18]. In the USA, Wise et al. [19] conducted a case-control study to evaluate 63,189 hepatitis C deaths using multiple-cause-of death data from 1999 to 2004 (during which effective ART was available). There was a strong association of HCV death with HIV infection, alcohol use and hepatitis B; approximately, 10.5% observed deaths due to HCV occurred with HIV coinfection. Likewise, several studies have reported rapid fibrosis progression in persons with HIV/HCV coinfection on paired liver biopsies. Sulkowski and colleagues [20] reported that significant fibrosis progression was observed over a 3-year period in ~24% of HIV/HCV coinfected persons with no or minimal fibrosis on first liver biopsy; ART exposure did not appear to be protective in this cohort. Similarly, Macias et al. [21] observed fibrosis progression of at least one stage over a 3-year period in 55% of 135 HIV/HCV coinfected who underwent two liver biopsies. Finally, Thein and coworkers [22] conducted a meta-analysis involving 27 studies on the natural history of HCV including 7,666 individuals (HIV/HCV coinfection, $n=2,636$; HCV monoinfection, $n=4,970$). The overall relative risk (RR) of cirrhosis among coinfected patients relative to monoinfected patients was 2.11 (95% CI 1.51–2.96). This increased risk of cirrhosis in patients with coinfection relative to those with monoinfection was similar in person taking ART (RR 1.72, 95% CI 1.06–2.80) and those not taking ART (RR 2.49, p5% CI 1.81–3.42) (Fig. 11.2). Furthermore, in meta-regression analysis, Thein et al. did not detect a significant association detected between ART and risk of cirrhosis. Thus, in these natural history studies, antiretroviral therapy did not appear to account fully for the more rapid disease progression in HIV/HCV coinfected persons.

Clearly, additional research is needed to fully understand the long-term effect of ART on HCV disease progression. Nonetheless, as a consequence of the high HCV prevalence, accelerated HCV disease progression and effective antiretroviral therapy, HCV-related morbidity and mortality is substantial in HIV-infected persons. In one study, Gebo and coworkers [23] evaluated rates of admission at an urban hospital from 1995 to 2000 among HIV-infected patients and found that admissions for liver-related complications among HCV-positive patients increased nearly fivefold from 5.4 to 26.7 admissions per 100 person-years during that time. Similarly, among 23,441 HIV-infected North American and European patients followed in the Data Collection on Adverse Events of Anti-HIV Drugs (DAD) study, liver disease was the second leading cause of death, with an incidence rate of 0.23 cases per 100 person-years follow-up behind HIV/AIDS (0.59 cases per 100 person-years) and ahead of cardiovascular disease (0.14 cases per 100 person-years) [24]. In a survey of 340 French HIV treatment centers, liver disease accounted for 15.4% of all deaths observed in 2005 and, among those dying from liver disease, 25% were due to hepatocellular carcinoma. By contrast, HBV-related liver deaths remained stable during the same time period [25]. Thus, in the context of effective treatment of HIV disease, HCV deaths due primarily to liver failure and hepatocellular will continue to be an important cause of mortality in HIV-infected persons. However, more effective

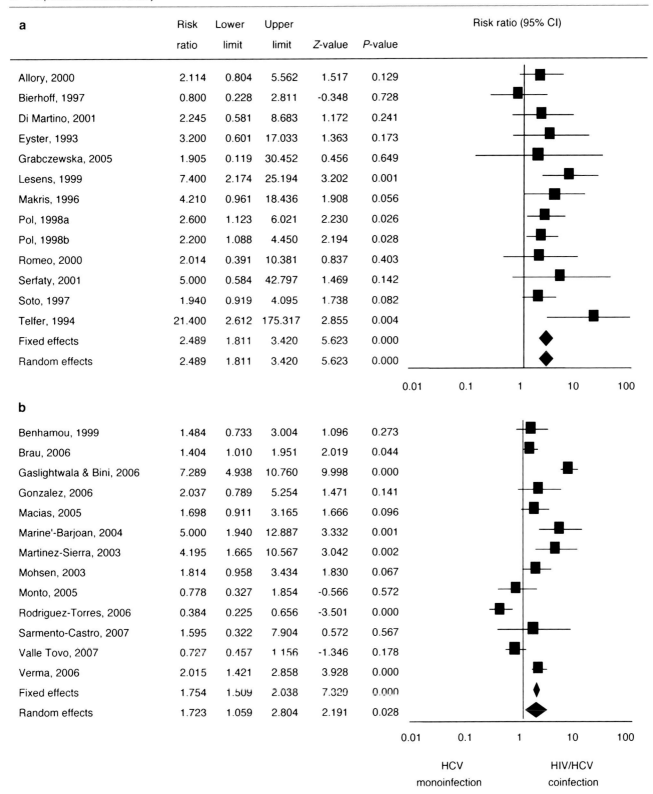

Fig. 11.2 Risk ratios of cirrhosis among individuals monoinfected with hepatitis C virus monoinfected and individuals coinfected with HIV/HCV. (**a**) Non-HAART group; and (**b**) HAART group. Adapted from Thein HH, Yi Q, Dore GJ, Krahn MD. Natural history of hepatitis C virus infection in HIV-infected individuals and the impact of HIV in the era of highly active antiretroviral therapy: a meta-analysis. AIDS 2008; 22(15):1979–1991 [22]

HCV treatment strategies may prevent liver mortality in this population. Berenguer and colleagues [26] reported that HIV/HCV coinfected patients who achieved a sustained viral response following treatment with interferon plus ribavirin were markedly less likely to die from liver disease compared to those without eradication of HCV. Thus, while not effective for all coinfected patients, the treatment of HCV infection in HIV-infected patients at risk for cirrhosis is strongly recommended [27].

Effect of HCV on HIV Infection

The effect of HCV infection on HIV disease progression is less clear than the effect of HCV. Indeed, in meta-analysis of 27 studies in the era of effective antiretroviral therapy, HCV was associated with an increased risk of overall mortality, but HCV coinfection was not associated with an increased risk for AIDS-defining events compared to HIV monoinfection (risk ratio 1.12; 95% CI, 0.82–1.51) [28]. Some studies report impaired immune reconstitution in patients with HIV/HCV coinfection treated with ART compared to those with HIV alone [29]; however, this effect has not been observed in other studies [30, 31]. In a meta-analysis of 8 studies, the mean increase in CD4 cell count following ART was slightly lower (−33.4 cells/mm^3) in coinfected persons compared to those monoinfected; this difference is not likely to be clinically relevant [32]. Patients with underlying viral hepatitis are more likely to experience hepatotoxicity on ART [33, 34]. However, for most persons, this does not impact ART delivery, since the majority (approximately 90%) of coinfected patients do not develop severe hepatotoxicity. In some studies, the risk of ART-associated hepatotoxicity is greater in coinfected persons with advanced hepatic fibrosis, suggesting that liver disease staging prior to initiating ART may be useful to stratify the risk of hepatotoxicity [35]. Interestingly, effective treatment of HCV infection has been associated with reduced risk of ART-associated liver injury, suggesting the effect is directly related to active HCV infection [36, 37].

Conclusion

In the era of effective antiretroviral therapy, HCV infection is an increasing cause of morbidity and mortality among HIV-infected persons. The factors underlying the increasing burden of liver disease due to HCV include (1) the markedly decreased impact of HIV/AIDS due to HAART, (2) the high prevalence of HCV infection due to shared modes of transmission, (3) the adverse effect of HIV infection on HCV disease progression. Treatment of HIV disease with safe, effective antiretroviral therapy appears to partially ameliorate the negative impact of HIV infection; however, the relative risk of cirrhosis and liver failure remain higher in persons with HIV/HCV coinfection compared to those with HCV monoinfection despite the advent of HAART. Successful HCV treatment with eradication of chronic infection is likely to have the greatest impact on the natural history of HCV in HIV-infected persons.

References

1. Thomas DL, Astemborski J, Rai RM, Anania FA, Schaeffer M, Galai N, et al. The natural history of hepatitis C virus infection: host, viral, and environmental factors. JAMA. 2000;284(4):450–6.
2. Eyster ME, Fried MW, Di Bisceglie AM, Goedert JJ. Increasing hepatitis C virus RNA levels in hemophiliacs: relationship to human immunodeficiency virus infection and liver disease. Blood. 1994;84: 1020–3.
3. Eyster ME, Diamondstone LS, Lien JM, Ehmann WC, Quan S, Goedert JJ. Natural history of hepatitis C virus infection in multitransfused hemophiliacs: effect of coinfection with human immunodeficiency virus. The Multicenter Hemophilia Cohort Study. J Acquir Immune Defic Syndr. 1993;6:602–10.
4. Goedert JJ, Eyster ME, Lederman MM, Mandalaki T, De Moerloose P, White GC, et al. End-stage liver disease in persons with hemophilia and transfusion-associated infections. Blood. 2002;100(5):1584–9.
5. Ge D, Fellay J, Thompson AJ, Simon JS, Shianna KV, Urban TJ et al. Genetic variation in IL28B predicts hepatitis C treatment-induced viral clearance. Nature 2009.
6. Thomas DL, Thio CL, Martin MP, Qi Y, Ge D, O'Huigin C, et al. Genetic variation in IL28B and spontaneous clearance of hepatitis C virus. Nature. 2009;461(7265):798–801.
7. Grebely J, Petoumenos K, Hellard M, Matthews GV, Suppiah V, Applegate T et al. Potential role for Interleukin-28B genotype in treatment decision-making in recent hepatitis C virus infection. Hepatology 2010.
8. Dore GJ, Hellard M, Matthews GV, Grebely J, Haber PS, Petoumenos K, et al. Effective treatment of injecting drug users with recently acquired hepatitis C virus infection. Gastroenterology. 2010;138(1):123–35.
9. Matthews GV, Hellard M, Haber P, Yeung B, Marks P, Baker D, et al. Characteristics and treatment outcomes among HIV-infected individuals in the Australian Trial in Acute Hepatitis C. Clin Infect Dis. 2009;48(5):650–8.
10. Graham CS, Baden LR, Yu E, Mrus JM, Carnie J, Heeren T, et al. Influence of human immunodeficiency virus infection on the course of hepatitis c virus infection: a meta-analysis. Clin Infect Dis. 2001;33(4):562–9.
11. Qurishi N, Kreuzberg C, Lüchters G, Effenberger W, Kupfer B, Sauerbruch T, et al. Effect of antiretroviral therapy on liver-related mortality in patients with HIV and hepatitis C coinfection. Lancet. 2004;362(9397):1708–13.
12. Brau N, Salvatore M, Rios-Bedoya CF, Fernandez-Carbia A, Paronetto F, Rodriguez-Orengo JF, et al. Slower fibrosis progression in HIV/HCV-coinfected patients with successful HIV suppression using antiretroviral therapy. J Hepatol. 2006;44(1):47–55.
13. Verma S, Wang CH, Govindarajan S, Kanel G, Squires K, Bonacini M. Do type and duration of antiretroviral therapy attenuate liver fibrosis in HIV-hepatitis C virus-coinfected patients? Clin Infect Dis. 2006;42(2):262–70.
14. Sherman KE, Andersen JW, Butt AA, Umbleja T, Alston B, Koziel MJ et al. Sustained long-term antiviral maintenance therapy in HCV/HIV-coinfected patients (SLAM-C). J Acquir Immune Defic Syndr. 2010.

15. Schuppan D, Stolzel U, Oesterling C, Somasundaram R. Serum assays for liver fibrosis. J Hepatol. 1995;22(2 Suppl):82–8.
16. Panel on Antiretroviral Guidelines for Adults and Adolescents. Guidelines for the use of antiretroviral agents in HIV-1-infected adults and adolescents. Department of Health and Human and Services. 2009:1–161.
17. Rockstroh JK, Bhagani S, Benhamou Y, Bruno R, Mauss S, Peters L, et al. European AIDS Clinical Society (EACS) guidelines for the clinical management and treatment of chronic hepatitis B and C coinfection in HIV-infected adults. HIV Med. 2008;9(2):82–8.
18. Smit C, van den Berg C, Geskus R, Berkhout B, Coutinho R, Prins M. Risk of hepatitis-related mortality increased among hepatitis C virus/HIV-coinfected drug users compared with drug users infected only with hepatitis C virus: a 20-year prospective study. J Acquir Immune Defic Syndr. 2008;47(2):221–5.
19. Wise M, Finelli L, Sorvillo F. Prognostic factors associated with hepatitis C disease: a case-control study utilizing U.S. multiple-cause-of-death data. Public Health Rep. 2010;125(3):414–22.
20. Sulkowski MS, Mehta SH, Torbenson MS, Higgins Y, Brinkley SC, de Oca RM, et al. Rapid fibrosis progression among HIV/hepatitis C virus-co-infected adults. AIDS. 2007;21(16):2209–16.
21. Macias J, Berenguer J, Japon MA, Giron JA, Rivero A, Lopez-Cortes LF, et al. Fast fibrosis progression between repeated liver biopsies in patients coinfected with human immunodeficiency virus/hepatitis C virus. Hepatology. 2009;50(4):1056–63.
22. Thein HH, Yi Q, Dore GJ, Krahn MD. Natural history of hepatitis C virus infection in HIV-infected individuals and the impact of HIV in the era of highly active antiretroviral therapy: a meta-analysis. AIDS. 2008;22(15):1979–91.
23. Gebo KA, Diener-West M, Moore RD. Hospitalization rates differ by hepatitis C satus in an urban HIV cohort. J Acquir Immune Defic Syndr. 2003;34(2):165–73.
24. Weber R, Sabin CA, Friis-Moller N, Reiss P, El Sadr WM, Kirk O, et al. Liver-related deaths in persons infected with the human immunodeficiency virus: the D:A:D study. Arch Intern Med. 2006;166(15):1632–41.
25. Salmon-Ceron D, Rosenthal E, Lewden C, Bouteloup V, May T, Burty C, et al. Emerging role of hepatocellular carcinoma among liver-related causes of deaths in HIV-infected patients: The French national Mortalite 2005 study. J Hepatol. 2009;50(4):736–45.
26. Berenguer J, Alvarez-Pellicer J, Martin PM, Lopez-Aldeguer J, Von-Wichmann MA, Quereda C, et al. Sustained virological response to interferon plus ribavirin reduces liver-related complications and mortality in patients coinfected with human immunodeficiency virus and hepatitis C virus. Hepatology. 2009;50(2):407–13.
27. Ghany MG, Strader DB, Thomas DL, Seeff LB. Diagnosis, management, and treatment of hepatitis C. Hepatology (in press).
28. Chen TY, Ding EL, Seage Iii GR, Kim AY. Meta-analysis: increased mortality associated with hepatitis C in HIV-infected persons is unrelated to HIV disease progression. Clin Infect Dis. 2009;49(10):1605–15.
29. Greub G, Ledergerber B, Battegay M, Grob P, Perrin L, Furrer H, et al. Clinical progression, survival, and immune recovery during antiretroviral therapy in patients with HIV-1 and hepatitis C virus coinfection: the Swiss HIV Cohort Study. Lancet. 2000; 356(9244):1800–5.
30. Sulkowski MS, Moore RD, Mehta SH, Chaisson RE, Thomas DL. Hepatitis C and progression of HIV disease. JAMA. 2002; 288(2):199–206.
31. Chung RT, Evans SR, Yang Y, Theodore D, Valdez H, Clark R, et al. Immune recovery is associated with persistent rise in hepatitis C virus RNA, infrequent liver test flares, and is not impaired by hepatitis C virus in co-infected subjects. AIDS. 2002;16(14): 1915–23.
32. Miller MF, Haley C, Koziel MJ, Rowley CF. Impact of hepatitis C virus on immune restoration in HIV-infected patients who start highly active antiretroviral therapy: a meta-analysis. Clin Infect Dis. 2005;41(5):713–20.
33. Sulkowski MS, Thomas DL, Chaisson RE, Moore RD. Hepatotoxicity associated with antiretroviral therapy in adults infected with human immunodeficiency virus and the role of hepatitis C or B virus infection. JAMA. 2000;283(1):74–80.
34. Nunez M. Hepatotoxicity of antiretrovirals: incidence, mechanisms and management. J Hepatol. 2006;44(1 Suppl):S132–9.
35. Aranzabal L, Casado JL, Moya J, Quereda C, Diz S, Moreno A, et al. Influence of liver fibrosis on highly active antiretroviral therapy-associated hepatotoxicity in patients with HIV and hepatitis C virus coinfection. Clin Infect Dis. 2005;40(4):588–93.
36. Labarga P, Soriano V, Vispo ME, Pinilla J, Martin-Carbonero L, Castellares C, et al. Hepatotoxicity of antiretroviral drugs is reduced after successful treatment of chronic hepatitis C in HIV-infected patients. J Infect Dis. 2007;196(5):670–6.
37. Soriano V, Puoti M, Sulkowski M, Cargnel A, Benhamou Y, Peters M. Care patients coinfected with HIV and hepatitis C virus: 2007 updated recommendations from the HCV–HIV International Panel. AIDS. 2007;21:1073–89.

Natural History of Hepatitis B Virus in HIV-Infected Patients

Chloe L. Thio

Introduction

Both human immunodeficiency virus-1 (HIV) and hepatitis B virus (HBV) are transmitted via mucosal and percutaneous routes, so approximately 10% of HIV-infected persons worldwide are coinfected with HBV. In the USA, the HIV Outpatient Study found that between 1996 and 2007, the prevalence of HBV was stable ranging from 7.8 to 8.6% with the greatest fraction being in men who have sex with men [1]. Thus, chronic HBV is a continuing important coinfection in the HIV-infected population.

Since HIV suppresses the immune system, it initially seems logical that HBV disease would be more severe in coinfected patients. Conversely, the weakened immune response from HIV may not accelerate liver disease progression since HBV-related liver disease is primarily immune mediated. Several natural history studies shed light on the balance between these opposing forces. In this chapter, we review these studies on the natural history of acute and chronic HBV in HIV-infected persons, including a few studies conducted during the era of potent antiretroviral therapy (ART).

Acute Hepatitis B Virus Infection

Insight into the incidence of acute HBV in HIV-infected individuals comes from the Adult/Adolescence Spectrum of HIV Project using data from 1998 to 2001 [2]. There were 316 cases of acute HBV among 16,248 HIV-infected patients yielding an incidence rate of 12.2/1,000 person-years (PYs), which is substantially higher compared to the rate in the general population (0.033 cases/1,000 PYs) [3]. The incidence was higher in black subjects (RR 1.4, 95% confidence interval (CI) 1.0–2.0), those with alcoholism (RR 1.7, 95% CI 1.2–2.3), those with active injection drug users (RR 1.6, 95% CI 1.1–2.4), and those with AIDS-defining conditions (RR 1.5, 95% CI 1.2–1.9). The incidence rate in those taking ART either with or without lamivudine was lower (RR 0.5) as was the rate in those who had received at least one dose of the HBV vaccine (RR 0.6, 95% CI 0.4–0.9). A study of US military and their dependents found that incident HBV infections in HIV-infected subjects were higher in the pre-ART era compared to the post-ART era (4 to 1.1 cases per 100 person-years, $P<0.001$); however, from 2000 to 2008, there was a trend toward an increased risk that was not statistically significant [4].

Several studies have investigated the risk of an acute infection developing into chronic HBV in HIV-infected individuals. Two studies from 1991 demonstrated that chronic HBV was more likely to occur in HIV-infected compared to HIV-uninfected men who have sex with men [5, 6]. Bodsworth et al. [5] found that after acute HBV, 23% of the HIV-infected compared to 4% of the HIV-uninfected men became chronically infected. Furthermore, among the HIV-infected men, the CD4+ T-cell counts were significantly lower in those who developed chronic HBV compared to those who did not (342 cells/mm^3 versus 547 cells/mm^3; $P<0.005$). In those who acquired HIV and HBV simultaneously, the risk of developing chronic HBV was twice as high at 40%. A more recent study reported similar numbers with a 2.62-fold (95% CI 1.78–3.85) increased risk of developing chronic HBV if HIV-infected compared to uninfected [7]. In this study, HIV-infected persons on ART at the time of an acute HBV infection, had a reduced risk of becoming chronically HBV infected compared to those who were not on ART (OR 0.18, 95% CI 0.04–0.79). Most subjects were on ART that included anti-HBV agents, so this study could not determine whether it was the ART, HBV active agents in ART, or both that led to the risk reduction. Thus, HIV increases the risk for developing chronic HBV (Table 12.1).

C.L. Thio (✉)
Department of Medicine, Johns Hopkins University School of Medicine, 855 N. Wolfe Street, Baltimore, MD 21205, USA
e-mail: cthio@jhmi.edu

Table 12.1 Known effects of HIV on the natural history of hepatitis B virus (HBV)

Effects on acute HBV
  Increases risk for becoming chronic
Effects on chronic HBV
  Lower HBeAg seroconversion
  Higher HBV DNA
  Increased cirrhosis
  Increased liver-related mortality
  Increased isolated anti-HBc
  Lower ALT
Effects of HAART
  Increased hepatotoxicity
  Unclear effects on liver disease

HAART highly active antiretroviral therapy, *anti-HBc* hepatitis B core antibody, *HBeAg* hepatitis B "e" antigen, *ALT* alanine aminotransferase

Chronic Hepatitis B

Once chronic HBV is established, HIV also affects hepatitis Be antigen (HBeAg) clearance, HBV replication, and liver disease. In a study of 150 men who have sex with men, the 82 HIV–HBV coinfected men were more likely to be HBeAg positive compared to the 68 HBV monoinfected men ($P<0.001$) [8]. Mai et al. [9] also demonstrated decreased HBeAg seroconversion in 56 HIV–HBV coinfected men compared to 43 HBV monoinfected men, but they also found more HBV replication as documented by increased likelihood of detectable HBV DNA ($P<0.0005$). CD4+ T-cell count was not associated with HBeAg status or detectable HBV DNA. Despite evidence of more HBV replication in the HIV–HBV coinfected subjects, their ALT levels were lower. Other studies have demonstrated similar findings of higher HBV DNA but lower ALT levels in HIV–HBV coinfected individuals [10].

Unfortunately, these lower ALT levels, which may be from a suppressed immune response, do not translate to less liver disease. In one cross-sectional study, cirrhosis on liver biopsy was found in 28% of the 65 HIV–HBV coinfected men who have sex with men compared to only 13% of the 67 HBV monoinfected men ($P=0.04$) [10]. Given the increased risk of cirrhosis, it is not surprising that increased liver-related mortality has been demonstrated in HIV–HBV coinfected individuals. In the MACS cohort where 5,293 men were studied, the 326 HIV–HBV coinfected men had a liver mortality rate of 14.2 per 1,000 person-years (PYs) compared to 0.8/1,000 PYs in HBV monoinfected, 1.7/1,000 PYs in HIV monoinfected, and 0/1,000 PYs in those without HIV or HBV [11]. In a clinic-based population followed from 1993 to 2001, liver deaths occurred in 15% of HIV–HBV coinfected subjects compared to 6% of HIV monoinfected subjects [12]. Thus, it is clear that HIV accelerates the progression of HBV-related liver disease despite an overall depressed immune system.

A fulminant form of chronic HBV known as *fibrosing cholestatic hepatitis*, which was first described in patients on immunosuppressive therapy, has also been found in HIV–HBV coinfected patients [13]. This form of hepatitis is uncommon. It is attributed to cytopathic injury of hepatocytes by HBV and is characterized histologically by ballooning of hepatocytes with evidence of significant cholestasis. It has also been described in a case of HBV reactivation in a patient with advanced HIV disease [14].

Effects of Acute HIV on Chronic Hepatitis B

Only one study has examined chronic HBV during acute HIV seroconversion. In this study of nine men with HBV, HBV DNA levels were determined before and after HIV seroconversion [15]. Interestingly, HBV DNA levels in five of the men decreased dramatically with a mean of 6.29 log copies/ml and loss of HBeAg. Three of the men had stable HBV DNA levels and only one man had an increase in HBV DNA. The authors hypothesized that this unexpected reduction in HBV DNA may have been due to release of cytokines (e.g., interferon) with acute HIV. In the one man who was followed until CD4 T-cell decline, the HBV DNA gradually increased above the original value. Thus, this is consistent with the above studies since in those studies the HBV DNA was likely determined years after HIV seroconversion.

Seroreversion

Seroreversion, which is defined as spontaneous loss of anti-HBs, occurs infrequently and is not clearly more common in the setting of HIV infection. In a study of 263 HIV-infected and 50 HIV un-infected individuals followed for a median of 21 and 13 months, respectively, the seroreversion rate was 1.8/100 PYs in both groups [16]. In the HIV Atlanta Veteran Affairs Cohort Study, 229 HIV-infected patients with anti-HBs had repeat testing and only six became anti-HBs negative for a rate of 0.019/100 PYs [17]. Combining their six cases with 18 others in literature, 45% of those who lost anti-HBs had a decline in CD4+ T-cell counts, 62% had transaminase elevations at the time of anti-HBs loss, and two had stopped lamivudine with subsequent loss of anti-HBs.

By contrast, some studies have shown a higher seroreversion rate in the setting of HIV infection. A study of hemophiliacs found that seroreversion occurred in 13% of HIV-infected individuals and in 0% of the HIV-negative patients [18]. Biggar et al. [19] followed 13 HIV-infected and 12 HIV-uninfected subjects, who had anti-HBs from a prior HBV infection, for 3 years. Of the HIV-infected subjects, 6 had undetectable (4 subjects) or borderline (2 subjects) anti-HBs levels, whereas only 1 HIV-uninfected subject had borderline levels ($P<0.05$).

Isolated Anti-HBc Serology

Isolated anti-HBc serological pattern is defined as negative HBsAg and anti-HBs but positive anti-HBc. It is more common in HIV-infected individuals with the prevalence ranging from 9 to 61.7%. A large study from Taiwan of 2,351 HIV-infected individuals found that 411 (17.5%) had isolated anti-HBc [20] and 963 (41%) had past infection, which was defined as anti-HBs and anti-HBc positive. Isolated anti-HBc was associated with older age, lower CD4 T-cell count, and higher HIV RNA levels than those with past infection. In contrast to other studies [21–23] isolated anti-HBc subjects were less likely to be infected with hepatitis C, but this may be attributable to more sexual transmission rather than injection drug use in this cohort. In the multivariate analysis, older age (OR 1.03, 95% CI 1.02–1.04) and CD4 T-cell counts <100 cells/mm^3 (OR 1.52, 95% CI 1.03–2.23) were associated with isolated anti-HBc. Serum HBV DNA was found in 8.3% of 277 subjects with isolated anti-HBc who were tested and in 14.3% of 56 subjects with anti-HBs who were tested. The median HBV DNA in the two groups was 3.67 and 4.35 log cp/ml, respectively.

Several other studies have investigated whether occult hepatitis B (detectable HBV DNA without HBsAg) is present in HIV-infected patients with isolated anti-HBc, but there is no consensus. The prevalence of detectable HBV DNA ranges from 0 to 89% with most studies reporting HBV DNA values $\leq 10^3$ IU/ml [24], as reviewed by Sun et al. [20]. The study by Hofer et al. [24] was at the upper limit of the prevalence range (89%), but the prospective design of that study was unique and may explain the high prevalence. In that study, a subject was counted as being HBV DNA positive if any one of the visits tested had a detectable HBV DNA. Thus, it is possible that low levels of HBV DNA are intermittently detectable supporting the hypothesis that these individuals have chronic HBV.

An important, unanswered question is whether isolated anti-HBc has clinical ramifications, which has been addressed in studies focusing on whether survival is different in patients with isolated anti-HBc. In one study, this serological pattern was not associated with lower survival [25]. By contrast, Hoffmann et al. [26] found a 3.6-fold increased risk of death in MACS men with isolated anti-HBc compared to those never infected with HBV. Surprisingly, of the 5 men with isolated anti-HBc who died, four died from cardiovascular causes suggesting that there are behavioral or environmental differences or perhaps higher levels of inflammation that increased the risk for cardiovascular disease. In HBV monoinfected subjects, there is some evidence that occult HBV increases the risk for development of hepatocellular carcinoma [27], but whether this is true for HIV-infected subjects has not been studied. Additional studies are needed to determine whether isolated anti-HBc has long-term consequences.

The etiology of the isolated anti-HBc pattern is not known but possibilities include decline in anti-HBs with immunosuppression, chronic HBV with low levels of HBsAg, and false positive serology. From the available studies, it is not clear which of these accounts for the majority of isolated anti-HBc cases. One longitudinal study from Taiwan of 179 patients followed subjects with isolated anti-HBc for a median of 5 years and found that 40.8% developed anti-HBs, 10.1% lost all markers, and 3.9% developed HBsAg. In a study of women at risk for HIV infection, 322 had isolated anti-HBc of whom 282 were HIV+ [25]. After a median of 7.5 years of follow-up, 20.2% acquired anti-HBs and 2.5% developed HBsAg. Acquisition of anti-HBs was associated with an increase in CD4 T-cell count and HAART use at >50% of the visits in univariate analysis, but only the latter remained in a multivariate analysis. HBsAg acquisition was associated with CD4 count <200 cells/mm^3 at study entry. These two studies would suggest that loss of anti-HBs, especially with decline in CD4 T-cell counts, was the most common cause for isolated anti-HBc. However, this hypothesis is not supported by several studies that have looked at the anamnestic response to HBV vaccine. A study from Thailand found that only 7% of 28 subjects with an isolated anti-HBc had an anamnestic response to HBV vaccine [23]. In another study, [28] 24% of subjects with isolated anti-HBc had an anamnestic to vaccine, although 47% of those that were anti-HBe positive had an anamnestic response compared to only 7% in the anti-HBe negative group. Thus, further studies are needed to determine the etiology of the isolated anti-HBc serological pattern.

Hepatocellular Carcinoma

There are limited data on whether HIV affects the development of hepatocellular carcinoma (HCC). One French study of 822 HIV-infected individuals of whom 8% were coinfected with HBV found that 22% of deaths in the HIV–HBV coinfected group were liver-related compared to 2% in the HIV monoinfected group [29]. The liver-related deaths in the monoinfected group were attributed to alcoholic cirrhosis. In the HIV–HBV coinfected group, 50% of the liver-related deaths were from HCC compared to 13% of the liver-related deaths in the HIV monoinfected group. This study suggests that HIV may accelerate the development of HBV-related HCC, although the ideal comparison group, which would be HBV monoinfected subjects, was not included in this study.

The Swiss HIV cohort study found that immunosuppression from HIV increased the risk for HCC among men who have sex with men, in whom the primary risk factor for HCC was HBV. They found that for every 100 cell/ml decrease in CD4 T-cell count, there was a 1.68-fold increased risk of developing HCC (95% CI 1.15–2.46) [30].

ART and Hepatitis B Natural History

We are just beginning to address the question of how ART affects the natural history of HBV. Several studies have demonstrated that HIV–HBV coinfected patients have an increased incidence of hepatotoxicity (defined as aminotransferase elevations) from ART compared to HIV monoinfected patients, especially those with high HBV DNA levels [31, 32]. However, it is not known if this hepatotoxicity translates into more liver disease. Sellier et al. [33] examined risk factors associated with advanced liver disease in a cohort of 107 HIV–HBV coinfected patients with 66% of African origin and the remainder of European origin. During the median 4.8 year follow-up, 78% received ART. Univariate analysis found multiple associations with advanced liver disease including male gender, higher HIV RNA and HBV DNA levels, and elevated transaminases. In multivariate analysis, AST level (HR per 10 unit increase 1.79, $P<0.001$) was the only one that remained associated with increased risk for advanced liver disease and lamivudine use was protective (HR per month of treatment, 0.96, $P<0.001$). Over a median 4.8 year follow-up period, there were 4 liver deaths giving an incidence of liver-related mortality of 0.7/1,000 person-years. In the EuroSIDA cohort, 9% of the 9,802 patients had chronic HBV. The liver mortality rate on ART was also 0.7/1,000 person-years and was significantly higher than in the HIV monoinfected subjects (0.2/1,000 person-years) [34]. However, the liver mortality rate prior to ART in that cohort is not known. This issue was addressed in the MACS cohort, where the liver mortality rate over a median 7-year follow-up on ART was higher than in these other cohorts (17/1,000 person-years), and surprisingly, it was not significantly lower than during the era prior to ART (14/1,000 person-years) [11, 26]. This difference in mortality rates compared to the other studies may be due to the longer follow-up in the MACS and development of lamivudine-resistant HBV. However, what this study cannot disentangle is whether the stable liver-mortality rate in the pre-ART and ART eras is a result of lack of impact of ART on liver disease or due to longer life expectancy and decreased death from AIDS-related causes.

Supporting the idea that the stable rate is due to the longer life expectancy, other studies have shown an improvement in liver-related death on ART that includes lamivudine. Puoti et al. [35] found a liver mortality rate of 7.5/1,000 PYs in HIV–HBV coinfected subjects, but the liver-related death per year of lamivudine use was reduced by 27% (OR 0.73 95% CI 0.59–0.9, $P=0.004$) over 4 years of follow-up. There are also data to support the hypothesis that ART has negative effects on the liver. In the D:A:D study, 23441 HIV-infected subjects of whom 6.8% had chronic hepatitis B were followed for a median of 3.5 years [36]. Those with chronic hepatitis B had an increased risk for liver-related death of 3.7 fold (95% CI 2.4–5.9). Multivariate showed increased risk of liver-related death for every year on mono or dual therapy before HAART. In addition, they found an 11% (95% CI 2–21%, $P=0.02$) increased risk for liver death for every year on ART after adjusting for CD4 T cell count.

Summary

Together, the studies clearly demonstrate that HIV has negative effects on HBV infection including decreased immune response to the virus and accelerated liver disease progression. ART leads to increased hepatotoxicity with chronic hepatitis B, but the longer-term effects of this are not yet clear. It is also not yet understood how HIV affects liver disease, but one intriguing idea is an increase in microbial translocation associated with HIV that leads to an increase in fibrosis [37]. It is not known if HBV modulates this process as well. Table 12.2 summarizes key questions related to HIV–HBV coinfection. Further work is needed to understand HIV and liver fibrosis as well as liver disease in HIV–HBV coinfected patients in the ART era.

Table 12.2 Outstanding questions on effect of HIV on natural history of hepatitis B virus (HBV)

Does HIV affect seroreversion?
Is occult hepatitis B more common in HIV infection?
What are the long-term consequences of isolated anti-HBc in HIV coinfection?
Why is the isolated anti-HBc prevalence higher in the setting of HIV infection?
Does HIV accelerate the development of hepatocellular carcinoma?
How does ART affect HBV-related liver disease?

anti-HBc hepatitis B core antibody

References

1. Spradling PR, Richardson JT, Buchacz K, Moorman AC, Brooks JT. Prevalence of chronic hepatitis B virus infection among patients in the HIV Outpatient Study, 1996–2007. J Viral Hepat. 2010; 17(12):879–86.
2. Kellerman SE, Hanson DL, McNaghten AD, Fleming PL. Prevalence of chronic hepatitis B and incidence of acute hepatitis B infection in human immunodeficiency virus-infected subjects. J Infect Dis. 2003;188:571–7.
3. Goldstein ST, Alter MJ, Williams IT, et al. Incidence and risk factors for acute hepatitis B in the United States, 1982–1998: implications for vaccination programs. J Infect Dis. 2002;185:713–9.
4. Chun HM, Fieberg AM, Hullsiek KH, et al. Epidemiology of Hepatitis B virus infection in a US cohort of HIV-infected individuals during the past 20 years. Clin Infect Dis. 2010;50:426–36.
5. Bodsworth NJ, Cooper DA, Donovan B. The influence of human immunodeficiency virus type 1 infection on the development of the hepatitis B carrier state. J Infect Dis. 1991;163:1138–40.
6. Hadler SC, Judson FN, O'Malley PM, et al. Outcome of hepatitis B virus infection in homosexual men and its relation to prior human immunodeficiency virus infection. J Infect Dis. 1991;163:454–9.
7. Landrum ML, Fieberg AM, Chun HM, et al. The effect of human immunodeficiency virus on hepatitis B virus serologic status in co-infected adults. PLoS One. 2010;5:e8687.
8. Bodsworth N, Donovan B, Nightingale BN. The effect of concurrent human immunodeficiency virus infection on chronic hepatitis B: a study of 150 homosexual men. J Infect Dis. 1989;160: 577–82.
9. Mai AL, Yim C, O'Rourke K, Heathcote EJ. The interaction of human immunodeficiency virus infection and hepatitis B virus infection in infected homosexual men. J Clin Gastroenterol. 1996;22:299–304.
10. Colin JF, Cazals-Hatem D, Loriot MA, et al. Influence of human immunodeficiency virus infection on chronic hepatitis B in homosexual men. Hepatology. 1999;29:1306–10.
11. Thio CL, Seaberg EC, Skolasky RL, et al. HIV-1, hepatitis B virus, and risk of liver-related mortality in the Multicenter AIDS Cohort Study (MACS). Lancet. 2002;360:1921–6.
12. Bonacini M, Louie S, Bzowej N, Wohl AR. Survival in patients with HIV infection and viral hepatitis B or C: a cohort study. AIDS. 2004;18:2039–45.
13. Fang JW, Wright TL, Lau JY. Fibrosing cholestatic hepatitis in patient with HIV and hepatitis B. Lancet. 1993;342:1175.
14. Poulet B, Chapel F, Deny P, et al. Fibrosing cholestatic hepatitis by B virus reactivation in AIDS. Ann Pathol. 1996;16:188–91.
15. Thio CL, Netski DM, Myung J, Seaberg EC, Thomas DL. Changes in hepatitis B virus DNA levels with acute HIV infection. Clin Infect Dis. 2004;38:1024–9.
16. Rodriguez Mendez ML, Gonzalez-Quintela A, Aguilera A, Barrio E. Prevalence, patterns, and course of past hepatitis B virus infection in intravenous drug users with HIV-1 infection. Am J Gastroenterol. 2000;95:1316–22.
17. Rouphael NG, Talati NJ, Rimland D. Hepatitis B reverse seroconversion in HIV-positive patients: case series and review of the literature. AIDS. 2007;21:771–4.
18. Drake JH, Parmley RT, Britton HA. Loss of hepatitis B antibody in human immunodeficiency virus-positive hemophilia patients. Pediatr Infect Dis J. 1987;6:1051–4.
19. Biggar RJ, Goedert JJ, Hoofnagle J. Accelerated loss of antibody to hepatitis B surface antigen among immunodeficient homosexual mean infected with HIV. N Engl J Med. 1987;318(10):630–1.
20. Sun HY, Lee HC, Liu CE et al. Factors associated with isolated anti-hepatitis B core antibody in HIV-positive patients: impact of compromised immunity. J Viral Hepat. 2010;17(8):578–87.
21. Gandhi RT, Wurcel A, McGovern B, et al. Low prevalence of ongoing hepatitis B viremia in HIV-positive individuals with isolated antibody to hepatitis B core antigen. J Acquir Immune Defic Syndr. 2003;34:439–41.
22. French AL, Operskalski E, Peters M, et al. Isolated hepatitis B core antibody is associated with HIV and ongoing but not resolved hepatitis C virus infection in a cohort of US women. J Infect Dis. 2007;195:1437–42.
23. Jongjirawisan Y, Ungulkraiwit P, Sungkanuparph S. Isolated antibody to hepatitis B core antigen in HIV-1 infected patients and a pilot study of vaccination to determine the anamnestic response. J Med Assoc Thai. 2006;89:2028–34.
24. Hofer M, Joller-Jemelka HI, Grob PJ, Luthy R, Opravil M. Frequent chronic hepatitis B virus infection in HIV-infected patients positive for antibody to hepatitis B core antigen only. Swiss HIV Cohort Study. Eur J Clin Microbiol Infect Dis. 1998;17:6–13.
25. French AL, Lin MY, Evans CT, et al. Long-term serologic follow-up of isolated hepatitis B core antibody in HIV-infected and HIV-uninfected women. Clin Infect Dis. 2009;49:148–54.
26. Hoffmann CJ, Seaberg EC, Young S et al. Hepatitis B and long-term HIV outcomes in co-infected HAART recipients. AIDS 2009; 23(14):1881–9.
27. Ikeda K, Kobayashi M, Someya T, et al. Occult hepatitis B virus infection increases hepatocellular carcinogenesis by eight times in patients with non-B, non-C liver cirrhosis: a cohort study. J Viral Hepat. 2009;16:437–43.
28. Gandhi RT, Wurcel A, Lee H, et al. Response to hepatitis B vaccine in HIV-1-positive subjects who test positive for isolated antibody to hepatitis B core antigen: implications for hepatitis B vaccine strategies. J Infect Dis. 2005;191:1435–41.
29. Salmon-Ceron D, Lewden C, Morlat P, et al. Liver disease as a major cause of death among HIV infected patients: role of hepatitis C and B viruses and alcohol. J Hepatol. 2005;42:799–805.
30. Clifford GM, Rickenbach M, Polesel J, et al. Influence of HIV-related immunodeficiency on the risk of hepatocellular carcinoma. AIDS. 2008;22:2135–41.
31. Hoffmann CJ, Charalambous S, Martin DJ, et al. Hepatitis B virus infection and response to antiretroviral therapy (ART) in a South African ART program. Clin Infect Dis. 2008;47:1479–85.
32. Audsley J, Seaberg E, Sasadeusz J et al. Factors associated with hepatotoxicity in an international HIV/HBV co-infected cohort on long-term HAART. 17th Conference on Retroviruses and Opportunistic Infections 2010. Abstract 691.
33. Sellier P, Schnepf N, Jarrin I, et al. Description of liver disease in a cohort of HIV/HBV coinfected patients. J Clin Virol. 2010; 47.13–7.
34. Konopnicki D, Mocroft A, De Wit S, et al. Hepatitis B and HIV: prevalence, AIDS progression, response to highly active antiretroviral therapy and increased mortality in the EuroSIDA cohort. AIDS. 2005;19:593–601.
35. Puoti M, Cozzi-Lepri A, Arici C, et al. Impact of lamivudine on the risk of liver-related death in 2,041 HBsAg- and HIV-positive individuals: results from an inter-cohort analysis. Antivir Ther. 2006;11: 567–74.
36. Weber R, Sabin CA, Friis-Moller N, et al. Liver-related deaths in persons infected with the human immunodeficiency virus: the D:A:D study. Arch Intern Med. 2006;166:1632–41.
37. Balagopal A, Philp FH, Astemborski J, et al. Human immunodeficiency virus-related microbial translocation and progression of hepatitis C. Gastroenterology. 2008;135:226–33.

Other Hepatitis Viruses and HIV Infection

José V. Fernández-Montero and Vincent Soriano

Introduction

Although hepatitis B virus (HBV) and hepatitis C virus (HCV) are the most frequent agents of liver disease in HIV-infected individuals, infection with other hepatitis viruses may lead to either acute episodes of liver damage (i.e., A and E) or chronic hepatic disease (i.e., Delta). Hepatotropic viruses other than B and C are often forgotten in the setting of HIV infection, and awareness and knowledge about their potential role as the cause of disease are important.

Hepatitis A in HIV

The hepatitis A virus (HAV) was identified in 1973 [1]. It displays a worldwide distribution (Fig. 13.1), causing only acute hepatitis, but being responsible for considerable morbidity and mortality, especially when infection is acquired in adulthood.

Virology

HAV is a 27-nm diameter particle, nonenveloped, icosahedral, which contains a positive-stranded RNA genome. The virus belongs to the *Heparnavirus* genus within the Picornaviridae family. The HAV genome comprised 7,474 nucleotides, which are divided into three regions: a 5′ untranslated region (742 nucleotides), a single long open reading frame (ORF) that encodes a 2,227 amino-acid polypeptide (6,681 nucleotides), and a 3′ noncoding region (63 nucleotides). The polypeptide encoded by the ORF is cotranslationally processed by a viral protease, resulting in four structural and seven nonstructural proteins. There is a single viral serotype, with four different genotypes, although no significant biological differences have been found among them [2].

The hepatocyte infection cycle begins when the virus binds to a receptor found in the cell surface. After infection, HAV acts as an mRNA, spending its entire vital cycle in the hepatocyte cytoplasm, where it experiences replication using a RNA-dependent RNA polymerase, coded by the virus itself. When enough viral RNA and virion proteins have been produced, viral assembly begins, forming mature virions. The whole replication cycle lasts for 5–10 h. Unlike other picornaviruses, HAV does not cause cytolysis when exiting the cell, and therefore, cytopathology is caused mainly by cellular immune responses.

Epidemiology

HAV spreads via the fecal–oral route and is more prevalent in low socioeconomic areas in which a lack of adequate sanitation and poor hygienic practices facilitate spreading of the virus. HAV infection can occur either sporadically or as epidemic outbreaks, showing a trend for cyclic infections. Worldwide around 1.4 million people get infected with HAV every year. In some developing countries, where hygienic conditions are poor, the lifelong risk for infection with HAV is above 90%, with most infections occurring in early childhood. Epidemic outbreaks are not frequent in developing countries, since adolescents and adults are already immune at those ages. In other areas where sanitary conditions are variable, infections are less common in the early childhood, with a higher incidence in adults, causing frequent epidemic outbreaks. Finally, in developed countries, where hygienic conditions are good, infection rates are low, and HAV infections are more common in adolescents and some high-risk groups, such as household and sexual contacts of infected persons, injecting and noninjecting drug users, men who have sex with men (MSM), people traveling to high-risk

J.V. Fernández-Montero (✉)
Department of Infectious Diseases, Carlos III Hospital,
Calle Sinesio Delgado 10, Madrid 28029, Spain
e-mail: jvicfer@gmail.com

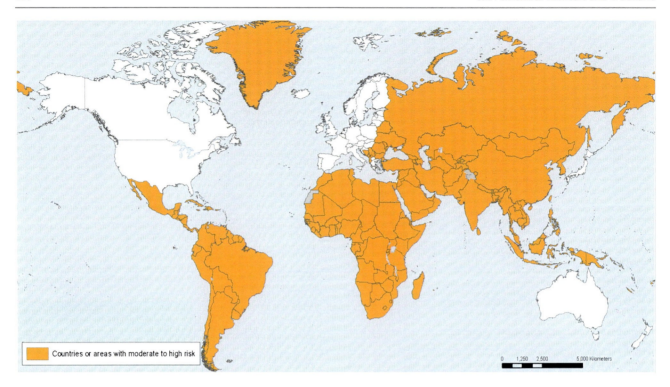

Fig. 13.1 Areas at risk of hepatitis A virus infection

areas, and persons with occupational exposure to HAV (such as laboratory or sewage workers).

Clinical Manifestations

HAV infection usually results in an acute, self-limited illness and only rarely leads to fulminant hepatic failure [3], which occurs more commonly in patients with underlying liver disease, particularly chronic hepatitis C. This was illustrated in a study of 163 patients with chronic hepatitis B and 432 with chronic hepatitis C who were prospectively followed for 7 years [4]. HAV superinfection was diagnosed in 27 patients. An uncomplicated course occurred in nine of the ten patients with hepatitis B in comparison with fulminant hepatic failure in 7 of the 17 patients with chronic hepatitis C; six of these patients died.

The manifestations also vary with age. HAV infection is usually silent or subclinical in children. By contrast, infection in adults presents with mild to severe forms. The incubation period ranges from 2 to 6 weeks, after which the illness begins in symptomatic patients. HAV is rarely associated with a relapsing or cholestatic clinical illness and may serve as a trigger for autoimmune hepatitis in genetically susceptible individuals. Morbidity and mortality differ significantly between age groups. HAV infection in the adulthood is associated with more severe symptoms and a higher mortality (1.8%). Hepatitis A does not appear to be worse in HIV-infected patients when compared to HIV-negative persons [5], although HAV-RNA viremia may be more prolonged [6].

Prevention

Individuals suffering from acute hepatitis A are contagious during the incubation period and remain so for about a week after jaundice appears [7]. Prevention of spread to others can be aided by adherence to sanitary practices such as handwashing, heating foods appropriately, and avoiding water and foods from endemic areas. Handwashing is highly effective in preventing the transmission of HAV, since the virus may survive for up to 4 h on the fingertips [8]. Chlorination and certain disinfecting solutions (household bleach 1:100 dilution) are enough to inactivate the virus. In hospitalized patients, use of gloves by health-care workers and an appropriate handling of biological material from patients are strongly recommended.

Apart from hygiene measures, the most important and efficacious was for preventing HAV infection is immunization. Inactivated and attenuated HAV vaccines have been developed and evaluated in human clinical trials [9]. However, only vaccines made from inactivated HAV have been evaluated for efficacy in controlled clinical trials [10]. The HAV vaccines currently licensed in the USA are the single-antigen vaccines HAVRIX® (manufactured by GlaxoSmithKline) and VAQTA® (manufactured by Merck) and the combination vaccine TWINRIX® (containing both HAV and HBV antigens; manufactured by GlaxoSmithKline). All are inactivated vaccines.

In HIV-negative persons, the HAV vaccine is highly immunogenic and efficacious. Protective levels of antibodies develop in 97–100% of individuals within 1 month of the first dose and in virtually all subjects after the second dose. The level of protection against clinical hepatitis is above 80% after a single dose [11]. The combined hepatitis A–hepatitis B vaccine is also highly efficacious [10]. Successful immunization in healthy persons is thought to confer protection for over 10 years, although immunity may be lifelong. Response rates are generally reduced in HIV-infected persons compared to HIV-negative persons, and correlate with the CD4 cell count at the time of vaccination [12]. Overall rates are 50–95%, but may be below 9% when CD4 counts are <200 cells/mL. By contrast, responses above 95% are seen in subjects with CD4 counts > 300–500 cells/mL. Plasma HIV RNA suppression on highly active antiretroviral therapy (HAART) is associated with improved anti-HAV antibody levels following vaccination [13]. Increasing the number of doses may also improve immunicity [14].

A trial involving 99 HIV-infected patients assessed the immunological efficacy and safety of a three-dose schedule of HAV vaccine in comparison with the standard two-dose schedule [15], showing an increase in antibody titers in the three-dose group. No significant differences in terms of adverse events were found. Duration of protection in HIV-infected persons is unknown, but might be shorter than in HIV-negative individuals. The low anti-HAV response rates in HIV-infected patients makes advisable to measure anti-HAV antibodies after vaccination, to ensure that the patient developed protective antibody titers. Supplementary vaccine doses might be advisable for nonresponders. IL-2 has been used as immune response enhancer in one study [16]; although the CD4 count rose significantly, no differences in terms of HAV-antibodies were found when comparing patients receiving HAART and those receiving HAART plus IL-2.

The HAV vaccine is safe and well tolerated in HIV-infected individuals [17] Injection site reactions are the most frequent side effects. Malaise and headache for 1–2 days may occur occasionally. Serious allergic reactions are very rare. Currently, HAV vaccination is recommended to all HAV-susceptible, HIV-infected persons. Certain patients, such as those with chronic liver disease, MSM, IDUs, or persons traveling to areas of intermediate or high endemicity are at special risk, and immunization should be particularly recommended in them. HIV-infected persons with CD4 counts >300 cells/mL may follow the standard vaccination schedule and receive two doses at 0 and 6–12 months. In those patients with CD4 counts <300 cells/mL a third dose may be considered. HIV-infected persons at risk for the infection should receive a boosting dose every 5 years. Finally, in patients with CD4 counts <200 cells/mL, human normal immunoglobin (HNIG) 500 mg might be considered together with the vaccine before travel.

Hepatitis D in HIV

Hepatitis D virus (HDV) is a unique defective RNA agent, first identified in 1977 [18], that requires the presence of HBV for its replication and expression. HDV infection can occur either simultaneously with HBV (coinfection) or as a superinfection in chronic HBV carriers. Infection with HDV is associated with higher rates of liver cirrhosis and, particularly in coinfection episodes, with fulminant hepatitis.

Virology

HDV has been classified in the *Deltavirus* genus [19]. It shares some similarities with viroids and plant satellite viruses, mainly in terms of genomic organization and replication mechanisms [20]. The HDV virion is a large particle, approximately 36 nm diameter, with an external lipoprotein envelope provided by HBV. Beneath this envelope, the viral capsid, formed by a structure of delta antigen (HDAg), can be found. This capsid contains the HDV genome, formed by a single-stranded, circular RNA, 1,700 nucleotides long.

The HDV RNA genome has six ORFs, three on the genomic strand and three on the antigenomic strand. One ORF encodes the HDAg, while the others do not seem to be actively transcribed. Two different antigens exist: a small 24-kDa HDAg, 155 amino acids long, and a large 27 kDa HDAg, 214 amino acids long. While the small HDAg accelerates HDV RNA synthesis, the large one inhibits it. Nevertheless, the presence of the large HDAg is necessary for virion morphogenesis [21]. HDV RNA replication occurs through a "double rolling circle model" in which the genomic strand is replicated by a host RNA polymerase to yield a multimeric linear structure that is autocatalytically cleaved into linear monomers and ligated into circular HDV RNA.

Epidemiology

Similarly to HBV, HDV is spread mainly through parenteral exposure. Worldwide, more than 350 million people are chronically infected with HBV, of whom around 15–20 million are superinfected with HDV [22]. Several regions, as the Mediterranean basin, the Middle East, Central Africa, and the northern countries of South America remain endemic for HDV (Fig. 13.2). In other countries with lower prevalence of HDV infection, viral transmission occurs in limited settings, such as within communities of IDUs.

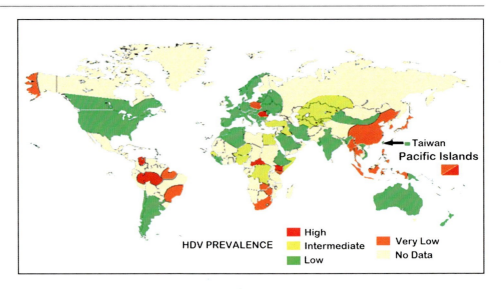

Fig. 13.2 Worldwide distribution of hepatitis delta virus

Several studies carried out in the 1980s and 1990s showed rates of HDV infection as high as 25% among HBsAg-positive individuals [23]. After the implementation of HBV vaccination programs, the prevalence of HDV infection has decreased dramatically in the Western world [24]. Improvements in socioeconomic conditions and an increased awareness of the risk of transmitting infectious diseases have contributed to this decrease as well. However, the decline appears to have stopped, and some resurgence of HDV has been noticed both in the Mediterranean area and in Central Europe, mainly as result of immigration flows from highly endemic regions.

At least eight HDV genotypes have been identified [19]. In terms of HDV genotype distribution, genotype 1 shows a global distribution, being the predominant variant both in Europe and in North America. Genotype 2 is found mainly in the Far East, while genotype 3 predominates in South America. Genotypes 4–8 have mostly been identified in African patients [25].

Clinical Manifestations

The clinical sequelae of HDV infection encompass a spectrum of manifestations from fulminant liver failure to the asymptomatic carrier state. Clinical features vary depending on the chronification of HDV infection. Acute HBV and HDV coinfection leads to complete viral clearance of both viruses in more than 90% of cases, but it may lead to severe acute hepatitis with the potential for a fulminant course. By contrast, only a minority of chronic HBsAg carriers experiencing HDV superinfection clear HDV [21]. Outbreaks of acute hepatitis D have been described worldwide [26, 27]. Nevertheless, the global incidence of acute HDV infection has significantly decreased in comparison with two decades ago largely due to the introduction of HBV vaccination programs.

Chronic HDV infection leads to more severe liver disease than chronic HBV monoinfection, and is associated with an accelerated course of liver fibrosis, an increased risk of hepatocellular carcinoma, and early decompensation in the setting of liver cirrhosis [28]. A study of 299 patients followed for up to 28 years found that persistent HDV replication was associated with annual rates of development of cirrhosis and liver cancer of 4% and 2.8%, respectively [29]. Overall, patients chronically infected with HDV suffer from a shorter survival [30].

Distinct HDV genotypes may be associated with different clinical outcomes. The genetic variability is significant in HDV [31]. Infection with HDV genotype 1 has shown a lower remission rate and more adverse outcomes [30] than infection with genotype 2. Genotypes 2 and 4 have been found in East Asia, causing relatively mild disease [32]. However, a genotype 2b variant has been found to be related with accelerated progression to cirrhosis [33]. HDV superinfection of HBV genotype F has particularly been associated with episodes of fulminant hepatitis [34]. Of note, while the genotype of HBV does not seem to affect the interaction of HBsAg with HDV, the HDV genotype may influence the efficiency of assembly of the HDV antigen with HBsAg to constitute virions. Finally, amino-acid sequence variations in HBsAg have shown to influence the assembly efficiency of HDV genotypes 2 and 4 [35].

Diagnosis

Due to the dependence of HDV from HBV, the presence of HBsAg is necessary for the diagnosis of HDV infection. The additional presence of IgM antibody to hepatitis B core antigen (IgM anti-HBc) is necessary for the diagnosis of acute HBV–HDV coinfection. All HIV-infected individuals positive for HBsAg should be tested for anti-HDV IgG antibodies. It is also advisable to repeat the test yearly or in case they develop an unexpected increase in ALT levels [36]. There is no evidence supporting direct HDV-RNA testing in the absence of anti-HDV antibodies as far as antibodies develop in almost every individual infected with HDV. It is important to consider, however, that a positive result for the presence of anti-HDV antibodies does not necessarily indicate active hepatitis D. Although waning of HDV-RNA has been reported in some individuals, indicating recovery from HDV infection, this is rarely seen in the HIV setting, and most anti-HDV patients with HIV infection display detectable HDV viremia.

Several laboratory techniques are currently available for the diagnosis of HDV infection. HDV-RNA can be detected in serum by either molecular hybridization or RT-PCR assays. Serum HDV-RNA is an early and sensitive marker of HDV replication in acute hepatitis D [37]. RT-PCR assays have shown higher sensitivity than hybridization tools [38]. It should be noticed, however, that due to extensive sequence heterogeneity of different HDV isolates with only a few conserved genomic regions, it is difficult to choose suitable primers for the amplification of HDV-RNA. Furthermore, the secondary and tertiary structures of the HDV-RNA may hamper efficient amplification even when highly conserved regions are targeted [39]. RT-PCR assays can also be useful for monitoring and assessing the eradication of HDV infection in patients with remission of liver disease after therapy [40]. A cross-sectional study conducted in a large series of chronic hepatitis delta patients [41] using real-time RT-PCR has allowed to assess the replicative profiles and mutual interactions between HBV and HDV in chronic carriers, showing a dynamic fluctuating profile, with different patterns of viral dominance over time.

Detection of anti-HDV antibodies, both IgM and IgG, can be detected by EIAs or RIAs. Total anti-HDV antibody may be recognized usually after 4 weeks of acute infection; thus, its clinical value is limited unless repeated testing is performed [42]. Nevertheless, anti-HDV seroconversion may be the only way to diagnose acute HDV infection in the absence of other markers of HDV infection. High titers of anti-HDV IgG are present in chronic HDV infection. Anti-HDV IgG shows a good correlation with HDV replication and may help in differentiating current from past HDV infection. Anti-HDV IgM can also be detected by EIAs or RIAs, but the availability of such techniques is limited. IgM anti-HDV is present during chronic HDV infection, and titers correlate with the level of HDV replication and potentially with severity of liver disease [43]. IgM anti-HDV gradually disappears from serum in patients who have persistent remission after successful therapy or liver transplantation.

Finally, both HDAg and HDV-RNA can be detected in liver tissues routinely processed for histopathologic evaluation. HDAg can be detected by direct immunofluorescence or immunohistochemical staining. However, as many as 50% of liver biopsy specimens from patients who have been infected with HDV for 10 or more years may be negative for HDAg, suggesting that HDV replication levels may decline with time [44].

From a clinical perspective, in countries with a high prevalence of HDV infection as well as in subjects with history of injection drug use who are HBsAg+, HDV testing should not be forgotten. Initial screening should begin with total anti-HDV. When possible, the diagnosis should be confirmed by immunohistochemical staining of liver biopsies for HDAg or by RT-PCR assays for HDV-RNA in serum. At this time, HDV-RNA quantitation is only useful if antiviral treatment is indicated, as far as there is no evidence that serum HDV-RNA levels correlate with any clinical marker of activity or liver disease staging [45]. Following success in the evaluation of liver fibrosis in chronic hepatitis B and C [46], noninvasive assessment of liver fibrosis in hepatitis delta using serum biomarkers or elastography is rapidly expanding in Europe. However, preliminary data with tests as APRI have shown poor correlation with liver fibrosis staging in delta hepatitis [47].

Treatment

The main aim of treatment of hepatitis D is to eradicate or to achieve long-term suppression of both HDV and HBV replication. Suppression of HDV replication is generally accompanied by normalization of serum aminotransferases and improvement of necroinflammatory activity on liver biopsy. Suppression of HDV replication is documented by loss of detectable HDV-RNA in serum and/or HDAg in the liver. A secondary end point is the eradication of HBV infection, with HBsAg to anti-HBs seroconversion. Eradication of HBV infection with development of anti-HBs will protect from re-infection with HBV as well as HDV. Patients who have cleared HDV but who remain HBsAg+ are still at risk for recurrence and/or re-infection with HDV.

Currently, there is no well-established treatment for HDV infection. Several therapeutic strategies have been proposed (Table 13.1). As far as different patterns of viral dominance between HDV and HBV and occasionally HCV exist, diverse therapeutic approaches can be explored. As previously mentioned, viral dominance may show a dynamic and complex pattern, hence adaptation of treatment during patient's follow-up is advisable.

Several nucleoside and nucleotide analogues have been assessed as possible therapy for HDV infection. Most have shown no activity against HDV. This is the case of famciclovir, which failed to provide antiviral activity during a 6-month

Table 13.1 Main clinical trials for the treatment of hepatitis delta

Trial	N	Clinical setting	Treatment	Outcome
Yurdaydin et al. [48]	15	CHD	FCV	No effect on serum HDV-RNA
Niro et al. [49]	31	CHD	LAM vs. placebo	No effect on serum HDV-RNA
Yurdaydin et al. [50]	39	CHD	LAM vs. LAM + IFNα-2a vs. IFNα-2a alone	SVR in 41%. No benefit of LAM addition
Sheldon et al. [53]	16	HDV–HIV coinfection	HAART	Slight HDV-RNA decline
Castelnau et al. [98]	14	CHD	PegIFNα-2b	SVR in 43%
Niro et al. [52]	38	CHD	PegIFNα-2b vs. PegIFNα-2b + RBV	SVR in 21%. No benefit of RBV addition

N number of patients, *CHD* chronic hepatitis D, *FCV* famciclovir, *LAM* lamivudine, *SVR* sustained virological response

period in a trial that enrolled 15 chronic hepatitis delta patients [48]. Lamivudine was also ineffective in trials that used the drug as monotherapy [49] and in combination with interferon alpha (IFNα) [50]. Although ribavirin has shown in vitro activity against HDV, no benefit has been seen in monotherapy [51] or in combination with pegIFNα [52].

More recently, a 6-year follow-up observational study involving 16 patients coinfected with HIV, HBV, and HDV [53], all of whom being under antiretroviral therapy including tenofovir, showed more promising results. Overall, 13 patients showed an average reduction in HDV viremia from 7 to 5.8 $\log_{10}$, and three subjects achieved undetectable serum HDV-RNA and normalized ALT. Clearance of serum HDV-RNA using tenofovir has also been confirmed in a more recent study [54]. Thus, prolonged treatment with potent HBV polymerase inhibitors could bring beneficial effects at least in a subset of patients with hepatitis D. These observations clearly warrant further investigation.

Interferon-based therapies are currently the recommended options for the treatment of HDV infection. The mechanism of action of IFNα in hepatitis D remains unknown. IFNα has not shown any antiviral activity against HDV when tested in vitro [55]. Thus, a possible mechanism of action for IFN therapy against HDV could be an indirect antiviral effect on the helper virus (HBV). The largest multicenter trial to date with IFN in hepatitis delta was carried out in Italy and involved 61 patients, who were randomly assigned to receive IFNα in doses of 5 MU/m^2 three times weekly for 4 months, followed by 3 MU/m^2 three times weekly for an additional 8 months, or placebo [56]. The patients were then followed for another 12 months. Although ALT normalization rates were significantly higher in the IFN group, the frequency of undetectable serum HDV-RNA or histological improvement rates at the end of the follow-up period did not differ significantly among groups.

Another smaller study involving 42 patients with chronic hepatitis D randomly assigned individuals to receive two different doses of IFNα (9 vs. 3 MU three times weekly) for 48 weeks or placebo [57]. Higher doses of IFNα were associated with higher rates of ALT normalization and undetectable serum HDV RNA at the end of treatment. Liver histology improvement, including reversal of cirrhosis, was also more frequent in the 9 MU group. Since 2006, pegIFN-α has been evaluated for the treatment of hepatitis D in several small trials. The largest published study has included 38 patients who were treated with pegIFN alfa-2b (1.5 MU/kg per week) alone or in combination with ribavirin for 48 weeks [50]. Most individuals on this trial had previously failed treatment with standard IFN. All patients were treated with pegIFN for an additional 24 weeks, and then followed off therapy for 24 weeks. The response rate was similar in the monotherapy and combination therapy groups, suggesting that ribavirin does not exert any benefit on HDV.

Finally, some trials have assessed the efficacy of pegIFN in combination with nucleoside analogues in hepatitis delta. One of the largest controlled trials included 90 patients with compensated chronic HDV infection who were randomly assigned to PegIFN alone or in combination with adefovir, or adefovir monotherapy [58]. After 48 weeks, both pegIFN groups demonstrated significant suppression of HBV replication. However, combination therapy appeared to offer no advantage while adefovir monotherapy had no effect on HDV replication. Patients receiving combination therapy had a significant decline in HBsAg levels with two clearing HBsAg.

Although many experts recommend treatment for chronic HDV infection with pegIFN-α for at least 1 year [21], extended treatment should be considered if patients are able to tolerate the adverse effects of therapy, show biochemical and virologic responses, and have a high probability of achieving clinical endpoints. Treatment with potent HBV polymerase inhibitors, such as tenofovir, may be considered only if IFN therapies are not feasible and there is high HBV replication. Newer experimental therapies, such as using prenylation inhibitors [59] or IFN-lambda are under investigation.

Hepatitis E in HIV

Similar to HAV, hepatitis E virus (HEV) spreads by the fecal–oral route. HEV was first isolated in 1955 during an outbreak of acute hepatitis in India. Among its clinical features, HEV has been characteristically associated with

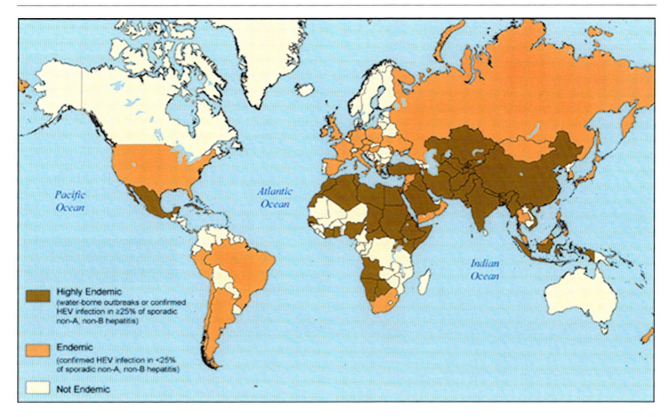

Fig. 13.3 Levels of endemicity for hepatitis E virus infection

fulminant hepatitis during pregnancy [60]. HEV infection is currently an important public health issue in developing countries and has recently emerged as an important pathogen in some immunosuppressed patients.

Virology

HEV is the sole member of genus hepevirus in the family Hepeviridae. HEV is an icosahedral, nonenveloped single stranded RNA virus that is approximately 27–34 nm in diameter. Its genome consists of a closed, positive, single RNA strand, around 7,200 kb long that contains three large ORFs. The ORF1 is located at the 5′ end of the genome and encodes viral nonstructural polyproteins that are involved in processing and in viral replication. It remains unclear whether the ORF1 polyprotein functions as a single protein with multiple functional domains or as individually cleaved smaller proteins [61]. The ORF2 is located at the 3′ end of the genome, and encodes the viral capsid protein and three potential glycosylation sites, which are crucial for the formation of infectious viral particles [62]. The ORF3 encodes a small cytoskeleton-associated phosphoprotein [63], as well as a protein that is essential for virus infectivity in vivo [64], although its expression is not required for virus replication, virion assembly, or infection in vitro [65].

Epidemiology

HEV is one of the most frequent agents of acute viral hepatitis worldwide. Although the real global burden of HEV infection has not been well established, up to one third of the world population has been infected with HEV [66]. Four different HEV genotypes have been described [67]. Genotypes 1 and 2 are restricted to humans and are mainly responsible for large waterborne epidemics in endemic regions [68], while genotypes 3 and 4 are found both in humans and several animal reservoirs, and are mainly responsible for sporadic cases of hepatitis E. Genotype 3 is found in Europe, the USA, and Japan, and genotype 4 is circualting in Asia [69]

HEV seroprevalence is higher in countries where water sanitation is poor, as in Central and South East Asia, North Africa, and the Middle East. There, HEV seroprevalence can be as high as 25% [70]. In Western countries, this figure in the general population is 1–3% in Europe and around 2% in the USA [71] (Fig. 13.3). However, recent estimates in the Unites States have reported significant higher rates of HEV seroprevalence in both natives and foreigners from endemic regions [72].

As being transmitted via the fecal–oral route, HEV infections may present as large outbreaks from waterborne infections or poorly cooked meat of animal reservoirs, such as swine, wild boar, or deer [73]. Occasionally, person-to-person transmission has been described in some outbreaks [74].

Clinical Manifestations

HEV generally causes a self-limited acute infection, although fulminant hepatitis can develop. Chronic hepatitis does not develop after acute HEV infection, except in the transplant setting, where unexpected reports of chronic liver disease associated with persistent HEV viremia have recently been described [75].

Self-limited, acute infection is the most common clinical condition associated with HEV infection. Although the main clinical features do not significantly differ between industrialized and developing countries, the mortality rate seems to be higher in the latter, where it can reach up to 11% [76]. Prior history of underlying liver disease or alcohol abuse predisposes to poor prognosis.

The incubation period of HEV infection ranges from 15 to 60 days. The clinical presentation may vary from asymptomatic forms to fulminant acute hepatitis. Clinical symptoms generally are nonspecific, including fever, pain, myalgia, anorexia, jaundice, or pruritus [77]. Infection with HEV genotype 4 is associated with more severe clinical manifestations [78]. HEV viremia and viral excretion in stools appear during the incubation period, 1–2 weeks before the onset of clinical symptoms. A few days to 2 weeks after the onset of symptoms, HEV-RNA is usually no longer detectable in the blood.

Chronic hepatitis E is an unexpected rare condition, which has been observed in immunocompromised patients, such as transplant recipients, individuals with hematological malignancies, and more recently in the setting of HIV infection [79, 80]. In transplant recipients, chronic HEV diagnosis was made during the course of the investigation of unexplained persistent liver enzyme elevations. Of note, half of the transplant recipients in whom chronic HEV infection was diagnosed were clinically asymptomatic. Symptomatic patients reported nonspecific symptoms, such as asthenia or joint pain. Patients with chronic hepatitis E showed elevated aminotransferases, persistent serum HEV-RNA, and histological inflammatory abnormalities.

In a Spanish study that examined 50 HIV-infected patients with CD4 counts <200 cells/μL and persistent unexplained elevated liver enzymes, HEV viremia was not recognized in any of them [81]. In a French series that included 245 HIV-infected individuals [82], 3 of them experienced acute HEV infection, but a total of 15 showed anti-HEV IgG, with an overall prevalence of anti-HEV IgG of around 6%. In Europe, the prevalence of anti-HEV IgG shows a geographical gradient, with the highest rates in Southern France. A case of persistent carriage of HEV in an HIV-infected patient with unexplained liver enzyme elevations has been reported [80]. The presence of HEV-RNA was demonstrated in serum and feces samples collected during the preceding 18 months. Further studies are needed testing HIV-infected subjects from distinct geographical regions stratified by diverse CD4 strata to assess the clinical relevance of chronic hepatitis E in the HIV setting.

Pregnant women are a population in which HEV infection remains an important health-care issue. For unknown reasons, fulminant hepatic failure occurs more frequently during pregnancy, resulting in an especially high mortality rate of up to 25%, primarily in women infected during the third trimester [83]. Pregnant women showing jaundice and acute viral hepatitis caused by HEV infection appear to have worse obstetric and fetal outcomes compared to pregnant women with jaundice and acute viral hepatitis due to other agents [84]. Of note, HEV infection during pregnancy has not been associated with higher mortality rates in other areas such as Egypt or Southern India [85]. Moreover, some studies have not shown any correlation between pregnancy and HEV disease severity [86]. Unknown variables such as HEV genotypes or subtypes could play a role in the severity of symptoms during pregnancy [87].

Diagnosis

The diagnosis of HEV infection is based upon the detection of HEV in serum or stools by PCR or by the detection of IgM antibodies to HEV [88]. Antibody tests against HEV alone are less accurate for diagnosis, since false positive and negative results have often been described [89]. Anti-HEV IgG and IgM assays are available for diagnosis.

HEV-RNA can be detected in stools approximately 1 week before the onset of illness and persists for as long as 2 weeks after. Because HEV is enterically transmitted, patients are infectious during fecal shedding. HEV viremia is generally transient, but persistence for up to 4 months has been described [90]. Anti-HEV IgM appears during the early phase of clinical illness and vanishes rapidly beyond 4–5 months [91]. The IgG response appears shortly after the IgM response, remaining positive for years after the acute episode. Anti-HEV IgM as measured by EIA has shown its good diagnostic accuracy in HEV outbreaks [92].

Serological and nucleic acid tests (qualitative and quantitative HEV-RNA) currently represent the gold standard for HEV testing and have been used for both epidemiological and diagnostic purposes. Compared to single and nested gel-based RT-PCR, the various real-time PCR assays have a higher sensitivity, are less laborious, save time, and are less prone to cross-contamination. Moreover, they are able to detect all four HEV genotypes [93].

Treatment

There is no specific treatment for HEV infection, being supportive therapy the only valid strategy considered for acute HEV infection. A pilot study has been carried out to assess the efficacy of ribavirin [94] in HIV-infected patients. In this study, six patients that received kidney transplants who were positive for HEV-RNA for more than 3 years received ribavirin monotherapy for 3 months at doses of 600–800 mg according to kidney function. After treatment, serum HEV-RNA became undetectable in all patients, and four of them showed sustained virological response, while the other two patients relapsed after therapy ended. ALT were normal at the end of treatment in all patients. In other solid organ transplant patients with chronic hepatitis E, treatment with pegylated interferon has similarly resulted in HEV clearance in some patients [95].

Several vaccines to prevent HEV infection are under development, with promising results [96]. The results a phase III trial using a recombinant HEV vaccine have recently been reported [97]. More than 110,000 individuals were recruited and randomized to receive either three doses of vaccine or placebo at weeks 0, 4, and 24. The rate of immunization was very high with relatively null or mild adverse events. There is no experience so far with HEV vaccines in HIV-infected persons. Whereas these vaccines arrive to the market, hygiene measures to reduce fecal–oral transmission must be implemented. Travelers to HEV endemic areas should be encouraged to keep safe practices that prevent infection, avoiding drinking water of unknown purity, uncooked shellfish, and uncooked fruits or vegetables.

References

1. Feinstone S, Kapikian A, Purcell R. Hepatitis A: detection by immune electron microscopy of a virus-like antigen associated with acute illness. Science. 1973;182:1026–31.
2. Lemon S, Jansen R, Brown F. Genetic, antigenic and biological differences between strains of hepatitis A virus. Vaccine. 1992;10 suppl 1:40–4.
3. Taylor R, Davern T, Munoz S. Fulminant hepatitis A virus infection in the United States: incidence, prognosis, and outcomes. Hepatology. 2006;44:1589–97.
4. Vento S, Garofano T, Renzini C, et al. Fulminant hepatitis associated with hepatitis A virus superinfection in patients with chronic hepatitis C. N Engl J Med. 1998;338:286–90.
5. Fonquernie L, Meynard JL, Charrois A, et al. Occurrence of acute hepatitis A in patients infected with HIV. Clin Infect Dis. 2001;32:297–9.
6. Ida S, Tachikawa N, Nakajima A, et al. Influence of HIV type 1 infection on acute hepatitis A virus infection. Clin Infect Dis. 2002;34:379–85.
7. Richardson M, Elliman D, Maguire H, et al. Evidence base of incubation periods, periods of infectiousness and exclusion policies for the control of communicable diseases in schools and preschools. Pediatr Infect Dis J. 2001;20:380–91.
8. Mbithi J, Springthorpe V, Boulet J, et al. Survival of hepatitis A virus on human hands and its transfer on contact with animate and inanimate surfaces. J Clin Microbiol. 1992;30:757–63.
9. D'Hondt E. Possible approaches to develop vaccines against hepatitis A. Vaccine. 1992;10 suppl 1:48–52.
10. Advisory Committee on Immunization Practices (ACIP). Prevention of hepatitis A through active or passive immunization: recommendations of the Advisory Committee on Immunization Practices (ACIP). MMWR Recomm Rep. 2006;55(7):1–23.
11. Geretti AM, British HIV. Association guidelines for immunization of HIV-infected adults 2008. HIV Med. 2008;9:795–848.
12. Shire N, Welge J, Sherman K. Efficacy of inactivated hepatitis A vaccine in HIV-infected patients: a hierarchical Bayesian meta-analysis. Vaccine. 2006;24:272–9.
13. Valdez H, Smith K, Landay A, et al. Response to immunization with recall and neoantigens after prolonged administration of an HIV-1 protease inhibitor-containing regimen. ACTG 375 team. AIDS. 2000;14:11–21.
14. Kemper C, Haubrich R, Frank I, et al. Safety and immunogenicity of hepatitis A vaccine in HIV-infected patients: a double-blind, randomized, placebo-controlled trial. J Infect Dis. 2003;187:1327–31.
15. Launay O, Grabar S, Gordien E, et al. Immunological efficacy of a three-dose schedule of hepatitis A vaccine in HIV-infected adults: HEPAVAC Study. J Acquir Immune Defic Syndr. 2008;49:272–5.
16. Valdez H, Mitsuyasu R, Landay A, et al. Interleukin-2 increases CD4+ lymphocyte numbers but does not enhance responses to immunization: results of A5046s. Infect Dis. 2003;187:320–5.
17. Wallace M, Brandt C, Earhart K, et al. Safety and immunogenicity of an inactivated hepatitis A vaccine among HIV-infected subjects. Clin Infect Dis. 2004;39:1207–13.
18. Rizzetto M, Canese M, Aricó S, et al. Immunofluorescence detection of a new antigen-antibody system (delta/anti-delta) associated with hepatitis B virus in liver and in serum of HBsAg carriers. Gut. 1977;18:997–1003.
19. Rizzetto M. Hepatitis D: thirty years after. J Hepatol. 2009;50:1043–50.
20. Bichko V, Netter H, Wu T. Pathogenesis associated with replication of hepatitis delta virus. Infect Agents Dis. 1994;3:94–7.
21. Wedemeyer H, Manns M. Epidemiology, pathogenesis and management of hepatitis D: update and challenges ahead. Nat Rev Gastroenterol Hepatol. 2010;7:31–40.
22. Hadziyannis S. Review: hepatitis delta. J Gastroenterol Hepatol. 1997;12:289–98.
23. Farci P. Delta hepatitis: an update. J Hepatol. 2003;39 suppl 1:212–9.
24. Gaeta G, Stroffolini T, Chiaramonte M, et al. Chronic hepatitis D: a vanishing Disease? An Italian multicenter study. Hepatology. 2000;32:824–7.
25. Makuwa M, Mintsa-Ndong A, Souquière S, et al. Prevalence and molecular diversity of hepatitis B virus and hepatitis delta virus in urban and rural populations in northern Gabon in central Africa. J Clin Microbiol. 2009;47:2265–8.
26. Manock S, Kelley P, Hyams K, et al. An outbreak of fulminant hepatitis delta in the Waorani, an indigenous people of the Amazon basin of Ecuador. Am J Trop Med Hyg. 2000;63:209–13.
27. Børresen M, Olsen O, Ladefoged K, et al. Hepatitis D outbreak among children in a hepatitis B hyper-endemic settlement in Greenland. J Viral Hepat. 2010;17:162–70.
28. Jardi R, Rodriguez F, Buti M. Role of hepatitis B, C, and D viruses in dual and triple infection: influence of viral genotypes and hepatitis B precore and basal core promoter mutations on viral replicative interference. Hepatology. 2001;34:404–10.
29. Romeo R, Del Ninno E, Rumi M, et al. A 28 year study of the course of hepatitis delta infection: a risk factor for cirrhosis and hepatocellular carcinoma. Gastroenterology. 2009;136:1629–35.

30. Su C, Huang Y, Huo T, et al. Genotypes and viremia of hepatitis B and D viruses are associated with outcomes of chronic hepatitis D patients. Gastroenterology. 2006;130:1625–35.
31. Dény P. Hepatitis delta virus genetic variability: from genotypes I, II, III to eight major clades? Curr Top Microbiol Immunol. 2006;307:151–71.
32. Wu J. Functional and clinical significance of hepatitis D virus genotype 2 infection. Curr Top Microbiol Immunol. 2006;307:173–86.
33. Watanabe H, Nagayama K, Enomoto N, et al. Chronic hepatitis delta virus infection with genotype II b variant is correlated with progressive liver disease. J Gen Virol. 2003;84:3275–89.
34. Smedile A, Rizzetto M, Gerin J. Advances in Hepatitis D virus biology and disease. In: Boyer JL, Ockner RK, editors. Progressin liver disease, vol. XII. Philadelphia: Saunders Company; 1994. p. 157–75.
35. Shih H, Jeng K, Syu W, et al. Hepatitis B surface antigen levels and sequences of natural hepatitis B virus variants influence the assembly and secretion of hepatitis D virus. J Virol. 2008;82:2250–64.
36. Brook G, Main J, Nelson M, et al. British HIV Association guidelines for the management of coinfection with HIV-1 and hepatitis B or C virus 2010. HIV Med. 2010;11:1–30.
37. Buti M, Esteban R, Roggendorf M, et al. Hepatitis D virus RNA in acute delta infection: serological profile and correlation with other markers of hepatitis D virus infection. Hepatology. 1988;8: 1125–9.
38. Madejon A, Castillo I, Bartolome J, et al. Detection of HDV-RNA by PCR in serum of patients with chronic HDV infection. J Hepatol. 1990;11:381–4.
39. Dinolfo L, Abate ML, Bertolo P, et al. Detection of hepatitis D virus RNA in serum by a reverse transcription, polymerase chain reaction-based assay. Int J Clin Lab Res. 1995;25:35–9.
40. Niro G, Casey J, Gravinese E, et al. Intrafamilial transmission of hepatitis delta virus: molecular evidence. J Hepatol. 1999;30: 564–9.
41. Schaper M, Rodríguez-Frías F, Jardi R, et al. Quantitative longitudinal evaluations of hepatitis delta virus RNA and hepatitis B virus DNA shows a dynamic, complex replicative profile in chronic hepatitis B and D. J Hepatol. 2010;52:658–64.
42. Aragona M, Macagno S, Caredda F, et al. Serological response to the hepatitis delta virus in hepatitis D. Lancet. 1987;1:478–80.
43. Smedile A, Lavarini C, Crivelli O, et al. Radioimmunoassay detection of IgM antibodies to the HBV-associated delta antigen: clinical significance in delta infection. J Med Virol. 1982;9:131–8.
44. Wu J, Chen T, Huang Y, et al. Natural history of hepatitis D viral superinfection: significance of viremia detected by polymerase chain reaction. Gastroenterology. 1995;108:796–802.
45. Zachou K, Yurdaydin C, Drebber U, et al. Quantitative HBsAg and HDV-RNA levels in chronic delta hepatitis. Liver Int. 2010;30: 430–7.
46. Kirk G, Astemborski J, Mehta S, et al. Assessment of liver fibrosis by transient elastography in persons with hepatitis C virus infection or HIV-hepatitis C virus coinfection. Clin Infect Dis. 2009;48: 963–72.
47. Zachou K, Yurdaydin C, Drebber U, et al. Quantitative HBsAg and HDV-RNA levels in chronic delta hepatitis. Liver Int. 2010;30:430–7.
48. Yurdaydin C, Bozkaya H, Gurel S, et al. Famciclovir treatment of chronic delta hepatitis. J Hepatol. 2002;37:266–71.
49. Niro GA, Ciancio A, Tillman H, et al. Lamivudine therapy in chronic delta hepatitis: a multicentre randomized-controlled pilot study. Aliment Pharmacol Ther. 2005;22:227–32.
50. Yurdaydin C, Bozkaya H, Onder F, et al. Treatment of chronic delta hepatitis with lamivudine vs lamivudine + interferon vs interferon. J Viral Hepat. 2008;15:314–21.
51. Garripoli A, Di Marco V, Cozzolongo R, et al. Ribavirin treatment for chronic hepatitis D: a pilot study. Liver. 1994;14:154–7.
52. Niro G, Ciancio A, Gaeta G, et al. Pegylated interferon alpha-2b as monotherapy or in combination with ribavirin in chronic hepatitis delta. Hepatology. 2006;44:713–20.
53. Sheldon J, Ramos B, Toro C, et al. Does treatment of hepatitis B virus (HBV) infection reduce hepatitis delta virus (HDV) replication in HIV-HB-VHDV coinfected patients? Antivir Ther. 2008;13:97–102.
54. Martin-Carbonero L, Teixeira T, Poveda E, et al. Clinical and virological outcomes in HIV-infected patients with chronic hepatitis B on long-term nucleos(t)ide analogues. AIDS. 2011;25(1):73–9.
55. McNair A, Cheng D, Monjardino J, et al. Hepatitis delta virus replication in vitro is not affected by interferon-alpha or -gamma despite intact cellular responses to interferon and dsRNA. J Gen Virol. 1994;75:1371–8.
56. Rosina F, Pintus C, Meschievitz C, et al. A randomized controlled trial of a 12-month course of recombinant human interferon-alpha in chronic delta (type D) hepatitis: a multicenter Italian study. Hepatology. 1991;13:1052–6.
57. Farci P, Mandas A, Coiana A, et al. Treatment of chronic hepatitis D with interferon alfa-2a. N Engl J Med. 1994;330:88–94.
58. Yurdaydin C, Wedemeyer H, Dalekos G, et al. A multicenter randomised study comparing the efficacy of pegylated interferon alfa-2A plus adefovir dipivoxil vs. pegylated interferon alfa-2A plus placebo vs. adefovir dipovoxil for the treatment of chronic delta hepatiticbrr: the intervention trial (HID-IT) (abstract). Hepatology. 2006;41(1):230.
59. Einav S, Glenn J. Prenylation inhibitors: a novel class of antiviral agents. J Antimicrob Chemother. 2003;52:883–6.
60. Meng X. Recent advances in hepatitis E virus. J Viral Hepat. 2010;17(8):598–9.
61. Ropp S, Tam A, Beames B, et al. Expression of the hepatitis E virus ORF1. Arch Virol. 2000;145:1321–37.
62. Graff J, Zhou Y, Torian U, et al. Mutations within potential glycosylation sites in the capsid protein of hepatitis E virus prevent the formation of infectious virus particles. J Virol. 2008;82:1185–94.
63. Zafrullah M, Ozdener M, Panda S, Jameel S. The ORF3 protein of hepatitis E virus is a phosphoprotein that associates with the cytoskeleton. J Virol. 1997;71:9045–53.
64. Graff J, Nguyen H, Yu C, et al. The open reading frame 3 gene of hepatitis E virus contains a cis-reactive element and encodes a protein required for infection of macaques. J Virol. 2005;79: 6680–9.
65. Emerson S, Nguyen H, Torian U, et al. ORF3 protein of hepatitis E virus is not required for replication, virion assembly or infection of hepatoma cells in vitro. J Virol. 2006;80:10457–64.
66. WHO. Viral hepatitis statement A62/22. http://apps.who.int/gb/ebwha/pdf_files/A62/A62_22-en.pdf. Accessed 9 Sept 2010.
67. Meng X. Hepatitis E virus: animal reservoirs and zoonotic risk. Vet Microbiol. 2010;140:256–65.
68. Purcell R, Emerson S. Hepatitis E: an emerging awareness of an old disease. J Hepatol. 2008;48:494–503.
69. Pavio N, Meng XJ, Renou C. Zoonotic hepatitis E: animal reservoirs and emerging risks. Vet Res. 2010;41:46–51.
70. Gomatos P, Monier M, Arthur R, et al. Sporadic acute hepatitis caused by hepatitis E virus in Egyptian adults. Clin Infect Dis. 1996;23:195–6.
71. Clemente-Casares P, Pina S, Buti M, et al. Hepatitis E virus epidemiology in industrialized countries. Emerg Infect Dis. 2003;9:448–54.
72. Faramawi MF, Johnson E, Chen S, Pannala P. The incidence of hepatitis E virus infection in the general population of the USA. Epidemiol Infect. 2010;72:1–6.
73. Krawczynski K, Hepatitis E. Hepatology. 1993;17:932–41.
74. Teshale E, Grytdal S, Howard C, et al. Evidence of person-to-person transmission of hepatitis E virus during a large outbreak in Northern Uganda. Clin Infect Dis. 2010;50:1006–10.

75. Bihl F, Negro F. Chronic hepatitis E in the immunosuppressed: a new source of trouble? J Hepatol. 2009;50:435–7.
76. Peron JM, Bureau C, Poirson H, et al. Fulminant liver failure from acute autochthonous hepatitis E in France: description of seven patients with acute hepatitis E and encephalopathy. J Viral Hepat. 2007;14:298–303.
77. Pavio N, Mansuy J. Hepatitis E in high-income countries. Curr Opin Infect Dis. 2010;23:521–7.
78. Ohnishi S, Kang J, Maekubo H, et al. Comparison of clinical features of acute hepatitis caused by hepatitis E virus (HEV) genotypes 3 and 4 in Sapporo, Japan. Hepatol Res. 2006;36: 301–7.
79. Kamar N, Selves J, Mansuy JM, et al. Hepatitis E virus and chronic hepatitis in organ-transplant recipients. N Engl J Med. 2008;358: 811–7.
80. Dalton H, Bendall R, Keane F, et al. Persistent carriage of hepatitis E virus in patients with HIV infection. N Engl J Med. 2009;361: 1025–7.
81. Madejón A, Vispo E, Bottecchia M, et al. Lack of hepatitis E virus infection in HIV patients with advanced immunodeficiency or idiopathic liver enzyme elevations. J Viral Hepat. 2009;16:895–6.
82. Renou C, Lafeuillade A, Cadranel J, et al. Hepatitis E virus in HIV-infected patients. AIDS. 2010;24:1493–9.
83. Asher L, Innis B, Shrestha M, et al. Virus-like particles in the liver of a patient with fulminant hepatitis and antibody to hepatitis E virus. J Med Virol. 1990;31:229–33.
84. Patra S, Kumar A, Trivedi S, et al. Maternal and fetal outcomes in pregnant women with acute hepatitis E virus infection. Ann Intern Med. 2007;147:28–33.
85. Navaneethan U, Shata M. Hepatitis E and pregnancy: understanding the pathogenesis. Liver Int. 2008;28:1190–9.
86. Bhatia V, Singhal A, Panda S, et al. A 20-year single-center experience with acute liver failure during pregnancy: is the prognosis really worse? Hepatology. 2008;48:1577–85.
87. Renou C, Pariente A, Nicand E, et al. Pathogenesis of Hepatitis E in pregnancy. Liver Int. 2008;28:1465.
88. Takahashi M, Kusakai S, Mizuo H, et al. Simultaneous detection of immunoglobulin A (IgA) and IgM antibodies against hepatitis E virus (HEV) is highly specific for diagnosis of acute HEV infection. J Clin Microbiol. 2005;43:49–56.
89. Zaki Mel S, Foud M, Mohamed A. Value of hepatitis E virus detection by cell culture compared with nested PCR and serological studies by IgM and IgG. FEMS Immunol Med Microbiol. 2009;56:73–9.
90. Clayson E, Myint K, Snitbhan R, et al. Viremia, fecal shedding, and IgM and IgG responses in patients with hepatitis E. J Infect Dis. 1995;172:927–33.
91. Favorov M, Fields H, Purdy M, et al. Serologic identification of hepatitis E virus infections in epidemic and endemic settings. J Med Virol. 1992;36:246–50.
92. Favorov M, Khudyakov Y, Mast E, et al. IgM and IgG antibodies to hepatitis E virus (HEV) detected by an enzyme immunoassay based on an HEV-specific artificial recombinant mosaic protein. J Med Virol. 1996;50:50–8.
93. Gyarmati P, Mohammed N, Norder H, et al. Universal detection of hepatitis E virus by two real-time PCR assays: TaqMan and Primer-Probe Energy Transfer. J Virol Methods. 2007;14:226–35.
94. Kamar N, Rostaing L, Abravanel F, et al. Ribavirin therapy inhibits viral replication in patients with chronic hepatitis E virus infection. Gastroenterology. 2010;139(5):1612–8.
95. Alric L, Bonnet D, Laurent G, Kamar N, Izopet J. Chronic hepatitis E virus infection: successful virologic response to pegylated interferon-alpha therapy. Ann Intern Med. 2010;153:135–6.
96. Shrestha M, Scott R, Joshi D, et al. Safety and efficacy of a recombinant hepatitis E vaccine. N Engl J Med. 2007;356:895–903.
97. Zhu F, Zhang J, Zhang X, et al. Efficacy and safety of a recombinant hepatitis E vaccine in healthy adults: a large-scale, randomised, double-blind, placebo-controlled, phase 3 trial. Lancet. 2010; 376(9744):895–902.
98. Castelnau C, Le Gal F, Ripault MP, Gordien E, Martinot-Peignoux M, Boyer N, et al. Efficacy of peginterferon alpha-2b in chronic hepatitis delta: relevance of quantitative RT-PCR for follow up. Hepatology. 2006;44(3):728–35.

Hepatitis B Virus: Replication, Mutation, and Evolution

Amy C. Sherman and Shyam Kottilil

Introduction

Hepatitis B Virus (HBV) is a DNA virus that utilizes a complex life cycle to replicate via an RNA intermediate transcript with the help of reverse transcriptase enzyme. Many steps in the life cycle of HBV have not been clearly understood mainly because of the lack of availability of culture systems that are permissive to full-length HBV genome replication. Chronic HBV infection can lead to liver cirrhosis and hepatocellular carcinoma. Effective treatments are available for chronic HBV that has been shown to significantly lower morbidity and mortality. However, the effectiveness of antiviral therapy is hampered by the development of mutations in the reverse transcriptase resulting in progressive liver disease. Mutagenesis also happens in the presence of host immune response and has resulted in the evolution of HBV across various species (avian, primate, and human) and geographical regions. This review focuses on a concise summary of HBV replication cycle, mutagenesis, and evolution.

HBV Replication

HBV belongs to the family hepadnaviridae and has a life cycle that is similar to that of other viruses in its family, producing approximately 10^{13} virions per day. However, certain characteristics of its replication mark the HBV cycle as distinct from other retroviruses and have allowed for the survival of viral material in infected cells. Lack of cell lines that permit HBV replication in vitro has hampered a clear understanding about the details of HBV life cycle. This review summarizes the most recent understanding about the step-wise process of HBV replication. The 3.2 kb HBV genome consists of four overlapping reading frames, PC-C (core), PS-S (surface), P (polymerase), X (Fig. 14.1). Transcription is controlled by four HBV promoters, Cp, PS1p, Sp, Xp, and two enhancers, enhancer I region and enhancer core domain. Briefly, infectious virions with partially double-stranded, circular DNA enter the host cell and shed their coating. Then, the partially double-stranded circular DNA is then converted to covalently closed circular (ccc)DNA within the host cell. Viral RNA is transcribed by RNA polymerase II and produces pregenomic RNA (pgRNA), which is packaged and then reverse transcribed into new relaxed coiled (RC-) DNA genomes. RCDNA is a small, partially double-stranded, relaxed circular DNA genome that needs to be converted to cccDNA, which serves as the template for all viral RNA transcription. The process is unique because the genetic code of HBV is stored in three different forms in two different locations in the cell: RC-DNA in the virions and both cccDNA and pgRNA within the cell [1]. Furthermore, translation of distinct entities of each gene products occurs instead of splicing from a single transcript. The distinct (−) strand DNA produced during replication is also a hallmark of HBV.

Genome Composition

The overlapping genome encodes for four regions: core, surface, viral DNA polymerase (P), and X. The core protein is responsible for pgRNA packaging and viral DNA replication, using three serine phosphorylation sites [2]. The precore (HBeAg) is a product of the core region. The surface proteins of HBV are largely involved in receptor binding and entry. Significantly, the PreS1 region of large surface protein (LHBs) has been demonstrated to be a direct component of viral attachment although no putative host receptor has been identified for HBV [3]. The P open reading frame (ORF) encodes the polymerase (pol), which is about 800 amino acids long and structured into four domains: the terminal protein (TP), the spacer domain, the reverse transcriptase (RT),

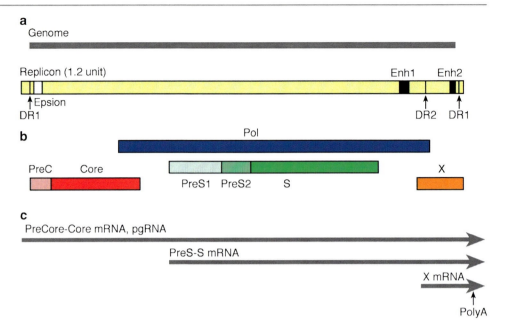

Fig. 14.1 The 3.2 kb HBV genome consists of four overlapping reading frames, PC-C (core), PS-S (surface), P (polymerase), X

and the ribonuclease H. The terminal protein plays a role in encapsidation and initiation of the (−)DNA strand, the spacer domain allows for mutations and assists in TP and RT function, the reverse transcriptase is involved in the synthesis of the genome, and the ribonuclease H is responsible for the degradation of pgRNA [4]. The X protein is involved in the regulation of several critical cellular pathways that are essential for HBV replication. Each of these elements of replication is described in greater detail below.

Viral Entry

The recent discovery of a functional model of HBV infection has led to increased knowledge about the mechanisms of Hepatitis B virion entry. HBV infectivity can now be studied using the hepatoma cell line HepaRG, which was derived from a liver tumor of a patient with chronic Hepatitis C infection [5]. Two types of viral particles are associated with HBV, the 22-nm-diameter spherical and the tubular subviral particles [6]. The 22-nm-diameter particle (Dane particle) is responsible for actual infection and replication. Three types of envelope glycoproteins (collectively called Hepatitis B surface antigen, or HBsAg) are essential for virion binding and entry: the large (LHBs), middle (MHBs), and small (SHBs) surface proteins. LHBs are more commonly expressed among infectious virions and are required for virion entry [7]. Large volumes of subviral particles are produced; however, most are essentially empty envelopes which are useful as a marker of HBV in serologic testing. The level of subviral particles may also be involved in regulating HBV replication.

Transcription

After entry into the cell and uncoating, the infectious virions are transported to the host cell nucleus where replication occurs within the viral capsids. The RC DNA is converted to cccDNA, which becomes the transcription template for new viral RNA particles. In order for conversion to occur, the following mechanistic steps must happen: both (+) and (−) strand DNA must be covalently ligated from the RC-DNA's complete (−)DNA strand and incomplete (+)DNA strand, the 5′ end of the (−)DNA must be detached from the P protein, and the RNA oligonucleotide primer at the 5′ end of the (+) DNA must be removed. The process and amplification of cccDNA occurs within the cell. During the late infection stage when a high amount of envelope proteins are present in the cell, the cccDNA amplification rate decreases, keeping the average cccDNA copy number between 1 and 50 in each nucleus [8]. However, before this occurs, cccDNA serves as a template to produce the transcript necessary for viral replication. RNA polymerase II transcribes genomic and subgenomic RNAs from cccDNA. pgRNA, which is one product of transcription, is then packaged and reverse transcribed into new RC-DNA genomes that are released from the cell.

Reverse Transcription

The mechanism for reverse transcription of Hepatitis B distinguishes HBV replication from other hepadnaviruses. Introduction of DHBV pgRNA into duck hepatocytes initiates infection with Woodchuck hepatitis virus, while for HBV, the ε stem-loop alone can mediate encapsidation,

Fig. 14.2 Two important regions of the HBV genome are the direct repeats DR1 and DR2, which are located in the 5′ ends of the (+)DNA. These are involved in DNA synthesis during replication

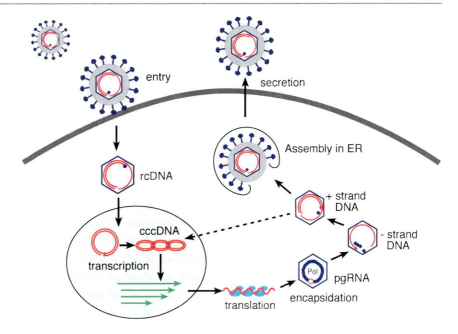

including packaging of heterologous RNAs [1]. In DHBV, the situation is more complex in that a second RNA element, called region II is required for pgRNA packaging [1]. As stated previously, one of the products transcribed from cccDNA is pgRNA. pgRNA is 3.4 kb, which is the length of the entire genome plus a terminal redundancy of the direct repeat 1 (DR1), e signal, and poly-A tail. pgRNA has two specific functions: (a) it is the mRNA for reverse transcriptase and the core protein, and (b) it is the template for the creation of new DNA genomes [9]. The reverse transcription process is also unique because it requires specific protein primers.

Release of Virions

The packaging of the pgRNA and reverse transcriptase into discrete capsids is an important step of HBV replication. The interaction of the encapsidation signal epsilon (ε) and the P protein on the pgRNA specifically allow for the packaging of the pgRNA and reverse transcriptase complex to occur; the binding of these two elements initiates the reverse transcription process. The interaction of the polymerase and epsilon RNA requires chaperones Hsp90 and p23 to function [10, 11]. These heat shock proteins (Hsp90) are responsible for forming the polymerase conformation needed for pgRNA to bind to epsilon RNA. Once the P protein is covalently linked to the first DNA nucleotide, the DNA transforms into a complete (−) strand DNA. (+) strand DNA can then be constructed from the (−) strand DNA, resulting in new RC-DNA. The reverse transcription process is completed before the genetic material leaves the cell, which differentiates HBV from other retroviruses.

Minus Strand (−)DNA Synthesis

Synthesis for the (−)DNA strand begins from the UUCA motif in the epsilon bulge [12], creating the complementary sequence 3′ AAGT at the 5′ end of (−)DNA in a stem-loop structure. Epsilon is a *cis*-acting element that acts as both a packaging signal for nucleocapsids and the initiation signal of reverse transcription [13]. Interestingly, this primer produced (3′AAGT5′) is then translocated to the 3′ proximal DR1* with the aid of specific factors φ, ε, and ω [14, 15]. From the acceptor DR1* site, elongation of the (−)DNA strand continues until the end of the pgRNA 3′ end. The bulk of the pgRNA template is degraded as part of the process of this elongation. The final RNase H cleavage occurs at 11–16 nt from the pgRNA 5′ end. This primer is then translocated (second strand jump) to the DR2 homologous site on the (−)DNA strand, resulting in a primer segment for the (+)strand DNA

Synthesis of (+)DNA, Noncovalently Closed Circular DNA

Two important regions of the HBV genome are the direct repeats DR1 and DR2, which are located in the 5′ ends of the (+)DNA. These are involved in DNA synthesis during replication, as described previously (Fig. 14.2). The (+)DNA is synthesized from the primer in DR2 and is completed when a third translocation occurs when the (+)DNA reaches the 5′ terminus of the minus strand DNA. At this point, the translocation from the 5′ end to the 3′ end of the (−)DNA yields a noncovalent closed, circular DNA molecule. Thus, the (+)DNA is only partially completed, resulting in the gapped yet double-stranded circular DNA that exists in the virions. At this stage, the nucleocapsid with RC-DNA is either (a) returned back to the nuclease where amplification of cccDNA occurs or (b) secreted out of the cell as a new infectious agent.

Protein X

Recent studies have examined the previously enigmatic function of the HBV X protein. The HBV X protein (HBx) is a small 154 amino-acid protein that regulates many cellular pathways, including cellular transduction, transcription, protein degradation, and calcium signaling. It also influences cell proliferation, apoptosis, and stimulation of HBV replication [16–18]. Of significance, it is believed to be a factor in HBV pathogenesis and hepatocellular carcinogenesis [19]. Studies have demonstrated that HBx regulation induces hepatocytes to commence the G1 phase of the cellular cycle, which may explain the linkage between HBV infection and the occurrence of hepatocellular carcinoma (HCC). Normally, the majority of hepatocytes are quiescent. However, when induced in vivo (in a rat model) by transfection with HBx, studies have shown that hepatocytes enter the G1 phase of the cell cycle and then fail to proceed to the S stage [18]. In the context of HBV replication, HBx acts to mediate cell cycle-regulatory proteins, such as p15, p16, and active G1-phase proteins p21, p27, cyclin D1, and cyclin E. HBx has also been shown to mobilize cytosolic calcium, which is necessary for HBV replication in HepG2 cultures [20, 21]. Furthermore, studies have demonstrated that quiescent hepatocytes are not suitable for HBV replication because this phenomenon is cell cycle dependent. There is an inverse correlation between expression of proliferating cell nuclear antigen and presence of episomal HBV DNA in individual hepatocytes in vivo [22]. Therefore, HBx's role of inducing hepatocytes to enter G1 is an essential part of successful HBV replication [18, 23, 24]. HBx promotes HIV-1 replication synergizing with Tat protein and T cell signal transduction pathways [25]. Studies have shown this to be in a NF-κB-dependent manner and a NF-AT-dependent manner. HBx mutants that fail to interact with the T cell signal transduction pathways lacked the ability to promote HIV-1 Long terminal repeat (LTR) transcription [25]. These studies suggest HBx can act as a nuclear coactivator and thereby enhance HIV replication in T cells [25].

HBV Mutation

HBV replication is associated with an increased rate of mutations, mainly due to the RT activity; however, this rate is much lower than retroviruses. It is estimated that the rate of evolution for HBV is $<2 \times 10^{-4}$ base substitutions per site per year, which is intermediate between the rates reported for other DNA and RNA viruses [26]. Interestingly, the rate of synonymous substitutions for HBV is 10^4 times higher than that has been reported for a host genome and it is 10^2 less than that of retroviral genes [27]. These closely related molecular variants play a major role in the evolution of HBV. In fact, eight genotypes of HBV have been identified, labeled A–H, which are defined by an 8% genetic difference and tend to display according to distinct geographical distributions. Within these genotypes, there are 24 subgenotypes. HBVs high rate of replication combined with a high error rate of the RT (due to a lack of proofreading) result in the possible occurrences of numerous single and double mutations on every nucleotide of the HBV genome. Furthermore, since HBV consists of overlapping genome domains, a mutation on one gene (e.g., the S gene) may affect changes on its overlapping gene (e.g., the polymerase gene). Yet, the overlapping genome simultaneously limits the number of viable mutations since many may generate nonviable virions [28]. The conservation of the direct repeats, promoters, and cis-acting elements must be conserved for replication to occur. Thus, the high mutation rate reported must occur to a greater degree in the pre-S domain, which is not as constrained.

The most common naturally occurring mutations are exhibited in both the precore and core domains. The most common precore variant results from a point mutation at nucleotide 1896 (G1896A) and displays to a higher degree in HBV genotype D. The mutation prevents the production of HBeAg, which allows the virus to escape immune recognition and persist within the host cells. Studies have demonstrated that the mutation arises during seroconversion [29]. Interestingly, the mutation is associated with a decreased risk of hepatocellular carcinoma. The most common variant of the core is a dual mutation at A1726T and G1764A, which results in downregulation of HBeAg synthesis of the precore mRNA. This mutation is more common among individuals with genotype C. Unlike the precore variant discussed, this mutation arises before seroconversion. Recently, there has been a significant shift from the occurrence of HBeAg+ to HBeAg− chronic hepatitis. The switch signifies the growing dominance of the precore and core variants over the wild-type form. The emergence of a greater HBeAg− population is most likely due to the effectiveness of the HBV vaccine. However, mutations have also arisen from the pervasive use of antiviral drugs. The development of drug resistance is initiated with mutations in the RT gene, followed by elevation in ALT levels and progression of liver disease [30]. Treatment of HBV infection with nucleoside and nucleotide analog therapies has encouraged selection of novel "escape" mutants. Three main areas are targeted as potential areas that would confer resistance: viral factors, host factors, and pharmacologic factors. In terms of viral factors, high HBV DNA serum levels before treatment and the presence of preexisting mutations are associated with increased risk of drug resistance. In terms of host receptivity, prior exposure to medications that select for the same resistance mutations and an increased immune pressure as indicated by high ALT levels leave patients more prone for resistance [31]. Furthermore, medication noncompliance or unfavorable pharmacogenetics can lead to antiviral drug-resistant mutations. Specific mutations and resistance to the most common anti-HBV agents are elucidated in greater detail below.

Resistance to Lamivudine

Lamivudine was the first nucleoside analog that was approved by the Food and Drug Administration (FDA) for treatment of chronic HBV. While it is effective and well tolerated, lamivudine is highly associated with viral resistance complications that result in a return of HBV DNA after initial suppression [32]. Resistance to lamivudine (LMV) has been identified to be associated with the YMDD locus of the catalytic domain of HBV pol. A specific mutation at position 204 (rtM204V/I) in the HBV polymerase decreases susceptibility 1,000-fold to lamivudine. At this position of the genome, valine or isoleucine substitutes methionine. In a longitudinal study, researchers demonstrated that genotypic resistance affected 15–25% of patients after year 1, and 70% of patients at 4–5 years [31].

Resistance to Adefovir

Adefovir dipivoxil is a nucleotide analog for treatment of HBeAg+, HBeAg−, and lamivudine-refractory chronic HBV infection. The substitution of alanine by threonine or valine at position 181 (rtA181T/V) and the substitution of asparagine by threonine or valine at position 236 (rtN235T/V) decrease susceptibility to adefovir by five- to tenfold [33]. Unlike lamivudine resistance, genotypic resistance was not observed in patients after 1 year. However, after 240 weeks (or, a little more than four and a half years), 29–30% of patients demonstrated adefovir resistance particularly among those who were previously treated with LMV monotherapy.

Resistance to Entecavir

Entecavir is a nucleoside analog for treatment of chronic Hepatitis B. Resistance to entecavir happens in a two-step mechanism. First, a mutation in the HBV polymerase at rtM204V or rtM204I results in a tenfold decrease in susceptibility to entecavir. If further mutations occur at rtThr184, rtSer202, or rtMet250, a decreased susceptibility by tenfold is observed [34]. Thus, in combination, mutations at both points cause a 100-fold decrease of susceptibility. In nucleoside-naïve patients, genotypic resistance was observed in about 1% of patients after 4–5 years. By contrast, in a cohort of lamivudine-refractory patients, about 51% experienced resistance to lamivudine after 5 years.

Resistance to Telbivudine

Telbivudine is a nucleoside analog. A mutation in the rtM204I region has been associated with genotypic resistance to Telbivudine. Among patients who are HBeAg+, about 5% show resistance after 1 year and 25% show resistance after 2 years. Among those patients who are HBeAg−, about 2% experience genotypic resistance after 1 year and 11% experience resistance after 2 years [35]. Studies have shown that patients with HBeAg+ have higher DNA levels, which suggests an explanation for the recorded higher risk of drug resistance.

Resistance to Tenofovir

Tenofovir is a nucleotide analog used for treatment of chronic Hepatitis B. Genotypic resistance has not been confirmed for tenofovir. Patients enrolled in a study who were taking tenofovir did not experience genotypic resistance after 2 years [36], but longer studies have not yet been performed. Certain studies suggest that HBeAg-negative patients may be more susceptible to developing tenofovir resistance because a mutation at rtA194T was associated with drug resistance for the mutant construct [37]. However, more research is needed to support this data. Previous studies have demonstrated that mutations associated with antiviral drug resistance can induce changes in the HBV surface region [38, 39]. These surface variants include rtV173L, which arises from the rtM204V or rtM204I mutations and causes reduced binding of HBsAg to the HBV surface antibody, and the stop codons Trp172X of the S protein, which arises from the rtA181T mutation and causes decreased virion secretion. These escape mutants of HBV potentially could result in antiviral drug associated potential vaccine escape mutants and lead to new infections in patients who may have protective anti-HBV antibody titers by previous vaccination.

Multidrug Resistance

Sequential monotherapy for HBV can promote the selection for multidrug-resistant strains of HBV (e.g., LMV followed by adefovir and LMV followed by entecavir (ETV)) due to the development of compensatory mutations that enhance replicative potential, but may also alter the binding characteristics of other agents at the polymerase binding site. These have been reported when there has been use of add-on strategies for patients who may have a partial response to initial antiviral therapy that does not result in rapid and complete suppression of HBV replication. High necroinflammatory activity in the liver as evidenced by high ALT levels usually allows a larger replication space for HBV to rapidly spread because of increased rates of hepatocyte replication in areas of injury. The lower rates of mutations observed with the use of tenofovir (TDF) and ETV may suggest their use as first-line agents. Close monitoring of patients undergoing therapy for HBV viral load is also necessary to make a switch of antiviral therapy before the occurrence of ALT flares to minimize the chances of selecting for MDR HBV strains. Such therapeutic strategies aimed at maximizing viral suppression and eradication rates ensure prevention of emergence of drug resistant HBV strains.

HBV Evolution

As described earlier, HBV undergoes several rounds of replication each day inside the infected host using an error prone RT enzyme. This process leads to the emergence of closely related molecular species termed quasi-species. A close molecular analysis of the heterogeneous HBV population helped us to understand the factors responsible for the diversity and the evolution of HBV across species and continents.

The rate of HBV evolution is estimated to be about 2×10^{-4} base substitutions per site per year, which is an intermediate rate between DNA virus and RNA virus rates [40]. This finding suggests that the origins of the virus began as a retrovirus or retrovirus-like particle and evolved through a process of deletion [41]. Evolution of the HBV virus occurs due to both genotypic variability and phenotypic variability. Genotypic variability results from the slow changes of the genome over time in the absence of selective pressure. By contrast, phenotypic variability arises due to specific selective pressures, such as host immune responses and vaccination, which leads to virus adaptations as demonstrated by the fairly conserved HBV genome observed in immunotolerant HBeAg-positive asymptomatic subjects with very high levels of replication. A fundamental mechanism of HBV evolution is dependent on the fixation of randomly generated mutations resulting in an improved replication fitness of the mutant variant [42]. In the case of HBV mutant strains that emerge during antiviral therapy, a major determinant is the presence of covalently closed circular DNA, which is maintained in the hepatocyte nuclei with a long half-life in infected cells [43]. Antiviral therapy is not able to prevent the formation of cccDNA resulting in new infection of hepatocytes in persistently viremic patients receiving therapy. In other words, HBV cccDNA serves as a reservoir of HBV responsible for relapse in patients receiving antiviral therapy. Apart from the persistence of cccDNA, there are other major mechanisms that facilitates emergence of HBV mutants. These include viral factors such as existence of quasi-species, high rate of HBV replication, error prone RT based life cycle, adaptive mutations with compensatory mutations. Host factors include compliance on antiviral therapy, immune response, enhanced hepatic inflammatory response, and host genetic background.

Genotypic Variability

Viral variability due to genetic changes can be classified using subtypes based on the molecular basis of HBsAg. The major subtype epitopes are known as the d/y and r/w determinants, which are distinguished by the amino acid at position 122 and 160 of HBsAg, respectively. However, with four different combinations of d, y, r, and w and other aminoacid presentations, there are a total of ten different subtypes [44]. Importantly, serotypes are distinct from genotypes, the latter of which was developed later to classify HBV types. However, some correlations have been discovered between serotype and genotype.

The geographical distribution of the genotypes provides interesting insights into the evolution of the Hepatitis B virus. Okamoto et al. [45] were the first to divide a collection of 18 full-length genomes into groups, identifying four distinct strains as A–D. Since their discovery, four additional genotypes have been identified. The eight genotypes, A–H, are present in discrete geographical regions. While genotype may be correlated with severity and progression of disease, no conclusive data has been reported. Genotype A is common worldwide, B and C are common in Asia, D is found in most places except Northern Europe and the Americas, E is present mainly in sub-Saharan Africa, F is common in South and Central America, G has been discovered in Europe, the USA, and Japan, and H is present in Central America and southern USA. The geographical separation seems to suggest that these HBV types evolved independently from each other. However, with increased migration and travel, these distinct types are beginning to be spread globally and heterogeneous genomes have been reported.

Recombination events are likely to occur due to the nature of HBV replication. The B2 and B3 subtypes, which are composed of a genotype B backbone and a core gene and core promoter of genotype C, yield interesting insights into the process of recombination. Since the promoter of genotype C is present in these subtypes, researchers have suggested that homologous recombination of cccDNA molecules occurs in which the two different HBV strains infect a single hepatocyte. If this is true, both genotype B and C would present in the cccDNA pool and additional recombinants would be produced by the chimerical pgRNA.

Phenotypic Variations

In contrast to genotypic variations, phenotypic variations emerge due to selective pressure from nature host immune responses, antiviral treatments, or vaccination. Phenotypic variations can be distinguished from genotypic variations because they are less fit and do not emerge in populations in the absence of selective pressures (e.g., drug-resistance mutations as described previously are lost when the therapy is stopped). Thus, although vaccination programs and use of nucleoside/nucleotide analogs have been largely successful in reducing the prevalence of HBV infection, we must now be aware that we are potentially increasing the rate of evolution of the virus. A recent shift to the precore and core mutations demonstrate that this mutation is more fit in a population pool that has received vaccination against the wild-type HBV.

Occult HBV

Occult HBV infection is defined as the presence of HBV DNA in the serum or liver tissue without the presence of the surface antigen (HBsAg). Mutations in the "a" determinant region of the S-gene have been associated with occult Hepatitis B. Studies have demonstrated that one of the mutations, T143M, may be the cause of HBsAg negativity [46]. If the gene is modified in such a way that it produces an antigenically altered surface protein, HBsAg would not be able to detect the protein [47].

In evolutionarily terms, it has been suggested that an accumulation of substitutions occurred in the core–surface protein interface. This evolutionary branch survived due to positive selection. In a comparison of the genome for occult infection with the genome of genotype D, van Hemert et al. [48] described that a 2986-202 RNA splicing event creates viral particles that lack the surface protein. The splicing does not effect a change in the polymerase, envelope, or X-protein functions.

Conclusion

In summary, HBV utilizes a complex, poorly understood process of life cycle using an error-prone RT enzyme, resulting in an enhanced rate of mutagenesis, which leads to selection of adapted strains influenced by the immune pressure and/or antiviral therapy. Existing molecular techniques to study HBV diversity is complex and labor-intensive, requiring novel molecular technology to be developed. Close analysis of HBV diversity has been helpful in providing valuable insights into our understanding of HBV origin, evolution, migration, and emergence of drug resistance. Availability of novel drugs that act at various stages of HBV life cycle, particularly in preventing the formation of cccDNA is imperative in preventing newer infections with multidrug-resistant HBV mutant strains in vaccinated subjects.

References

1. Nassal M, Hepatitis B. Hepatitis B viruses: reverse transcription a different way. Virus Res. 2008;134(1–2):235–49.
2. Lan YT, Li J, Liao W, Ou J. Roles of the three major phosphorylation sites of hepatitis B virus core protein in viral replication. Virology. 1999;259(2):342–8.
3. Xie Y, Zhai J, Deng Q, Tiollais P, Wang Y, Zhao M. Entry of hepatitis B virus: mechanism and new therapeutic target. Pathol Biol (Paris). 2010;58:301–7.
4. Liang TJ, Hepatitis B. The virus and disease. Hepatology. 2009;49 (5 Suppl):S13–21.
5. Gripon P, Rumin S, Urban S, et al. Infection of a human hepatoma cell line by hepatitis B virus. Proc Natl Acad Sci USA. 2002;99(24): 15655–60.
6. Lee WM. Hepatitis B virus infection. N Engl J Med. 1997;337(24): 1733–45.
7. Bruss V, Lu X, Thomssen R, Gerlich WH. Post-translational alterations in transmembrane topology of the hepatitis B virus large envelope protein. EMBO J. 1994;13(10):2273–9.
8. Tuttleman JS, Pourcel C, Summers J. Formation of the pool of covalently closed circular viral DNA in hepadnavirus-infected cells. Cell. 1986;47(3):451–60.
9. Beck J, Nassal M. Hepatitis B virus replication. World J Gastroenterol. 2007;13(1):48–64.
10. Hu J, Toft DO, Seeger C. Hepadnavirus assembly and reverse transcription require a multi-component chaperone complex which is incorporated into nucleocapsids. EMBO J. 1997;16(1):59–68.
11. Hu J, Seeger C. Hsp90 is required for the activity of a hepatitis B virus reverse transcriptase. Proc Natl Acad Sci USA. 1996;93(3): 1060–4.
12. Nassal M, Rieger A. A bulged region of the hepatitis B virus RNA encapsidation signal contains the replication origin for discontinuous first-strand DNA synthesis. J Virol. 1996;70(5):2764–73.
13. Pollack JR, Ganem D. An RNA stem-loop structure directs hepatitis B virus genomic RNA encapsidation. J Virol. 1993;67(6): 3254–63.
14. Tang H, McLachlan A. A pregenomic RNA sequence adjacent to DR1 and complementary to epsilon influences hepatitis B virus replication efficiency. Virology. 2002;303(1):199–210.
15. Oropeza CE, McLachlan A. Complementarity between epsilon and phi sequences in pregenomic RNA influences hepatitis B virus replication efficiency. Virology. 2007;359(2):371–81.
16. Bouchard MJ, Schneider RJ. The enigmatic X gene of hepatitis B virus. J Virol. 2004;78(23):12725–34.
17. Seeger C, Zoulim F, Mason WS. Hepadnaviruses. In: Knipe DM, Howley P, editors. Fields virology, No. 2. Philadelphia: Lippincott Williams and Wilkins; 2007.
18. Gearhart TL, Bouchard MJ. The hepatitis B virus X protein modulates hepatocyte proliferation pathways to stimulate viral replication. J Virol. 2010;84(6):2675–86.
19. Wei Y, Neuveut C, Tiollais P, Buendia MA. Molecular biology of the hepatitis B virus and role of the X gene. Pathol Biol. 2010;58:267–72.
20. McClain SL, Clippinger AJ, Lizzano R, Bouchard MJ. Hepatitis B virus replication is associated with an HBx-dependent mitochondrion-regulated increase in cytosolic calcium levels. J Virol. 2007;81(21):12061–5.

21. Bouchard MJ, Wang LH, Schneider RJ. Calcium signaling by HBx protein in hepatitis B virus DNA replication. Science. 2001;294(5550):2376–8.
22. Ozer A, Khaoustov VI, Mearns M, et al. Effect of hepatocyte proliferation and cellular DNA synthesis on hepatitis B virus replication. Gastroenterology. 1996;110(5):1519–28.
23. Friedrich B, Wollersheim M, Brandenburg B, Foerste R, Will H, Hildt E. Induction of anti-proliferative mechanisms in hepatitis B virus producing cells. J Hepatol. 2005;43(4):696–703.
24. Guidotti LG, Matzke B, Chisari FV. Hepatitis B virus replication is cell cycle independent during liver regeneration in transgenic mice. J Virol. 1997;71(6):4804–8.
25. Gomez-Gonzalo M, Carretero M, Rullas J, et al. The hepatitis B virus X protein induces HIV-1 replication and transcription in synergy with T-cell activation signals: functional roles of NF-kappaB/NF-AT and SP1-binding sites in the HIV-1 long terminal repeat promoter. J Biol Chem. 2001;276(38):35435–43.
26. Domingo E, Mas A, Yuste E, et al. Virus population dynamics, fitness variations and the control of viral disease: an update. Prog Drug Res. 2001;57:77–115.
27. Orito E, Mizokami M, Ina Y, et al. Host-independent evolution and a genetic classification of the hepadnavirus family based on nucleotide sequences. Proc Natl Acad Sci USA. 1989;86(18):7059–62.
28. Morozov V, Pisareva M, Groudinin M. Homologous recombination between different genotypes of hepatitis B virus. Gene. 2000;260(1–2):55–65.
29. Lok AS, Akarca U, Greene S. Mutations in the pre-core region of hepatitis B virus serve to enhance the stability of the secondary structure of the pre-genome encapsidation signal. Proc Natl Acad Sci USA. 1994;91(9):4077–81.
30. Bessesen M, Ives D, Condreay L, Lawrence S, Sherman KE. Chronic active hepatitis B exacerbations in human immunodeficiency virus-infected patients following development of resistance to or withdrawal of lamivudine. Clin Infect Dis. 1999;28(5):1032–5.
31. Lai CL, Dienstag J, Schiff E, et al. Prevalence and clinical correlates of YMDD variants during lamivudine therapy for patients with chronic hepatitis B. Clin Infect Dis. 2003;36(6):687–96.
32. Dienstag JL, Schiff ER, Wright TL, et al. Lamivudine as initial treatment for chronic hepatitis B in the United States. N Engl J Med. 1999;341(17):1256–63.
33. Angus P, Vaughan R, Xiong S, et al. Resistance to adefovir dipivoxil therapy associated with the selection of a novel mutation in the HBV polymerase. Gastroenterology. 2003;125(2):292–7.
34. Tenney DJ, Levine SM, Rose RE, et al. Clinical emergence of entecavir-resistant hepatitis B virus requires additional substitutions in virus already resistant to Lamivudine. Antimicrob Agents Chemother. 2004;48(9):3498–507.
35. Liaw YF, Gane E, Leung N, et al. 2-Year GLOBE trial results: telbivudine is superior to lamivudine in patients with chronic hepatitis B. Gastroenterology. 2009;136(2):486–95.
36. Marcellin P, Heathcote EJ, Buti M, et al. Tenofovir disoproxil fumarate versus adefovir dipivoxil for chronic hepatitis B. N Engl J Med. 2008;359(23):2442–55.
37. Amini-Bavil-Olyaee S, Herbers U, Sheldon J, Luedde T, Trautwein C, Tacke F. The rtA194T polymerase mutation impacts viral replication and susceptibility to tenofovir in hepatitis B e antigen-positive and hepatitis B e antigen-negative hepatitis B virus strains. Hepatology. 2009;49(4):1158–65.
38. Torresi J, Earnest-Silveira L, Deliyannis G, et al. Reduced antigenicity of the hepatitis B virus HBsAg protein arising as a consequence of sequence changes in the overlapping polymerase gene that are selected by lamivudine therapy. Virology. 2002;293(2):305–13.
39. Warner N, Locarnini S. The antiviral drug selected hepatitis B virus rtA181T/sW172* mutant has a dominant negative secretion defect and alters the typical profile of viral rebound. Hepatology. 2008;48(1):88–98.
40. Jazayeri SM, Alavian SM, Carman WF. Hepatitis B virus: origin and evolution. J Viral Hepat. 2010;17(4):229–35.
41. Miller RH, Robinson WS. Common evolutionary origin of hepatitis B virus and retroviruses. Proc Natl Acad Sci USA. 1986;83(8):2531–5.
42. Carman WF, Thomas HC. Implications of genetic variation on the pathogenesis of hepatitis B virus infection. Arch Virol Suppl. 1993;8:143–54.
43. Zoulim F. New insight on hepatitis B virus persistence from the study of intrahepatic viral cccDNA. J Hepatol. 2005;42(3):302–8.
44. Norder H, Courouce AM, Coursaget P, et al. Genetic diversity of hepatitis B virus strains derived worldwide: genotypes, subgenotypes, and HBsAg subtypes. Intervirology. 2004;47(6):289–309.
45. Okamoto H, Imai M, Shimozaki M, et al. Nucleotide sequence of a cloned hepatitis B virus genome, subtype ayr: comparison with genomes of the other three subtypes. J Gen Virol. 1986;67(Pt 11):2305–14.
46. Kumar GT, Kazim SN, Kumar M, et al. Hepatitis B virus genotypes and hepatitis B surface antigen mutations in family contacts of hepatitis B virus infected patients with occult hepatitis B virus infection. J Gastroenterol Hepatol. 2009;24(4):588–98.
47. Jeantet D, Chemin I, Mandrand B, et al. Cloning and expression of surface antigens from occult chronic hepatitis B virus infections and their recognition by commercial detection assays. J Med Virol. 2004;73(4):508–15.
48. van Hemert FJ, Zaaijer HL, Berkhout B, Lukashov VV. Occult hepatitis B infection: an evolutionary scenario. Virol J. 2008;5:146.

Hepatitis C Virus Treatment in HIV

Raymond Chung and Gyanprakash Avinash Ketwaroo

Introduction

Since the introduction of highly active antiretroviral therapy (HAART), HIV has been successfully converted into a chronic condition. In place of traditional opportunistic infections, Hepatitis C Virus (HCV)-related liver disease has emerged as a significant cause of morbidity and mortality in HIV infected persons [1]. HIV–HCV coinfected patients have an accelerated rate of fibrosis, developing cirrhosis more rapidly than those with HCV alone [2]. Among those with HCV-related decompensated liver disease, HIV coinfection also increases liver-related mortality [3]. Efforts to treat HCV are, therefore, warranted to forestall these complications.

Viral eradication is reflected by achievement of a sustained virologic response (SVR), defined as an undetectable HCV RNA 24 weeks after the end of a course of treatment. SVR is a particularly robust endpoint, with nearly 100% of patients remaining free of circulating HCV up to 18 years after achieving SVR [4]. In coinfected patients, accomplishment of SVR is associated with improved natural history, with reduced liver injury and lower overall mortality [5]. SVR, therefore, remains the gold standard, representing a clinical cure.

Initiation of Treatment

The treatment of chronic HCV infection in the HIV(+) person is best managed by a multidisciplinary team that includes hepatologists and infectious disease specialists who can anticipate and monitor response to treatment, drug interactions, and toxicities of treatment regimens. HIV–HCV coinfected patients who exhibit evidence of liver disease in the form of serum aminotransferase elevation and/or pathologic changes on liver biopsy should be considered for treatment. Since it is the development of fibrosis that indicates a trajectory toward cirrhosis and liver failure, this is typically used as an indication for treatment. Those with mild disease, or stage 0–1 fibrosis, are usually deferred for treatment in the presence of negative predictors of response to therapy, such as genotype 1 or 4 infection. In general, chronic hepatitis C with any stage of fibrosis is eligible for therapy, but the presence of moderate fibrosis (at least stage 2) should prompt the recommendation for treatment. Some patients with a high likelihood of achieving an SVR, especially those with HCV genotypes 2 or 3, may be offered treatment without liver biopsy to assess for fibrosis. Patients who are not offered treatment should be reassessed every 3 years, in part because of the more rapid progression of hepatic fibrosis in the HIV–HCV cohort [6–10].

Persistently Normal Alanine Aminotransferase

The liver biopsy, or a surrogate noninvasive marker of liver fibrosis, is particularly important in those HIV–HCV infected persons with persistently normal alanine aminotransferase (PNALT), since up to one third of these patients may have enough fibrosis to justify treatment [11, 12]. In a study of mostly genotype 1 patients, 10.5% of coinfected patients with PNALT had advanced liver fibrosis and nearly 30% had a Metavir score of at least F2 [13]. HIV–HCV patients with PNALT should, therefore, be considered for liver biopsy or noninvasive assessment of fibrosis. Empiric treatment may also be considered in those with genotype 2 or 3 infection.

R. Chung (✉)
Department of Gastroenterology, Massachusetts General Hospital,
55 Fruit St, Boston, MA 02114, USA
e-mail: Rtchung@partners.org

Regimen

Background

The currently recommended treatment regimen for chronic HCV monoinfection is a combination of pegylated-interferon alpha (PegIFN) and ribavirin (RBV) for 24–48 weeks, depending on viral genotype.

The precise mechanism by which interferon alpha suppresses HCV has not been fully elucidated. It is known that the interferon alpha molecule binds to interferon-receptor subunits on cells activating the janus kinase (*JAK*)-signal transducer and activator of transcription (STAT) pathway of downstream protein kinases. This results in the upregulation of several hundred interferon-stimulated genes. It is thought that the proteins expressed by these genes have antiviral properties, including inhibition of the translation of viral proteins and replication of viral RNA. Interferon alpha may also promote the adaptive immune response to hepatitis C infection [14].

Initial therapy with standard interferon alpha was of limited utility, with only about 8–20% in the treated monoinfected cohort achieving SVR [15]. The addition of ribavirin resulted in an improvement in treatment results, with SVR approaching 43% among patients of all genotypes [16]. Ribavirin is a synthetic guanosine analog, and the mechanism by which it enhances viral eradication in combination with interferon alpha, is also unclear. It is thought that it may directly inhibit the HCV polymerase, modulate the immune response, or may enhance viral mutagenesis during interferon therapy [14]. However, recent data suggest that ribavirin increases interferon stimulated gene induction [17].

Pegylation of the interferon-alpha (IFN) molecule reduces its rate of renal clearance, thus prolonging steady state duration of therapeutic levels of IFN. This enables PegIFN to be given weekly. In HCV monoinfection, combination PegIFN and RBV produces an SVR of 40–45% for genotypes 1 and 4 after 48 weeks of therapy, and about 70–80% for genotypes 2 and 3, after 24 weeks or therapy [18]. Two types of pegylated-interferon alpha can be used: PegIFN alpha 2a at 180 µg/week or PegIFN alpha 2b at 1.5 µg/kg per week. Both forms of pegylated interferon alpha are thought to be comparable in efficacy with similar side-effect profiles [19].

Treatment

The use of PegIFN and RBV for treatment of the HIV–HCV coinfected population has been studied extensively during the HAART era. In 2004, three landmark studies demonstrated the safety and efficacy of PegIFN and RBV in treating chronic HCV infection in HIV–HCV coinfected patients (Table 15.1) [22, 23]. While these studies showed that SVR could be accomplished in this group of patients, these rates are decidedly diminished compared to those seen in HCV monoinfected persons. In the ACTG trial, PegIFN alpha 2a in combination with RBV achieved an SVR of 27% compared

Table 15.1 Comparison of PegIFN + RBV regimens in major trials in HIV–HCV coinfection

	APRICOT (PegIFN Alpha 2a + RBV) [23]	ACTG (PegIFN Alpha 2a + RBV) [20]	RIBAVIC (PegIFN Alpha 2b + RBV) [21]	PRESCO (PegIFN Alpha 2a + weight-based RBV) [22]
Number patients, n	289	66	205	389
Age (year)	39.7 (± 7.9)	45 (Median)	39.5 (± −5.5)	40 (Median)
Male (%)	80	79	77	74
Race (%)	80% White, 11% black	50% White, 32% black	Not recorded	Not recorded
IVDA/no. (%)	180 (62%)	Not recorded	165 (80%)	348 (89.5%)
Mean serum HCV RNA (IU/ml)	5,600,000 ± 6,400,000	6,200,000 ± 400,000	937,000,000 (median)	Not recorded
HCV genotype 1 (%)	61	77	48	49
Cirrhosis/advanced fibrosis (%)	15	11	39	Not recorded
Antiretroviral Rx (%)	84	85	83	74
HIV-1 RNA mean (log 10 copies/ml)	2.3 ± 1.0	Not recorded	3.6 (Median)	<2 (Median)
Undetect HIV-1 RNA (%)	60	61	70	71.5
Mean CD4+ cells – (no./mm^3)	520 ± 277	495 (Median)	477 (Median)	546 (Median)
RBV regimen	400 mg po BID	Dose escalation	400 mg po BID	Weight-based
EVR (%)	71	44	Not recorded	Not recorded
ETVR (%)	47	41	35	50
SVR – overall (%)	40	27	27	67
SVR – Gt 1/4 (%)	29	14	17	35
SVR – Gt 2/3 (%)	62	73	44	72

EVR early virological response, *ETVR* end of treatment virological response

with only 12% in patients receiving interferon alpha 2a and RBV [20]. Significantly, in the PegIFN alpha 2a group, 73% of genotype 2/3 patients attained SVR, in contrast to only 14% of genotype 1 patients. In the larger APRICOT trial, treatment with PegIFN alpha 2a and RBV resulted in an SVR of 40% compared with 12% in the IFN and RBV group. Similar advantages over interferon alpha were replicated in HIV–HCV patients treated with PegIFN alpha2b, in the RIBAVIC study [21]. As in HCV monoinfected patients, there appears to be no statistical difference in efficacy and adverse events between PegIFN alpha 2a and PegIFN alpha 2b in the HIV–HCV coinfected cohort [24].

Ribavirin is essential for enhancing the rates of SVR in HIV–HCV coinfected patients. In the APRICOT trial, among genotype 1 patients, an SVR of 29% was achieved with both PegIFN and RBV compared with an SVR of only 14% in the nonribavirin arm; in genotypes 2 and 3, the SVR increased from 36 to 62% with the addition of RBV to the treatment regimen [23]. The dose of ribavirin is also important for ensuring viral eradication. In the monoinfected population, a weight based regimen of 1,000 mg/day or 1,200 mg/day is superior to 800 mg/day dosing in genotype 1 patients [25]. Lower doses of ribavirin were used in these early trials in HIV–HCV coinfection due to concerns over side effects, though there is now data to suggest that a weight-based RBV dosing regimen improves virologic response among the HIV–HCV cohort [22, 26]. A recent retrospective analysis in HIV–HCV patients found that a ribavirin concentration of <2.5 μg/ml at week 4 was associated with increased HCV relapse; however, the routine use of ribavirin concentrations has not been adopted in clinical practice because of concerns regarding assay quality control [27]. Currently, the HIV–HCV International Panel recommends a weight based dose of ribavirin of 1,000 mg/day for patients <75 kg or 1,200 mg/day for patients >75 kg, although a recent multicenter trial failed to detect improved efficacy with weight-based ribavirin dosing in genotype 1 HIV-coinfected patients [10, 28].

Viral Kinetics

During therapy with PegIFN and RBV, viral loads should be followed closely, since they predict response to therapy, and can determine treatment duration. An early virological response (EVR) is defined as at least a 2 log fall in HCV viral load after 12 weeks of therapy. As in monoinfected patients, EVR has a very high negative predictive value of 98–100% in HIV–HCV coinfection, that is, if an EVR is not attained, treatment should be discontinued for virologic futility [23]. Likewise, patients with viral RNA positivity at 24 weeks should also discontinue treatment [10]. By contrast, patients who clear HCV at 4 weeks of treatment, thereby achieving a rapid virologic response (RVR), appear more likely to accomplish SVR [29].

Attempts have been made to further tailor treatment duration based on EVR and RVR, but there are few randomized control trials [30]. There has also been the suggestion that patients may benefit from extending therapy to 72 weeks, though recent data do not support this [31]. Currently, the 2007 HIV–HCV International Panel recommends 48 weeks of therapy for all genotypes [10].

In summary, PegIFN alpha 2a or PegIFN alpha 2b with RBV 800–1,200 mg/day have demonstrated SVR rates of 38–75% in genotypes 2 and 3, and 14–33% in genotypes 1 or 4 [32]. Unlike monoinfected patients, persons with HCV genotypes 2 or 3 should be treated for 48 weeks. Overall, the HIV–HCV coinfected cohort appears to be less responsive to therapy, especially among genotype 1 or 4 patients.

Adverse Effects of Treatment

Treatment discontinuation and adherence can significantly lower SVR. In HCV monoinfected patients, genotype 1 subjects who received at least 80% of their PegIFN and RBV doses had a higher SVR than those who received less than 80% [33]. The HCV treatment regimen is not benign and can be associated with significant side effects that influence adherence and treatment discontinuation rates.

Side effects occur in almost 80% of patients who receive combination PegIFN and ribavirin therapy. Anemia is commonly encountered and is caused by hemolysis secondary to ribavirin, as well as suppression of the bone marrow by PegIFN. The mechanism by which RBV causes hemolysis is not completely understood. RBV appears to accumulate within red blood cells, resulting in a relative ATP deficiency and may thus increase the susceptibility of the erythrocyte to oxidative stress and extravascular hemolysis [34]. The hemolytic anemia is ribavirin dose dependent and stabilizes or resolves with dose reduction or discontinuation. Patients with a deficiency in inosine triphosphatase, an enzyme that degrades the competitive nucleotide inosine triphosphate, appear to tolerate ribavirin more readily; specifically, such patients have a reduced incidence of hemolytic anemia [35]. Erythropoietin may be used to ensure adequate hemoglobin concentrations during treatment to help maintain ribavirin doses [36].

The most frequent adverse events of interferon treatment are flu-like symptoms including myalgias, headaches, and low-grade fevers, seen in over 80% of patients. They are more severe within the first 48 hr of interferon administration. Interferon may also cause neutropenia, thrombocytopenia, fatigue, emotional lability, autoimmune thyroiditis, and ophthalmologic disorders, including ischemic retinopathy. Significant depression occurs in about 26% of patients using interferon and should be anticipated in those with mood and anxiety symptoms prior to treatment with PegIFN [37]. This is particularly important in the HIV–HCV cohort, where there is a high rate of drug use and baseline neurocognitive or psychiatric disorders. Psychiatric evaluation before and during HCV treatment should not be deferred if there is any suggestion of a mood disorder.

Because of the potential toxicity of PegIFN and RBV, those being considered for routine treatment should have a hemoglobin of at least 12 g/dL (men) or 11 g/dL (women), an absolute neutrophil count >1,500, and absence of retinopathy on funduscopic exam. However, each of these parameters is not absolute and should be considered in the context of individual risk and benefit. Interferon causes abortion in pregnant rhesus monkeys and ribavirin is teratogenic. Pregnancy is, therefore, contraindicated with combination therapy and women of child-bearing age, or men, should use two forms of barrier contraception with sexual activity. Given the common exacerbation of depression with interferon, and the real risk of suicide, active psychiatric illnesses must be stabilized before receiving treatment. Those with already decompensated liver failure with evidence of ascites, variceal bleeding, jaundice, coagulopathy, or encephalopathy do not tolerate interferon well,and should be considered for liver transplantation before consideration of a course of PegIFN/RBV, which can exacerbate decompensation. Such patients are best treated by specialists with experience in hepatic decompensation management. While being treated, patients should be frequently monitored (typically, every 4 weeks) for development of side effects. It is also recommended that HIV be suppressed before starting anti-HCV therapy. Most studies have enrolled patients with no opportunistic infections, a CD4 count greater than 200 cells/mm^3 and an HIV viral load of less than 50,000 copies/ml.

A large proportion of HIV–HCV individuals in the USA are injection drug users. These patients are thought to be at risk of jeopardizing treatment success due to ongoing or recent substance abuse. However, prior studies suggest that these patients may be successfully treated for HCV infection, provided they receive adequate medical and peer support [38]. Treatment for such patients should be decided on an individual basis, with attempts to ensure appropriate counseling, and psychiatric evaluation, as well as enrollment in the appropriate abstinence programs.

Predictors of Response

For those who are able to initiate and successfully complete therapy, there are several factors that predict response. In particular, an HCV RNA level of less than 800,000 IU/ml, absence of prior intravenous drug abuse, and genotypes 2 or 3 have been associated with an improved chance of attaining SVR [20, 21, 23]. Baseline HCV quasi-species complexity was an independent predictor of response in an HCV/HIV coinfected cohort, but this assay is not clinically available [39]. Other factors associated with poor treatment response include presence of cirrhosis, African-American or Hispanic race, and high body mass index (BMI).

With such low success rates in genotypes 1 and 4, improved tools for predicting response to therapy are needed to identify those who would most benefit. Genome wide association studies have identified a genetic variation in the *IL28B* gene as being highly associated with the likelihood of success of PegIFN and RBV therapy [40]. The *IL28B* locus encodes for interferon lambda-3, and research into how the *rs8099917* minor allele of the *IL28B* locus is associated with failure in genotypes 1 and 4 is ongoing. If the presence of an unfavorable genotype is confirmed, this information may be used to justify delaying the start of therapy in genotype 1 patients, particularly as we await the introduction of new treatment options.

Drug Interactions

Special considerations in the coinfected population include the interactions of HCV medications with HAART. Zidovudine should be avoided during HCV treatment, as it can exacerbate the anemia caused by ribavirin [22]. Ribavirin enhances didanosine exposure, resulting in higher risk of mitochondrial toxicity from this nucleoside reverse transcriptase inhibitor [41]. Coadministration of didanosine and ribavirin is, therefore, contraindicated.

The Future

Given the low SVR and high toxicities affecting PegIFN and RBV therapy in HIV–HCV coinfection, there is a major need for new therapies. On the horizon are several new direct acting antiviral agents (DAAs) for hepatitis C. The most promising DAAs are the protease inhibitors, which include ciluprevir, telaprevir and boceprevir. These drugs inhibit the viral NS3/4A serine protease responsible for processing the HCV polyprotein into mature viral proteins. Ciluprevir was associated with a 100–1,000-fold reduction in HCV viral load after only 2 days of treatment [42]. While studies of this drug were halted due to cardiotoxicity in animal trials, telaprevir continues to show promise in phase 2 trials of HCV monoinfected patients [43, 44]. In a recent multicenter, randomized control phase 2b trial, the addition of telaprevir permitted truncation of therapy to 24 weeks, at the same time enhancing SVR. Patients who received ribavirin and PegIFN for 24 weeks with telaprevir added to the treatment regimen for the first 12 weeks, achieved an SVR of 61%, compared with 42% in the standard of care regimen using ribavirin and PegIFN for 48 weeks [44].

While this class of drugs holds significant promise, there is the real risk of selecting for resistant variants. In nonresponders and relapsers in this study who had been treated with telaprevir, the selection of telaprevir-resistant mutants was demonstrated. It is anticipated that the development of such resistance may be minimized by the use of future drug cocktails similar to HAART therapy, where the HCV and the host machinery are attacked at multiple targets with non-overlapping resistance patterns. Other DAA targets include the viral RNA polymerase as well as the NS5A protein.

There are a number of intriguing host factor inhibitors that offer promise because they have a high barrier to viral resistance, since they do not apply direct selection pressure against the virus. Cyclophilins are cofactors that facilitate HCV replication, as they regulate RNA binding of the viral polymerase. There has been interest in using selective inhibitors of these cyclophilins as another means of reducing viral replication. Alisporivir (Debio-025) is a cyclosporine A derivative that inhibits host cell cyclophilins, without immunosuppressive activity. In phase II trials and animal models, alisporivir alone or in combination with PegIFN has been shown to reduce the HCV viral load [45]. Interestingly, alisporivir also has anti-HIV activity and is thus an attractive candidate for future trials involving HIV–HCV patients [46].

In summary, the effectiveness of recent DAAs and ongoing clinical trials of others surely will mean transformation of the standard of care for HCV. Trials involving groups with disappointing SVR rates, such as HIV–HCV coinfected patients, are eagerly anticipated. It is expected that a larger combination regimen or drug cocktail, with increased efficacy, will soon be available.

Nonresponders/Relapsers

With the low rates of SVR after initial treatment of HCV in the HIV–HCV coinfected population, we can anticipate a particularly large number of relapsers and nonresponders. Patients who develop a recurrence of HCV after having become HCV RNA negative at end of treatment are considered relapsers. Retreatment with the same regimen usually results in a second relapse and thus alternative dosing, duration, or regimens should be considered. Nonresponders, or patients with persistent HCV viral load during and at the end of treatment, have a poor prognosis. If initially treated with standard of care combination therapy, they are likely to have a poor response to retreatment with PegIFN and RBV.

There had been some suggestion that nonresponders or relapsers have a mortality or histologic benefit to treatment despite not achieving SVR [47, 48]. Efforts to investigate whether maintenance PegIFN therapy could produce histologic benefit in the absence of viral clearance were made.

However, the long-term use of weekly, maintenance peg-IFN has recently been shown to have no clinical advantage in monoinfection [49]. Similarly, the SLAM-C trial in HCV-HIV coinfection failed to demonstrate a difference for maintenance PegIFN in altering fibrosis progression, although the observation arm in the study experienced little fibrosis progression [50].

Relapsers and nonresponders who were initially treated with a suboptimal regimen could derive significant benefit from retreatment. In a small study of patients initially treated with interferon monotherapy, interferon and RBV, or PegIFN plus RBV 800 mg/day, an overall SVR of 30.8% was attained with PegIFN and weight based RBV retreatment [51]. An SVR of 72.7% was obtained for genotypes 2 and 3 and 19.5% for genotypes 1 and 4. In the subset of prior PegIFN and RBV failures, SVR was 27% overall: 16% in prior nonresponders and 35% in relapsers. In the specific group of genotype 1 prior nonresponders, SVR was a dismal 9%. While genotype is notably associated with response to retreatment, multivariate analysis also highlighted the importance of maintaining an adequate RBV plasma concentration [51]. It is anticipated that the introduction of the protease inhibitors will improve retreatment SVR. Preliminary results show that the addition of telaprevir to a retreatment regimen may increase SVR from 20 to 73% for prior relapsers and from 9 to 39% for prior nonresponders [52]. Thus it is hoped that the introduction of protease inhibitors will offer a real treatment option for coinfected patients who have failed prior PegIFN and RBV treatment. This benefit must be weighed against the risk of selecting out and enriching for protease inhibitor-resistant variants.

Acute Hepatitis C Virus: Treatment

Acute HCV is defined as infection with HCV of less than 6 months' duration [53]. Patients with acute HCV are usually asymptomatic, and given the lack of a reliable IgM-based diagnostic test, or clear distinction between laboratory findings of acute and chronic hepatitis C, often remain undiagnosed. In clinical practice, acute HCV is diagnosed when a patient with recent risk of exposure presents with an elevated ALT > 10 times the upper limit of normal in the setting of a positive HCV RNA test. In HCV monoinfected patients, a 98% SVR with interferon therapy has been reported in acute HCV [54]. In the HIV–HCV population, data on the success of treatment are limited, though several studies report an SVR of 59–94% with 24 weeks of PegIFN and RBV therapy [55, 56]. Current guidelines suggest initiating therapy 12 weeks after the date of estimated exposure to allow for spontaneous clearance, and then to treat with 24 weeks of Peg-IFN and weight-based ribavirin [10]. In summary, because acute HCV is highly treatable and success rates are substantially higher than in those patients who move on to chronic HCV, the need for providers to identify these patients with HIV coinfection is great.

Summary

HCV is a significant cause of morbidity and mortality in the HIV-infected population. While treating HCV with PegIFN and RBV in HIV–HCV coinfected persons is not as effective as in HCV monoinfected patients, appreciable SVR rates can be accomplished. In those patients chronically coinfected with HCV genotypes 2 or 3, clinical cure rates are substantial, approaching those of monoinfected persons. HCV genotypes 1 and 4 remain difficult to treat, and new treatment options, including viral protease inhibitors, are of particular promise for this group. It is also anticipated that protease inhibitors and perhaps other classes of small molecule agents will significantly improve SVR when added to standard PegIFN and RBV for treating prior relapsers and nonresponders. Furthermore, the development of a new treatment regimen that ultimately combines oral direct acting antiviral and host cofactor inhibitors is eagerly awaited.

References

1. Monga HK, Rodriguez-Barradas MC, Breaux K, et al. Hepatitis C virus infection-related morbidity and mortality among patients with human immunodeficiency virus infection. Clin Infect Dis. 2001; 33(2):240–7.
2. Benhamou Y, Bochet M, Di Martino V, et al. Liver fibrosis progression in human immunodeficiency virus and hepatitis C virus coinfected patients. The Multivirc Group. Hepatology. 1999;30(4): 1054–8.
3. Pineda JA, Romero-Gómez M, Díaz-García F, et al. HIV coinfection shortens the survival of patients with hepatitis C virus-related decompensated cirrhosis. Hepatology. 2005;41(4):779–89.
4. Maylin S, Martinot-Peignoux M, Moucari R, et al. Eradication of hepatitis C virus in patients successfully treated for chronic hepatitis C. Gastroenterology. 2008;135(3):821–9.
5. Berenguer J, Alvarez-Pellicer J, Martín PM, et al. Sustained virological response to interferon plus ribavirin reduces liver-related complications and mortality in patients coinfected with human immunodeficiency virus and hepatitis C virus. Hepatology. 2009; 50(2):407–13.
6. Bonnard P, Lescure FX, Amiel C, et al. Documented rapid course of hepatic fibrosis between two biopsies in patients coinfected by HIV and HCV despite high CD4 cell count. J Viral Hepat. 2007; 14(11):806–11.
7. Regev A, Berho M, Jeffers LJ, et al. Sampling error and intraobserver variation in liver biopsy in patients with chronic HCV infection. Am J Gastroenterol. 2002;97(10):2614–8.
8. Shaheen AA, Myers RP. Systematic review and meta-analysis of the diagnostic accuracy of fibrosis marker panels in patients with HIV/hepatitis C coinfection. HIV Clin Trials. 2008;9(1):43–51.
9. Vergara S, Macías J, Rivero A, et al. The use of transient elastometry for assessing liver fibrosis in patients with HIV and hepatitis C virus coinfection. Clin Infect Dis. 2007;45(8):969–74.
10. Soriano V, Puoti M, Sulkowski M, et al. Care of patients coinfected with HIV and hepatitis C virus: 2007 updated recommendations from the HCV-HIV International Panel. AIDS. 2007;21(9): 1073–89.
11. Uberti-foppa C, Bona AD, Galli L, et al. Liver fibrosis in HIV-positive patients. Liver. 2006;41(1):63–7.
12. Sánchez-Conde M, Berenguer J, Miralles P, et al. Liver biopsy findings for HIV-infected patients with chronic hepatitis C and persistently normal levels of alanine aminotransferase. Clin Infect Dis. 2006;43(5):640–4.
13. Martin-Carbonero L, de Ledinghen V, Moreno A, et al. Liver fibrosis in patients with chronic hepatitis C and persistently normal liver enzymes: influence of HIV infection. J Viral Hepat. 2009;16(11): 790–5.
14. Feld JJ, Hoofnagle JH. Mechanism of action of interferon and ribavirin in treatment of hepatitis C. Nature. 2005;436(7053):967–72.
15. Carithers RL, Emerson SS. Therapy of hepatitis C: meta-analysis of interferon alfa-2b trials. Hepatology. 1997;26(3 Suppl 1):83S–88.
16. McHutchison JG, Gordon SC, Schiff ER, et al. Interferon alfa-2b alone or in combination with ribavirin as initial treatment for chronic hepatitis C. Hepatitis Interventional Therapy Group. N Engl J Med. 1998;339(21):1485–92.
17. Feld JJ, Lutchman GA, Heller T, et al. Ribavirin improves early responses to peginterferon through enhanced interferon signaling. Gastroenterology. 2010;139(1):154–62.e4.
18. Dienstag JL, McHutchison JG. American Gastroenterological Association technical review on the management of hepatitis C. Gastroenterology. 2006;130(1):231–64. quiz 214–7.
19. McHutchison JG, Lawitz EJ, Shiffman ML, et al. Peginterferon alfa-2b or alfa-2a with ribavirin for treatment of hepatitis C infection. N Engl J Med. 2009;361(6):580–93.
20. Chung RT, Andersen J, Volberding P, et al. Peginterferon Alfa-2a plus ribavirin versus interferon alfa-2a plus ribavirin for chronic hepatitis C in HIV-coinfected persons. N Engl J Med. 2004;351(5): 451–9.
21. Carrat F, Bani-Sadr F, Pol S, et al. Pegylated interferon alfa-2b vs standard interferon alfa-2b, plus ribavirin, for chronic hepatitis C in HIV-infected patients: a randomized controlled trial. JAMA. 2004;292(23):2839–48.
22. Núñez M, Miralles C, Berdún MA, et al. Role of weight-based ribavirin dosing and extended duration of therapy in chronic hepatitis C in HIV-infected patients: the PRESCO trial. AIDS Res Hum Retroviruses. 2007;23(8):972–82.
23. Torriani FJ, Rodriguez-Torres M, Rockstroh JK, et al. Peginterferon Alfa-2a plus ribavirin for chronic hepatitis C virus infection in HIV-infected patients. N Engl J Med. 2004;351(5):438–50.
24. Berenguer J, González-García J, López-Aldeguer J, et al. Pegylated interferon {alpha}2a plus ribavirin versus pegylated interferon {alpha}2b plus ribavirin for the treatment of chronic hepatitis C in HIV-infected patients. J Antimicrob Chemother. 2009;63(6): 1256–63.
25. Hadziyannis SJ, Sette H, Morgan TR, et al. Peginterferon-alpha2a and ribavirin combination therapy in chronic hepatitis C: a randomized study of treatment duration and ribavirin dose. Ann Intern Med. 2004;140(5):346–55.
26. Ramos B, Núñez M, Rendón A, et al. Critical role of ribavirin for the achievement of early virological response to HCV therapy in HCV/HIV-coinfected patients. J Viral Hepat. 2007;14(6):387–91.
27. Morello J, Soriano V, Barreiro P, et al. Plasma ribavirin trough concentrations at week 4 predict HCV relapse in HIV/HCV-coinfected patients treated for chronic hepatitis C. Antimicrob Agents Chemother. 2010;54(4):1647–9.
28. Rodriguez-Torres M, Slim J, Bhatti L, et al. Standard versus high dose ribavirin in combination with peginterferon alfa-2a (40 kD) in genotype 1 (G1) HCV patients coinfected with HIV: final results of the PARADIGM study. Program and abstracts of the 60th Annual

Meeting of the American Association for the Study of Liver Diseases; October 30–November 3, 2009; Boston, MA; 2009. Abstract 1561.
29. Ferenci P, Laferl H, Scherzer T, et al. Peginterferon alfa-2a and ribavirin for 24 weeks in hepatitis C type 1 and 4 patients with rapid virological response. Gastroenterology. 2008;135(2):451–8.
30. Van den Eynde E, Crespo M, Esteban JI, et al. Response-guided therapy for chronic hepatitis C virus infection in patients coinfected with HIV: a pilot trial. Clin Infect Dis. 2009;48(8):1152–9.
31. Buti M, Lurie Y, Zakharova N. Extended treatment duration in chronic hepatitis C genotype 1 infected slow-responders: final results of the SUCCESS study. In: 44th Annual Meeting of the European Association for the Study of the Liver (EASL 2009). Copenhagen, Denmark; 2009.
32. Iorio A, Marchesini E, Awad T, Gluud LL. Antiviral treatment for chronic hepatitis C in patients with human immunodeficiency virus. *Cochrane Database Syst Rev.* 2010;(1):CD004888.
33. Raptopoulou M, Tsantoulas D, Vafiadi I, et al. The effect of adherence to therapy on sustained response in daily or three times a week interferon alpha-2b plus ribavirin treatment of naive and nonresponder chronic hepatitis C patients. J Viral Hepat. 2005;12(1):91–5.
34. De Franceschi L, Fattovich G, Turrini F, et al. Hemolytic anemia induced by ribavirin therapy in patients with chronic hepatitis C virus infection: role of membrane oxidative damage. Hepatology. 2000;31(4):997–1004.
35. Fellay J, Thompson AJ, Ge D, et al. ITPA gene variants protect against anaemia in patients treated for chronic hepatitis C. Nature. 2010;464(7287):405–8.
36. Afdhal N. Epoetin alfa maintains ribavirin dose in HCV-infected patients: a prospective, double-blind, randomized controlled study. Gastroenterology. 2004;126(5):1302–11.
37. Raison CL, Demetrashvili M, Capuron L, Miller AH. Neuropsychiatric adverse effects of interferon-alpha: recognition and management. CNS Drugs. 2005;19(2):105–23.
38. Sylvestre DL. Treating hepatitis C virus infection in active substance users. Clin Infect Dis. 2005;40 Suppl 5:S321–4.
39. Sherman KE, Rouster SD, Stanford S, et al. Hepatitis C virus (HCV) quasispecies complexity and selection in HCV/HIV-coinfected subjects treated with interferon-based regimens. J Infect Dis. 2010;201(5):712–9.
40. Rauch A, Kutalik Z, Descombes P, et al. Genetic variation in IL28B is associated with chronic hepatitis c and treatment failure: a genome-wide association study. Gastroenterology. 2010;138(4):1338–45.
41. Fleischer R, Boxwell D, Sherman KE. Nucleoside analogues and mitochondrial toxicity. Clin Infect Dis. 2004;38(8):e79–80.
42. Lamarre D, Anderson PC, Bailey M, et al. An NS3 protease inhibitor with antiviral effects in humans infected with hepatitis C virus. Nature. 2003;426(6963):186–9.
43. Hézode C, Forestier N, Dusheiko G, et al. Telaprevir and peginterferon with or without ribavirin for chronic HCV infection. N Engl J Med. 2009;360(18):1839–50.
44. McHutchison JG, Everson GT, Gordon SC, et al. Telaprevir with peginterferon and ribavirin for chronic HCV genotype 1 infection. N Engl J Med. 2009;360(18):1827–38.
45. Watashi K. Alisporivir, a cyclosporin derivative that selectively inhibits cyclophilin, for the treatment of HCV infection. Curr Opin Investig Drugs. 2010;11(2):213–24.
46. Paeshuyse J, Kaul A, De Clercq E, et al. The non-immunosuppressive cyclosporin DEBIO-025 is a potent inhibitor of hepatitis C virus replication in vitro. Hepatology. 2006;43(4):761–70.
47. Nishiguchi S, Shiomi S, Nakatani S, et al. Prevention of hepatocellular carcinoma in patients with chronic active hepatitis C and cirrhosis. Lancet. 2001;357(9251):196–7.
48. Imazeki F, Yokosuka O, Fukai K, Saisho H. Favorable prognosis of chronic hepatitis C after interferon therapy by long-term cohort study. Hepatology. 2003;38(2):493–502.
49. Di Bisceglie AM, Shiffman ML, Everson GT, et al. Prolonged therapy of advanced chronic hepatitis C with low-dose peginterferon. N Engl J Med. 2008;359(23):2429–41.
50. Sherman KE, Andersen JW, Butt AA, Umbleja T, Alston B, Koziel MJ, Peters MG, Sulkowski M, Goodman ZD, Chung RT; for the Aids Clinical Trials Group A5178 Study Team. Sustained Long-Term Antiviral Maintenance Therapy in HCV/HIV-Coinfected patients (SLAM-C). J Acquir Immune Defic Syndr. 2010;55(5):597–605.
51. Labarga P, Vispo E, Barreiro P, et al. Rate and predictors of success in the retreatment of chronic hepatitis C virus in HIV/HCV-coinfected patients with prior nonresponse or relapse. J Acquir Immune Defic Syndr. 2010;53(3):364–8.
52. McHutchison JG, Manns MP, Muir AJ, et al. Telaprevir for previously treated chronic HCV infection. N Engl J Med. 2010;362(14):1292–303.
53. Low E, Vogel M, Rockstroh J, Nelson M. Acute hepatitis C in HIV-positive individuals. AIDS Rev. 2008;10(4):245–53.
54. Jaeckel E, Cornberg M, Wedemeyer H, et al. Treatment of acute hepatitis C with interferon alfa-2b. N Engl J Med. 2001;345(20):1452–7.
55. Dominguez S, Ghosn J, Valantin M, et al. Efficacy of early treatment of acute hepatitis C infection with pegylated interferon and ribavirin in HIV-infected patients. AIDS. 2006;20(8):1157–61.
56. Corey KE, Ross AS, Wurcel A, et al. Outcomes and treatment of acute hepatitis C virus infection in a United States population. Clin Gastroenterol Hepatol. 2006;4(10):1278–82.

Treatment of Hepatitis B in HIV-Infected Persons

Ellen Kitchell and Mamta K. Jain

Introduction

Hepatitis B virus (HBV) is a potentially controllable infection, but it is rarely eliminated from the body. During HBV replication, a covalently closed circular DNA molecule is formed, which remains intracellular and serves as a persistent reservoir that can cause reactivation of HBV infection years after a patient discontinues therapy.

Because HBV is rarely eradicated from its host, the goals of treatment are to prevent complications of hepatic disease, including cirrhosis and hepatocellular carcinoma. The most significant factor associated with liver dysfunction and disease progression is elevated HBV DNA levels [1, 2]; thus, the goal of therapy is HBV DNA suppression.

Previous clinical trials have established that decreases in serum HBV DNA levels, normalization of transaminases, and loss of hepatitis B e antigen (HBeAg) and hepatitis B surface antigen (HBsAg) are associated with improved liver histology and clinical outcomes. Recent trials evaluating HBV treatments typically report the above noninvasive markers as surrogates for clinical response.

Two major categories of medications, interferon and nucleos(t)ide analog inhibitors, are available for treatment of HBV. Interferon preparations used for treatment of HBV include IFN-α-2b and pegylated IFN-α-2a. Nucleos(t)ide analogs active against hepatitis B include lamivudine, entecavir, adefovir, tenofovir, and telbivudine. A summary of currently available HBV medications is provided in Table 16.1.

E. Kitchell (✉)
Department of Internal Medicine, Southwestern Medical Center,
University of Texas, 5323 Harry Hines Blvd, Dallas, TX 75390, USA
e-mail: ellen.kitchell@utsouthwestern.edu

Interferon α and Pegylated Interferon α

Interferon-α was the first Food and Drug Administration (FDA)-approved drug for treatment of chronic hepatitis B infection. Interferon interferes with viral replication and activates the immune system, but the exact mechanism is unknown. Standard interferon, given three times weekly, can lead to loss of HBsAg, with 5–10% of HBV-monoinfected patients developing HBsAb within 1 year of treatment. HBeAg loss as a result of interferon-α treatment is more durable than that seen after discontinuation of lamivudine, with up to 80% maintaining negative HBeAg 5 years after discontinuation of treatment [3]. Patients with positive HBeAg, elevated alanine transaminase (ALT) levels, and low serum HBV-DNA titers at baseline have the highest rates of response to interferon [4].

Early studies of patients coinfected with HIV showed lower rates of response to interferon therapy than monoinfected patients [5–8]; however, these studies were performed in patients with severe immunocompromise prior to the advent of antiretroviral therapy (ART). One reason for the decreased response of HIV/HBV-coinfected patients to interferon may be related to lower baseline transaminases; in one small study, HIV patients with elevated transaminases at baseline had improved response to interferon therapy as compared to those with lower ALT [9].

For the most part, standard interferon has been replaced by pegylated interferon, which can be dosed once weekly, and has improved efficacy at converting HBeAg to HBeAb and normalization of LFTs in HBV monoinfected patients [10]. No studies using pegylated interferon in HIV/HBV coinfected patients have been conducted.

Interferon therapy may appeal to select HIV-coinfected patients because it can be administered for a finite period of time, 4–12 months, and HBeAg seroconversion achieved is

Table 16.1 Medication for the treatment of HBV–HIV coinfection, dosage, effectiveness, and side effects

Medication	Dosage	Log HBV drop at 1 y	HBeAg loss at 1 y, %	Side effects
Interferon-α-2b	5–10 MU 3×/week × 16 week	0–27% undetectable HBV DNA	0–8.3	Flu-like symptoms, cytopenias, thyroid dysfunction, psychiatric
Pegylated-IFN-α-2a[a]	180 μg/week	4.5 (32% undetectable HBV DNA)[a]	32[a]	As above
Lamivudine	300 mg/day	2.7 (40–87% undetectable HBV DNA)	22–29	Nausea, diarrhea, skin rash, rare lactic acidosis/steatosis
Emtricitabine	200 mg/day	3 (50% undetectable HBV DNA)	50	Nausea, diarrhea, rash; rare lactic acidosis/steatosis
Adefovir	10 mg/day	4.6 (25% undetectable HBV DNA)	8	Nausea, fatigue, headache, rare renal toxicity, Fanconi's syndrome
Tenofovir	300 mg/day	4–5.5 (65% undetectable HBV DNA)	0–25	Rash, nausea/vomiting, diarrhea, headache, rare renal toxicity, Fanconi's syndrome; possible osteopenia; lactic acidosis/steatosis
Entecavir	0.5 mg/day for lamivudine-naïve pts; 1 mg/day for lamivudine-experienced pts	3.6–4.2 (80% undetectable HBV DNA)	2	Headache, fatigue, dizziness, rare lactic acidosis
Telbivudine[a]	600 mg/day	6 (56% undetectable HBV DNA)	16–33%	Fatigue, mild elevation in CK levels; rare lactic acidosis

MU million units, *y* year, *HBV DNA* hepatitis B DNA levels, *CK* creatine kinase
[a]No data available for HIV-coinfected patients, data shown are from HBV-monoinfected patients

more durable than nucleos(t)ide analogs after discontinuation of therapy. However, the use of interferon has been limited by its numerous side effects, which include flu-like symptoms, bone marrow suppression, thyroid dysfunction, and depression. It is contraindicated in patients with decompensated liver disease (e.g., ascites or encephalopathy).

Lamivudine

Lamivudine is an oral cytosine nucleoside analog with both anti-HBV and anti-HIV activities; 100 mg/day is needed to suppress HBV, but 300 mg/day is needed for HIV suppression. In several studies, the addition of lamivudine to ART in HIV/HBV-coinfected patients led to a 2–3 log reduction in HBV DNA levels in 1 year. Forty to eighty-seven percent achieved HBV DNA suppression at 12–17 months, and 22–29% had HBeAg seroconversion in 1–2 years [11–13]. Response to lamivudine may be related to baseline CD4 count; patients with CD4 > 200 cells/μL had an average 2 log decrease in serum HBV DNA levels after 6 months of therapy as compared to no decrease in patients with CD4 < 200 cells/μL [14].

With long-term use of lamivudine, development of HBV resistance is common. Mutations of the HBV DNA polymerase in the YMDD region (rtL80V/I, rtV173L, rtL180M, and rtM204I/V) are often responsible for resistance to lamivudine. Viral resistance is seen in up to 90% of HIV–HBV coinfected patients after 4 years [15, 16]. Development of resistance to lamivudine may be accompanied by rebounds in serum HBV DNA, worsening of liver histology, and liver enzyme flares [17–19]. Continuation of lamivudine in patients who have developed HBV-resistance provides no benefit [20, 21] and may lead to accumulation of compensatory mutations that generate higher levels of resistance to other agents.

Lamivudine is generally well-tolerated; mild side effects include nausea, diarrhea, and skin rash. Lactic acidosis and severe hepatomegaly with steatosis, including fatal cases, have been reported with the use of lamivudine and other nucleoside analogs used alone or in combination.

Emtricitabine

Emtricitabine (FTC) is a cytosine analog similar to lamivudine with antiviral activity against HBV and HIV. Analysis of HBV DNA levels in HIV treatment trials using FTC showed up to 3 log copies/mL reduction in serum HBV DNA in coinfected patients, and almost half of the patients had undetectable serum HBV DNA at week 48 [22].

Emtricitabine is frequently used in combination with tenofovir as a coformulation, Truvada® (Gilead Sciences, Foster

City, CA, USA), for the treatment of both HIV and HBV in coinfected patients. Because of its activity against HIV, it should be used in combination with other HIV-active agents. Lamivudine and FTC share almost total cross-resistance, and FTC should not be used after resistance to lamivudine has developed.

Adefovir Dipivoxil

Adefovir, a nucleotide analog of adenosine, also inhibits HBV DNA polymerase. It was first developed as anti-HIV therapy at doses of 60–120 mg/day; however, it frequently caused renal toxicity. At a dose of 10 mg/day, it is effective against HBV but not HIV, and renal side effects are rare. Multiple randomized, controlled studies in monoinfected patients have shown its efficacy compared to lamivudine or placebo in both HBeAg positive and negative patients [23–27], including in patients with lamivudine-resistant virus [28]. However, it has low viral potency at suppressing HBV DNA when compared to other HBV-active agents when the 10 mg daily oral dose is utilized.

An open-label study in HIV/HBV infected patients with baseline lamivudine resistance demonstrated that adefovir added to an ART regimen lowered serum HBV DNA by a median 5.9 log copies/mL at 144 weeks. Approximately 25% (7/35) developed undetectable HBV DNA during the course of the study, and three patients converted HBeAg to HBeAb. HIV replication was not inhibited, and no new HIV mutations were seen at the 10 mg/day dose used in the study [29]. Induction of the K65R mutation in HIV, which was noted at the 120 mg/day doses of adefovir, has not been observed clinically [30–32] at the 10 mg dose.

Patients who have been treated previously with lamivudine may develop resistance mutations that confer cross-resistance to adefovir (rtA181T/V) [33]; however, adefovir is usually effective in most patients with history of lamivudine exposure and/or resistance. Other genetic polymorphisms that render HBV resistant to adefovir are I233V and L217R [34]. A mutation in codon 236 within the DNA polymerase gene may also reduce susceptibility to adefovir [35].

Adefovir is generally well tolerated, with nausea, fatigue, and headache being the most frequently reported side effects. Renal toxicity and Fanconi's syndrome have been rarely reported.

Tenofovir Disoproxil Fumarate

Tenofovir, an adenosine nucleotide analog active against HBV DNA polymerase and HIV, has one of the highest potencies and clinical efficacy against HBV. In patients with HIV, several studies examining the use of tenofovir within ART regimens have shown reduction of HBV DNA levels of 4–5 log copies/mL [36, 37] and HBeAg seroconversion of 7–25% [38–40]. In a study of patients with lamivudine-resistant HBV, tenofovir demonstrated a significant reduction in HBV DNA level compared to adefovir (mean HBV DNA 5.5 log copies/mL vs. 2.8 log copies/mL, respectively) in both mono- and coinfected patients [41].

In a randomized, controlled study evaluating the addition of tenofovir or adefovir to a stable anti-HIV regimen, tenofovir was noninferior to adefovir at suppressing HBV replication in HIV–HBV coinfected patients (4.4 log copies/mL vs. 3.2 log copies/mL, respectively) at 48 weeks [42]. A larger double-blind, placebo-controlled trial in HBV-monoinfected patients demonstrated superior efficacy of tenofovir in suppressing HBV DNA levels, HBeAg seroconversion, and histologic improvement as compared to adefovir [43].

HBV resistance to tenofovir is rare, even in patients who have baseline resistance to lamivudine. In two studies, the development of A194T resulted in a tenfold decrease in susceptibility to tenofovir [32, 44]. In addition, adefovir-resistance mutations rtA181V and rtN236T decrease susceptibility to tenofovir [45]. However, tenofovir has been used effectively in patients who have developed clinical failure of both lamivudine and adefovir [46].

The most commonly reported adverse effects in patients treated with tenofovir include rash, diarrhea, headache, and nausea. Renal impairment and Fanconi's syndrome are reported in some patients treated with tenofovir. Analysis of patients treated with tenofovir in cohort studies have shown small decreases in glomerular filtration rate as compared to those treated with other antiretrovirals, although no changes in creatinine or renal dysfunction were noted [47]. Patients with pre-existing renal impairment or those receiving other nephrotoxic agents are at increased risk for nephrotoxicity. Evaluation of renal function (including serum creatinine, serum phosphorus, and urinalysis) is recommended for patients receiving tenofovir, especially in patients with baseline renal impairment.

Tenofovir use has been associated with an increased loss of bone mineral density in patients with HIV during the first several months of therapy, although it stabilizes over time. Lactic acidosis, hepatomegaly, and steatosis have been rarely reported with tenofovir.

Entecavir

Entecavir, a guanosine analog, inhibits HBV replication at multiple steps, including priming, reverse transcription, and positive strand synthesis. Entecavir is more effective than adefovir and lamivudine, reducing HBV DNA by 7 log copies/mL in monoinfected patients, and is effective against lamivudine- and adefovir-resistant virus [48, 49]. In one study evaluating the effect of adding entecavir to a stable ART regimen in HIV-infected patients with baseline lamivudine resistance, entecavir reduced HBV DNA by a mean 3.65 log copies/mL as compared to placebo over 24 weeks [50].

Development of HBV viral resistance against entecavir is rare in HBV-treatment naïve patients. Entecavir resistance usually results from the accumulation of multiple mutations in the DNA polymerase, with cross-resistance with lamivudine (including the rtL180M and rtM204V/I) [51]. Other entecavir mutations in the polymerase region of HBV include rtT184V/A/I/L, rtS202G/C, and rtM250I/V. In patients who are lamivudine-resistant, 1 mg/day rather than 0.5 mg/day of entecavir is recommended. If entecavir resistance has developed, lamivudine should not be utilized. Entecavir and adefovir have not been shown to have cross-resistance and could be substituted for one another or combined [35].

Entecavir was previously thought not to have activity against HIV; however, recent studies have shown that it can produce reductions in HIV RNA of 1- to 2-log copies/mL [52, 53]. Use of entecavir has been associated with development of the M184V mutation in HIV in coinfected patients; in one study, 6/17 patients developed a de novo M184V mutation on therapy [54]. Entecavir should be used only in combination with a fully suppressive regimen against HIV in coinfected patients. Entecavir is generally well-tolerated; most commonly reported side effects include diarrhea, headache, indigestion, nausea, and fatigue.

Telbivudine

A newer medication for treatment of HBV is telbivudine, an L-nucleoside analog of thymidine that specifically inhibits HBV polymerase. The GLOBE trial in monoinfected HBV patients showed higher anti-HBV potency compared with lamivudine with decrease in HBV viral load than lamivudine (6 log copies/mL vs. 4.5 log copies/mL) [55]. Telbivudine was found to be more potent and effective against HBV in comparison with adefovir, as well [56].

No clinical trials of telbivudine have been performed in HIV–HBV coinfected patients to evaluate for efficacy or generation of resistance mutations within HIV. Previous treatment guidelines for patients with HIV/HBV have reflected the thought that telbivudine does not have activity against HIV; however, recently published case reports demonstrated transient reductions in HIV-1 RNA in patients treated with telbivudine. No HIV-genotypic resistance mutations were identified in these studies [57, 58].

Telbivudine has a low rate of inducing HBV resistance. Commonly noted mutations include rtM204I, rtL180M, and rtL80V/I, which cause cross-resistance to lamivudine. Telbivudine does not appear to be effective in lamivudine-resistant virus [59], and there is no benefit of combining lamivudine with telbivudine. There is no evidence yet of cross-resistance between adefovir or tenofovir and telbivudine. Telbivudine is generally well tolerated; however, elevated creatine kinase levels may rarely be seen.

Combination Therapy

Multiple medications included in a regimen to treat HBV could prevent resistance or have additive or synergistic effects against the virus; however, few studies have investigated combination therapy in clinical practice.

Interferon + Nucleoside Therapy

Most studies examining the effect of interferon combined with lamivudine show no improvement in HBV DNA suppression or ability to convert HBeAg compared with pegylated interferon monotherapy [60, 61]. However, several studies have shown that adding interferon to lamivudine monotherapy decreases the rate of lamivudine resistance mutations [62, 63].

Adefovir Versus Adefovir/Lamivudine

Studies of adefovir combination therapy in HBV-monoinfected patients have shown mixed results. One trial comparing the use of adefovir alone to adefovir plus emtricitabine showed a greater suppression of HBV DNA and normalization of ALT in the combination group. Rates of HBeAg conversion were similar between the two groups [64]. Another trial evaluating the addition of lamivudine to patients with persistently high HBV DNA levels on adefovir therapy showed improved virologic response once lamivudine was added [65]. However, another study comparing lamivudine plus adefovir to adefovir alone showed no increase in effectiveness [66].

Emtricitabine/Tenofovir

Several retrospective studies have examined the use of lamivudine/tenofovir combination in HIV-positive patients as part of ART. One study comparing lamivudine therapy alone, those initiated on lamivudine and tenofovir at beginning of therapy, or later addition of tenofovir therapy to a regimen containing lamivudine showed higher rate of undetectable HBV viral load and HBeAg seroconversion when lamivudine and tenofovir were combined in the initial regimen; however, the study was underpowered to show statistical significance [67].

Table 16.2 Treatment guidelines for patients with CD4 > 350–500 cells/μL

Organization	HBeAg	ALT	HBV DNA
European Consensus Conference [77]	Positive	N/A	>20,000 IU/mL if fibrosis present on biopsy
European Consensus Conference [77]	Negative	N/A	>2,000 IU/mL if fibrosis present on biopsy
European AIDS Clinical Society (EACS) [78]	N/A	–	>2,000 IU/mL if ALT elevated or liver biopsy showing disease activity
CDC OI Guidelines [79]	Positive	Abnormal	>20,000 IU/mL
CDC OI Guidelines [79]	Negative	Abnormal	>2,000 IU/mL
British HIV Association (if CD4 > 500 cells/μL) [80]	Positive	N/A	>2,000 IU/mL or fibrosis on noninvasive testing
HIV-Hepatitis B Virus International Panel [81]	–	–	>2,000 IU/mL if elevated ALT or significant fibrosis on biopsy

HBeAg hepatitis B e antigen, *ALT* alanine transaminase, *HBV DNA* hepatitis B Virus DNA, *OI* opportunistic infection

In a retrospective analysis of ART naïve patients enrolled in randomized clinical trials of tenofovir in HIV, which was added to a backbone of efavirenz and lamivudine, HBV-positive patients experienced a mean 4.5 log copies/mL decrease in HBV DNA in the tenofovir/lamivudine arm as compared to a decrease of 1.9 log copies/mL group treated with lamivudine alone [37]. All of the patients receiving lamivudine monotherapy developed resistance mutations by 144 weeks of therapy, as compared to one sixth on combination therapy.

Several small pilot studies of lamivudine/tenofovir combination therapy in HIV patients showed potent suppression of HBV viral load [68], and superior efficacy at achieving undetectable HBV viral load as compared to lamivudine or tenofovir monotherapy [69, 70]. However, a recent prospective study in ART-naïve HIV-HBV coinfected patients showed no difference in decrease in HBV DNA over 48 weeks of combination lamivudine/tenofovir therapy (4.73 log copies/mL) versus tenofovir alone (4.57 copies/mL). Tenofovir was more effective than lamivudine monotherapy at decreasing HBV viral load. No episodes of HBV resistance were noted in the tenofovir arms compared to the lamivudine monotherapy arm [71].

When to Start Treatment for HBV Infection in HIV-Coinfected Patients

The threshold for treatment of HIV–HBV coinfected patients is unclear. No studies have demonstrated the specific HBV DNA levels associated with increased risk of liver damage in HIV-infected patients, or whether elevated liver enzymes or HBeAg status is associated with worse prognosis in this subgroup. Given the more aggressive nature of hepatitis B in HIV-infected patients, it is typically recommended to start therapy at lower HBV DNA levels than in monoinfected patients.

Traditionally, the decision to treat HBV with antiviral therapy has depended heavily on the decision whether to start patients on medications for HIV. If patients meet criteria for ART initiation by other means (e.g., CD4 < 350 cells/μL), initiation of therapy active against hepatitis B as part of ART is indicated. In patients who do not meet criteria for ART initiation, many recommendations on the optimal timing of HBV treatment exist. Table 16.2 indicates some of the guidelines released by national and international committees.

More recent recommendations have reflected the shift toward earlier initiation of ART in patients with HBV. As HIV infection is associated with more rapid progression of hepatitis B infection, ART may slow development of liver complications by conserving and reestablishing HBV-specific immune function or by suppressing HIV-associated immune activation. In addition, the treatment options for patients not receiving a fully suppressive ART regimen are limited (i.e., interferon and adefovir). In recent HIV treatment guidelines, HBV is considered a relative indication to initiate ART, regardless of CD4 count [72].

Management of Patients with Hepatitis B and HIV Coinfection

Initial assessment of patients with HIV and HBV (see Fig. 16.1) should include HBeAg, HBsAg, HBeAb, HBV DNA, CBC, liver function tests, CD4 count, and HIV viral load. Patients should be counseled regarding the risks of transmission of HBV and other hepatitis viruses, and should receive hepatitis A vaccine if not immune. Treatment recommendations are summarized in Fig. 16.1 for HIV/HBV patients who are naïve to ART.

No data exists on what role liver biopsy should play in HIV–HBV coinfected patients. However, given the significant mortality associated with HBV in this population, a liver biopsy should be considered to stage severity of liver fibrosis,

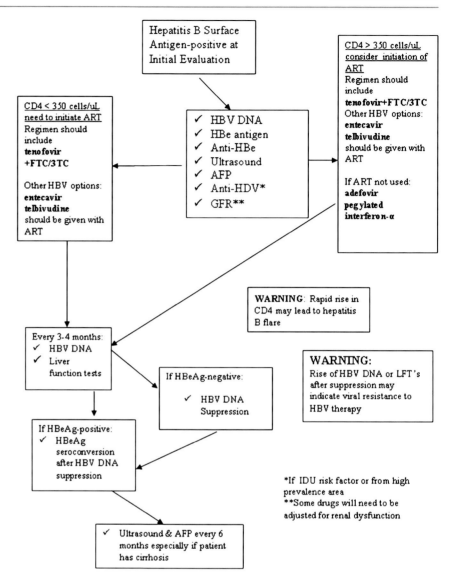

Fig. 16.1 Evaluation and management of an HIV–HBV coinfected patient (Note: *HBV DNA* hepatitis B viral load, *HBeAg* hepatitis Be antigen, *anti-HBe* hepatitis Be antibody, *AFP* alpha-fetoprotein, *anti-HDV* hepatitis D antibody, *GFR* glomerular filtration rate, *TDF* tenofovir disoproxil fumarate, *FTC* emtricitabine, *3TC* lamivudine, *ART* antiretroviral therapy, *LFT's* liver function tests, *HBV* hepatitis B, *IDU* injection drug use)

especially in those who are not initiated on ART. The degree of liver fibrosis could impact treatment decisions and monitoring for HCC.

In HIV/HBV patients with a history of lamivudine use, it should be assumed that HBV isolates are lamivudine-resistant. Either tenofovir or entecavir at an increased dose of 1 mg/day, should be used in this group.

Once a patient has started therapy, HBV DNA levels should be obtained every 3–4 months, similar to how HIV RNA levels are monitored during therapy, to evaluate for response [73]. Once a patient is found to have response to treatment, HBeAg and anti-HBe should be monitored periodically. In HIV-infected patients, the response to HBV therapy may be delayed. In one study, 20% of patients on tenofovir did not reach undetectable viremia after 52 weeks of therapy, although most of those patients later became undetectable after 20 months [74]. If patients do not demonstrate decreasing HBV viral load, addition or substitution of another HBV-active agent should be considered.

There is no consensus on discontinuation of HBV active therapy in HIV-infected patients; most providers choose to continue medications indefinitely. As HBsAg seroconversion is durable, discontinuation of HBV therapy may be considered if HBsAg loss occurs. If a patient develops virologic failure of HIV and medication regimen switch is considered, medications active against HBV should be continued unless a patient has developed HBV resistance.

An increase in the HBV viral load >1 log copies/mL compared with the lowest level achieved previously on therapy may indicate nonadherence or development of HBV resistance. Drug discontinuation or mutation-associated viral breakthrough may be associated with a flare in serum ALT levels, and hepatic decompensation among those with advanced fibrosis/cirrhosis [17]. Polymerase mutation testing of the YMDD mutation may be helpful in cases of possible lamivudine resistance. For patients failing lamivudine, emtricitabine, or telbivudine, a change to tenofovir or adefovir is indicated. Higher-dose entecavir may also be considered, although in patients with lamivudine resistance, risk for developing entecavir resistance is high. In patients failing entecavir, tenofovir or adefovir should be started. Tenofovir may also be effective in patients failing adefovir [46].

Control of HBV replication can be beneficial to those who have cirrhosis or hepatocelluar carcinoma, resulting in decreased rates of liver decompensation and increased survival [75]. Select patients may also be candidates for transplantation in some centers, as posttransplant survival is similar in HIV-coinfected patients and those with HBV alone [76].

References

1. Chen CJ, Yang HI, Su J, et al. Risk of hepatocellular carcinoma across a biological gradient of serum hepatitis B virus DNA level. JAMA. 2006;295(1):65–73.
2. Iloeje UH, Yang HI, Su J, Jen CL, You SL, Chen CJ. Predicting cirrhosis risk based on the level of circulating hepatitis B viral load. Gastroenterology. 2006;130(3):678–86.
3. Krogsgaard K. The long-term effect of treatment with interferon-alpha 2a in chronic hepatitis B. The Long-Term Follow-up Investigator Group. The European Study Group on Viral Hepatitis (EUROHEP). Executive team on anti-viral treatment. J Viral Hepat. 1998;5(6):389–97.
4. Lok AS, McMahon BJ. Chronic hepatitis B. Hepatology. 2007;45(2):507–39.
5. Brook MG, Chan G, Yap I, et al. Randomised controlled trial of lymphoblastoid interferon alfa in Europid men with chronic hepatitis B virus infection. BMJ. 1989;299(6700):652–6.
6. McDonald JA, Caruso L, Karayiannis P, et al. Diminished responsiveness of male homosexual chronic hepatitis B virus carriers with HTLV-III antibodies to recombinant alpha-interferon. Hepatology. 1987;7(4):719–23.
7. Nunez M, Puoti M, Camino N, Soriano V. Treatment of chronic hepatitis B in the human immunodeficiency virus-infected patient: present and future. Clin Infect Dis. 2003;37(12):1678–85.
8. Wong DK, Cheung AM, O'Rourke K, Naylor CD, Detsky AS, Heathcote J. Effect of alpha-interferon treatment in patients with hepatitis B e antigen-positive chronic hepatitis B. A meta-analysis. Ann Intern Med. 1993;119(4):312–23.
9. Di Martino V, Thevenot T, Boyer N, Degos F, Marcellin P. Serum alanine transaminase level is a good predictor of response to interferon alfa therapy for chronic hepatitis B in human immunodeficiency virus-infected patients. Hepatology. 2000;31(4):1030–1.
10. Cooksley WG, Piratvisuth T, Lee SD, et al. Peginterferon alpha-2a (40 kDa): an advance in the treatment of hepatitis B e antigen-positive chronic hepatitis B. J Viral Hepat. 2003;10(4):298–305.
11. Dore GJ, Cooper DA, Barrett C, Goh LE, Thakrar B, Atkins M. Dual efficacy of lamivudine treatment in human immunodeficiency virus/hepatitis B virus-coinfected persons in a randomized, controlled study (CAESAR). The CAESAR Coordinating Committee. J Infect Dis. 1999;180(3):607–13.
12. Benhamou Y, Katlama C, Lunel F, et al. Effects of lamivudine on replication of hepatitis B virus in HIV-infected men. Ann Intern Med. 1996;125(9):705–12.
13. Hoff J, Bani-Sadr F, Gassin M, Raffi F. Evaluation of chronic hepatitis B virus (HBV) infection in coinfected patients receiving lamivudine as a component of anti-human immunodeficiency virus regimens. Clin Infect Dis. 2001;32(6):963–9.
14. Haverkamp M, Smit M, Weersink A, Boucher CA, Hoepelman AI. The effect of lamivudine on the replication of hepatitis B virus in HIV-infected patients depends on the host immune status (CD4 cell count). AIDS. 2003;17(10):1572–4.
15. Benhamou Y, Bochet M, Thibault V, et al. Long-term incidence of hepatitis B virus resistance to lamivudine in human immunodeficiency virus-infected patients. Hepatology. 1999;30(5):1302–6.
16. Matthews GV, Bartholomeusz A, Locarnini S, et al. Characteristics of drug resistant HBV in an international collaborative study of HIV-HBV-infected individuals on extended lamivudine therapy. AIDS. 2006;20(6):863–70.
17. Bessesen M, Ives D, Condreay L, Lawrence S, Sherman KE. Chronic active hepatitis B exacerbations in human immunodeficiency virus-infected patients following development of resistance to or withdrawal of lamivudine. Clin Infect Dis. 1999;28(5):1032–5.
18. Pillay D, Cane PA, Ratcliffe D, Atkins M, Cooper D. Evolution of lamivudine-resistant hepatitis B virus and HIV-1 in co-infected individuals: an analysis of the CAESAR study. CAESAR co-ordinating committee. AIDS. 2000;14(9):1111–6.
19. Yuen MF, Chow DH, Tsui K, et al. Liver histology of Asian patients with chronic hepatitis B on prolonged lamivudine therapy. Aliment Pharmacol Ther. 2005;21(7):841–9.
20. Jang JW, Choi JY, Bae SH, et al. Stopping lamivudine therapy after biochemical breakthrough may be a feasible option in selected HBeAg-positive patients. J Med Virol. 2005;77(3):367–73.
21. Kim YJ, Kim BG, Jung JO, Yoon JH, Lee HS. High rates of progressive hepatic functional deterioration whether lamivudine therapy is continued or discontinued after emergence of a lamivudine-resistant mutant: a prospective randomized controlled study. J Gastroenterol. 2006;41(3):240–9.
22. Raffi F, Snow A, Borroto-Esoda K, et al. Anti-HBV activity of emtricitabine (FTC) in patients co-infected with HIV and hepatitis B virus. [Oral presentation]. Paper presented at: 2nd International AIDS Conference on Pathogenesis and Treatment; July 13–16, 2003. Paris, France; 2003.
23. Hadziyannis SJ, Tassopoulos NC, Heathcote EJ, et al. Long-term therapy with adefovir dipivoxil for HBeAg-negative chronic hepatitis B for up to 5 years. Gastroenterology. 2006;131(6):1743–51.
24. Hadziyannis SJ, Tassopoulos NC, Heathcote EJ, et al. Adefovir dipivoxil for the treatment of hepatitis B e antigen-negative chronic hepatitis B. N Engl J Med. 2003;348(9):800–7.
25. Kim do Y, Kim HJ, Lee CK, et al. Efficacy of adefovir dipivoxil in the treatment of lamivudine-resistant hepatitis B virus genotype C infection. Liver Int. 2007;27(1):47–53.
26. Marcellin P, Chang TT, Lim SG, et al. Adefovir dipivoxil for the treatment of hepatitis B e antigen-positive chronic hepatitis B. N Engl J Med. 2003;348(9):808–16.
27. Zeng M, Mao Y, Yao G, et al. A double-blind randomized trial of adefovir dipivoxil in Chinese subjects with HBeAg-positive chronic hepatitis B. Hepatology. 2006;44(1):108–16.
28. Peters MG, Hann Hw H, Martin P, et al. Adefovir dipivoxil alone or in combination with lamivudine in patients with lamivudine-resistant chronic hepatitis B. Gastroenterology. 2004;126(1):91–101.
29. Benhamou Y. Treatment algorithm for chronic hepatitis B in HIV-infected patients. J Hepatol. 2006;44(1 Suppl):S90–4.
30. Benhamou Y, Bochet M, Thibault V, et al. Safety and efficacy of adefovir dipivoxil in patients co-infected with HIV-1 and

lamivudine-resistant hepatitis B virus: an open-label pilot study. Lancet. 2001;358(9283):718–23.
31. Delaugerre C, Marcelin AG, Thibault V, et al. Human immunodeficiency virus (HIV) Type 1 reverse transcriptase resistance mutations in hepatitis B virus (HBV)-HIV-coinfected patients treated for HBV chronic infection once daily with 10 milligrams of adefovir dipivoxil combined with lamivudine. Antimicrob Agents Chemother. 2002;46(5):1586–8.
32. Sheldon J, Camino N, Rodes B, et al. Selection of hepatitis B virus polymerase mutations in HIV-coinfected patients treated with tenofovir. Antivir Ther. 2005;10(6):727–34.
33. Karatayli E, Karayalcin S, Karaaslan H, et al. A novel mutation pattern emerging during lamivudine treatment shows cross-resistance to adefovir dipivoxil treatment. Antivir Ther. 2007;12(5):761–8.
34. Schildgen O, Sirma H, Funk A, et al. Variant of hepatitis B virus with primary resistance to adefovir. N Engl J Med. 2006;354(17):1807–12.
35. Angus P, Vaughan R, Xiong S, et al. Resistance to adefovir dipivoxil therapy associated with the selection of a novel mutation in the HBV polymerase. Gastroenterology. 2003;125(2):292–7.
36. Benhamou Y, Piketty C, Katlama C, et al. Anti-hepatitis B virus (HBV) activity of tenofovir dispoproxil fumarate (TDF) in human immunodeficiency virus (HIV) co-infected patients [abstract]. Hepatology. 2003;38(4):712A–3.
37. Dore GJ, Cooper DA, Pozniak AL, et al. Efficacy of tenofovir disoproxil fumarate in antiretroviral therapy-naive and -experienced patients coinfected with HIV-1 and hepatitis B virus. J Infect Dis. 2004;189(7):1185–92.
38. Nelson M, Portsmouth S, Stebbing J, et al. An open-label study of tenofovir in HIV-1 and Hepatitis B virus co-infected individuals. AIDS. 2003;17(1):F7–10.
39. Ristig MB, Crippin J, Aberg JA, et al. Tenofovir disoproxil fumarate therapy for chronic hepatitis B in human immunodeficiency virus/hepatitis B virus-coinfected individuals for whom interferon-alpha and lamivudine therapy have failed. J Infect Dis. 2002;186(12):1844–7.
40. Stephan C, Berger A, Carlebach A, et al. Impact of tenofovir-containing antiretroviral therapy on chronic hepatitis B in a cohort co-infected with human immunodeficiency virus. J Antimicrob Chemother. 2005;56(6):1087–93.
41. van Bommel F, Wunsche T, Mauss S, et al. Comparison of adefovir and tenofovir in the treatment of lamivudine-resistant hepatitis B virus infection. Hepatology. 2004;40(6):1421–5.
42. Peters MG, Andersen J, Lynch P, et al. Randomized controlled study of tenofovir and adefovir in chronic hepatitis B virus and HIV infection: ACTG A5127. Hepatology. 2006;44(5):1110–6.
43. Marcellin P, Heathcote EJ, Buti M, et al. Tenofovir disoproxil fumarate versus adefovir dipivoxil for chronic hepatitis B. N Engl J Med. 2008;359(23):2442–55.
44. Audsley J, Arrifin N, Yuen LK, et al. Prolonged use of tenofovir in HIV/hepatitis B virus (HBV)-coinfected individuals does not lead to HBV polymerase mutations and is associated with persistence of lamivudine HBV polymerase mutations. HIV Med. 2009;10(4):229–35.
45. Qi X, Xiong S, Yang H, Miller M, Delaney WE. In vitro susceptibility of adefovir-associated hepatitis B virus polymerase mutations to other antiviral agents. Antivir Ther. 2007;12(3):355–62.
46. van Bommel F, Zollner B, Sarrazin C, et al. Tenofovir for patients with lamivudine-resistant hepatitis B virus (HBV) infection and high HBV DNA level during adefovir therapy. Hepatology. 2006;44(2):318–25.
47. Gallant JE, Winston JA, DeJesus E, et al. The 3-year renal safety of a tenofovir disoproxil fumarate vs. a thymidine analogue-containing regimen in antiretroviral-naive patients. AIDS. 2008;22(16):2155–63.
48. Chang TT, Lai CL. Hepatitis B virus with primary resistance to adefovir. N Engl J Med. 2006;355(3):322–3. author reply 323.
49. Lai CL, Shouval D, Lok AS, et al. Entecavir versus lamivudine for patients with HBeAg-negative chronic hepatitis B. N Engl J Med. 2006;354(10):1011–20.
50. Pessoa MG, Gazzard B, Huang AK, et al. Efficacy and safety of entecavir for chronic HBV in HIV/HBV coinfected patients receiving lamivudine as part of antiretroviral therapy. AIDS. 2008;22(14):1779–87.
51. Tenney DJ, Levine SM, Rose RE, et al. Clinical emergence of entecavir-resistant hepatitis B virus requires additional substitutions in virus already resistant to Lamivudine. Antimicrob Agents Chemother. 2004;48(9):3498–507.
52. Jain MK, Zoellner CL. Entecavir can select for M184V of HIV-1: a case of an HIV/hepatitis B (HBV) naive patient treated for chronic HBV. AIDS. 2007;21(17):2365–6.
53. McMahon MA, Jilek BL, Brennan TP, et al. The HBV drug entecavir – effects on HIV-1 replication and resistance. N Engl J Med. 2007;356(25):2614–21.
54. Sasadeusz J, Audsley J, Mijch A, et al. The anti-HIV activity of entecavir: a multicentre evaluation of lamivudine-experienced and lamivudine-naive patients. AIDS. 2008;22(8):947–55.
55. Liaw YF, Gane E, Leung N, et al. 2-Year GLOBE trial results: telbivudine is superior to lamivudine in patients with chronic hepatitis B. Gastroenterology. 2009;136(2):486–95.
56. Chan HL, Heathcote EJ, Marcellin P, et al. Treatment of hepatitis B e antigen positive chronic hepatitis with telbivudine or adefovir: a randomized trial. Ann Intern Med. 2007;147(11):745–54.
57. Low E, Cox A, Atkins M, Nelson M. Telbivudine has activity against HIV-1. AIDS. 2009;23(4):546–7.
58. Milazzo L, Caramma I, Lai A, et al. Telbivudine in the treatment of chronic hepatitis B: experience in HIV type-1-infected patients naive for antiretroviral therapy. Antivir Ther. 2009;14(6):869–72.
59. Lai CL, Gane E, Liaw YF, et al. Telbivudine versus lamivudine in patients with chronic hepatitis B. N Engl J Med. 2007;357(25):2576–88.
60. Kaymakoglu S, Oguz D, Gur G, et al. Pegylated interferon Alfa-2b monotherapy and pegylated interferon Alfa-2b plus lamivudine combination therapy for patients with hepatitis B virus E antigen-negative chronic hepatitis B. Antimicrob Agents Chemother. 2007;51(8):3020–2.
61. Lau GK, Piratvisuth T, Luo KX, et al. Peginterferon Alfa-2a, lamivudine, and the combination for HBeAg-positive chronic hepatitis B. N Engl J Med. 2005;352(26):2682–95.
62. Sarin SK, Kumar M, Kumar R, et al. Higher efficacy of sequential therapy with interferon-alpha and lamivudine combination compared to lamivudine monotherapy in HBeAg positive chronic hepatitis B patients. Am J Gastroenterol. 2005;100(11):2463–71.
63. Shi M, Wang RS, Zhang H, et al. Sequential treatment with lamivudine and interferon-alpha monotherapies in hepatitis B e antigen-negative Chinese patients and its suppression of lamivudine-resistant mutations. J Antimicrob Chemother. 2006;58(5):1031–5.
64. Hui CK, Zhang HY, Bowden S, et al. 96 weeks combination of adefovir dipivoxil plus emtricitabine vs. adefovir dipivoxil monotherapy in the treatment of chronic hepatitis B. J Hepatol. 2008;48(5):714–20.
65. Wang LC, Chen EQ, Cao J, et al. Combination of lamivudine and adefovir therapy in HBeAg-positive chronic hepatitis B patients with poor response to adefovir monotherapy. J Viral Hepat. 2010;17(3):178–84.
66. Sung JJ, Lai JY, Zeuzem S, et al. Lamivudine compared with lamivudine and adefovir dipivoxil for the treatment of HBeAg-positive chronic hepatitis B. J Hepatol. 2008;48(5):728–35.
67. Jain MK, Comanor L, White C, et al. Treatment of hepatitis B with lamivudine and tenofovir in HIV/HBV-coinfected patients: factors associated with response. J Viral Hepat. 2007;14(3):176–82.

68. Bani-Sadr F, Palmer P, Scieux C, Molina JM. Ninety-six-week efficacy of combination therapy with lamivudine and tenofovir in patients coinfected with HIV-1 and wild-type hepatitis B virus. Clin Infect Dis. 2004;39(7):1062–4.
69. Nelson M, Bhagani S, Fisher M, et al. A 48-week study of tenofovir or lamivudine or a combination of tenofovir and lamivudine for the treatment of chronic hepatitis B in HIV/HBV co-infected individuals. Paper presented at: Conference on Retroviruses and Opportunisitic Infections; February 5–8, 2006. Denver, Colorado; 2006.
70. Matthews GV, Seaberg E, Dore GJ, et al. Combination HBV therapy is linked to greater HBV DNA suppression in a cohort of lamivudine-experienced HIV/HBV coinfected individuals. AIDS. 2009;23(13):1707–15.
71. Matthews GV, Avihingsanon A, Lewin SR, et al. A randomized trial of combination hepatitis B therapy in HIV/HBV coinfected antiretroviral naive individuals in Thailand. Hepatology. 2008;48(4): 1062–9.
72. Guidelines for the use of antiretroviral agents in HIV-1-infected adults and adolescents. Department of Health and Human Services; 2008. Accessed 1 June 2010.
73. Jain MK, Opio CK, Osuagwu CC, Pillai R, Keiser P, Lee WM. Do HIV care providers appropriately manage hepatitis B in coinfected patients treated with antiretroviral therapy? Clin Infect Dis. 2007; 44(7):996–1000.
74. Benhamou Y, Fleury H, Trimoulet P, et al. Anti-hepatitis B virus efficacy of tenofovir disoproxil fumarate in HIV-infected patients. Hepatology. 2006;43(3):548–55.
75. Chuma M, Hige S, Kamiyama T, et al. The influence of hepatitis B DNA level and antiviral therapy on recurrence after initial curative treatment in patients with hepatocellular carcinoma. J Gastroenterol. 2009;44(9):991–9.
76. Roland ME, Barin B, Carlson L, et al. HIV-infected liver and kidney transplant recipients: 1- and 3-year outcomes. Am J Transplant. 2008;8(2):355–65.
77. Alberti A, Clumeck N, Collins S, et al. Short statement of the first European Consensus Conference on the treatment of chronic hepatitis B and C in HIV co-infected patients. J Hepatol. 2005;42(5): 615–24.
78. Rockstroh JK, Bhagani S, Benhamou Y, et al. European AIDS Clinical Society (EACS) guidelines for the clinical management and treatment of chronic hepatitis B and C coinfection in HIV-infected adults. HIV Med. 2008;9(2):82–8.
79. Kaplan JE, Benson C, Holmes KH, Brooks JT, Pau A, Masur H. Guidelines for prevention and treatment of opportunistic infections in HIV-infected adults and adolescents: recommendations from CDC, the National Institutes of Health, and the HIV Medicine Association of the Infectious Diseases Society of America. MMWR Recomm Rep. 2009;58(RR-4):1–207. quiz CE201–204.
80. Brook G, Main J, Nelson M, et al. British HIV Association guidelines for the management of coinfection with HIV-1 and hepatitis B or C virus 2010. HIV Med. 2010;11(1):1–30.
81. Soriano V, Puoti M, Peters M, et al. Care of HIV patients with chronic hepatitis B: updated recommendations from the HIV-Hepatitis B Virus International Panel. AIDS. 2008;22(12):1399–410.

Prevention of Hepatitis Infection in HIV-Infected Patients

Edgar Turner Overton and Judith A. Aberg

Introduction

For HIV-infected persons with access to potent antiretroviral therapy (ART), HIV infection can be controlled, and medically managed like other chronic medical conditions such as diabetes and hypertension [1, 2]. Despite the spectacular advances in therapy, there remain significant challenges for HIV care providers. Coinfection with viral hepatitis is one of these challenges, as liver-related diseases now are the leading significant cause of non-AIDS related deaths among HIV-infected patients [3, 4]. While there are numerous etiologies for liver injury among HIV-infected patients, coinfection with hepatitis viruses poses the greatest risk due to shared routes of transmission and immunosuppression, which may limit their ability to spontaneously clear these infections. As with many other diseases, prevention is the key! In this chapter, we review strategies to prevent coinfection with hepatitis viruses among HIV-infected individuals. Topics covered include routine screening and education of patients, behavioral interventions, and the aggressive utilization of available hepatitis vaccines.

Knowledge Is Power

Despite the recognition that HIV shares routes of transmission with the hepatitis viruses, particularly hepatitis B (HBV) and hepatitis C (HCV), many providers fail to screen their HIV-infected patients for evidence of coinfection. For example, a recent French study reported that ¼ of all HIV providers did not check HBV serologies in their HIV-infected patients [5]. Another recent survey of US providers found that >90% correctly identified risk factors for HCV, yet only 59% routinely ask patients about HCV risk factors and 30% do not test those persons with risk factors for HCV [6]. Serologic testing allows not only for screening for these important comorbidities but also to identify persons who will benefit from hepatitis A virus (HAV) and HBV vaccination, and importantly to create the environment to discuss important behavioral prevention strategies.

Hepatitis A

While HAV does not cause chronic hepatitis, it is the most common cause of viral hepatitis in the USA [7]. This virus is traditionally associated with contaminated water or food; however, sexual transmission is also common, specifically for persons engaging in anal sex (see Table 17.1) [8]. With more than 50% of incident cases of HIV in the USA occurring in men who have sex with men (MSM), HAV screening and vaccination remain a priority for secondary prevention [9]. Despite there being no risk for chronic HAV infection, acute HAV may lead to temporary interruption of ART with negative consequences regarding subsequent HIV viral suppression [10]. Additionally, previous research has found that HIV-infected persons have higher levels of HAV viremia and take longer to clear the HAV virus [11]. These findings have implications from a public health perspective and may result in higher risk of transmission of HAV by HIV-infected persons with acute HAV.

Hepatitis B

Given that HIV and HBV share routes of infection and there is a safe, effective HBV vaccine, proactive screening for HBV is essential [12, 13]. Worldwide, HBV is the leading cause of cirrhosis and hepatocellular carcinoma [14].

E.T. Overton (✉)
Department of Internal Medicine/Infectious Diseases Division,
Washington University School of Medicine,
660 S. Euclid Ave, Campus Box 8051, St. Louis, MO 63110, USA
e-mail: toverton@dom.wustl.edu

Table 17.1 Persons at increased risk of HAV infection

- Men who have sex with men (MSM)
- Persons with chronic liver disease (specifically hepatitis B or C)
- Illicit drug users, particularly injection drug users
- Persons with clotting factor disorsers (i.e., hemophiliacs)
- Travelers to areas of high HAV endemicity
- Persons at occupational risk for infection

There are estimated to be 1.25 million chronic carriers of HBV in the USA currently with approximately 5,000 attributable deaths annually [15, 16]. HBV is more efficiently transmitted by blood-borne exposure than HIV and can be shed in body fluids, such as saliva and sweat, which do not normally transmit HIV. While 90–95% of immunocompetent adults will spontaneously clear HBV infection, clearance rates are lower for HIV-infected persons. In US-based surveillance, coinfection is most common in MSM and injection drug users (5–10%), although reported in approximately 4% of HIV-infected women, as well [17, 18].

HIV modulates the disease caused by HBV. The incidence of acute hepatitis is lower in coinfected patients, but chronic infection occurs more often in this population [19]. The latter point has been shown with decreased clearance of HBV e antigen in HIV-infected patients when compared with that of HIV-negative patients (12% vs. 49% clearance at 5 years) [20]. Furthermore, in prospective studies of MSM, coinfection with HIV and HBV was associated with a 15-fold increase in mortality when compared with HBV alone [21]. Additional data suggest that HBV accelerates the course of HIV infection; however, this finding has not been proven in larger epidemiologic studies [22, 23].

Hepatitis C

In the USA, HCV is the leading etiology for liver transplantation [24]. An estimated four million Americans are currently living with chronic HCV infection and as many as 75% are unaware of this chronic comorbidity [25, 26]. Parenteral transmission is the primary route for HCV transmission. With the advent of screening of blood products in 1985, the incidence of HCV declined precipitously and now injection drug use accounts for at least 60% of all incident HCV infections [27, 28]. Sexual transmission also occurs and there have been a number of recent reported outbreaks among MSM, specifically when other risk factors were also reported: coinfection with other sexually transmitted diseases (STI)s, sharing drugs via anal or intranasal routes, unprotected anal intercourse, and certain anal–oral and anal–hand contact during sexual encounters [29, 30]. Long-term studies have found that monogamous partners of HCV-infected individuals have a slightly increased risk of acquiring HCV although the overall rate remains quite low (1.5%) [31]. Perinatal transmission is rare but is higher for babies born to mothers coinfected with HIV and HCV [32].

Clearly, HIV-infected persons are at risk for coinfection with hepatitis viruses. With the success of current HIV treatment strategies, HIV providers should aggressively screen for hepatitis coinfection, counsel patients on risk reduction strategies, and offer timely vaccination for HAV and HBV.

Laboratory Testing

A baseline assessment of liver function should be performed for all HIV-infected persons, including measurement of hepatic inflammation with transaminases, AST and ALT. While there are numerous other causes, a low platelet counts may indicate end stage liver disease. Similarly, low albumin or elevated international normalized ratio (INR)/partial thromboplastin time (PTT) may suggest impaired liver synthetic function and warrants further evaluation.

The most recent guidelines from the HIV Medicine Association (HIVMA) and European AIDS Clinical Society are consistent in their recommendation to evaluate baseline liver function and hepatitis serologies at the initial visit for HIV care [33, 34]. Initial testing should include HAV antibody (anti-HAV total), HCV antibody (anti-HCV), HBV surface antigen (HBsAg), HBV core antibody (anti-HBc total), and HBV surface antibody (anti-HBs). This testing will identify the majority of patients with chronic HBV and HCV as well as those persons who are immune from HAV and HBV, whether from vaccination or past infection (see Table 17.2). Persons who are negative for HBsAg and antibody to HBsAg but positive for HBV total core antigen antibody should be screened for chronic HBV infection by determination of HBV DNA. HCV RNA should also be performed in HCV-seronegative patients with a history of injection drug use or with unexplained increased serum transaminases, as approximately 3% of HIV-infected persons with undetectable HCV antibodies have chronic HCV infection [35, 36]. Persons who are seronegative for HAV and HBV should be offered vaccination (see section below). Baseline HCV Ab screening is a recommended performance indicator in the quality standards established by the two major authorities on quality of HIV care in the USA [9, 37]. In addition, the New York State AIDS Institute Guidelines recommend annual HCV screening for HIV-infected persons who are seronegative but have ongoing risky behaviors, i.e., injection drug use, MSM, and those with multiple sexual partners.

Table 17.2 Hepatitis serologies

		Hepatitis A		Hepatitis B						Hepatitis C		
	Sero-negative state	Acute HAV	Past HAV/vaccination	Acute HBV	Inactive carrier	Occult infection[a]	Chronic infection	Cleared infection	Vaccination	Acute HCV	Chronic HCV	Cleared HCV[b]
HAV Ab IgG	−	−	+									
HAV Ab IgM	−	+	−									
HBV sAg	−			+	+	−	+	−	−			
HBV sAb	−			−	−	−	−	+	+			
HBV cAb IgG[c]	−			±	+	±	+	+	−			
HBV cAb IgM	−			+	±	±	−	−	−			
HBV eAg	−			+	−	−	+	−	−			
HBV eAb	−			−	+	−	−	+	−			
HBV viral load	−			+	+	+	+	−	−			
HCV Ab	−									±	+	+
HCV viral load	−									+	+	−

[a] See the text for discussion of isolated HBcAb positivity
[b] An isolated HCV Ab with two negative HCV RNA tests separated by 6 months is most consistent with past infection. It may also reflect a false positive antibody which can be confirmed with a HCV recombinant immunoblot assay (RIBA) test
[c] Also referred to as HBV Total cAb

Behavioral Prevention and Intervention

After completing serologic testing, care providers should review the results and interpretations with patients. All HIV-infected patients should receive counseling about the modes of transmission for the hepatitis viruses, highlighting that all three can be transmitted sexually so safe sexual practices including consistent condom use remain a high priority to prevent acquisition of the hepatitis viruses. Specifically for HBV and HCV, patients should also be counseled about the risk for household transmission through shared use of toothbrushes and razors, and more importantly through sharing of drug using equipment, most notably needle-sharing but also intranasal drug paraphernalia (see Table 17.3). While the artistry of tattooing and body piercing remains a topic of debate, providers should also counsel patients of the risk for acquisition of both HBV and HCV, particularly when equipment is not sterile or tattoo dye is reused on multiple persons.

HIV care providers must use a risk reduction strategy to help patients improve their health [38]. The first step is having an open discussion with patients about illicit drug as well as alcohol use. Data from the HIV Cost and Services Utilization Study cohort reports high prevalence of consumption of alcohol (50%), cocaine or heroin (17%), amphetamines (15%), and marijuana or hashish (34%) [39]. Prescription drug use and heavy alcohol use were strongly associated with HIV risk behavior in a study of men who were clients at commercial sex venues, suggesting prevention efforts should be focused on misuse of prescription and atypical drugs of abuse in addition to illicit substance [40]. Unfortunately, illicit drug users who are living with HIV are often marginalized and fail to seek care due to poor socioeconomic status and stigmatization. Furthermore, many persons will fail to disclose the use of illicit drugs given the perceived stigma [41]. Views on personal privacy vary by gender, race, ethnicity, and age, so prevention messages must be adapted to accommodate specific populations [42]. Therefore, routine screening and education with all patients will significantly reduce stigma and raise awareness only if tailored individually as is done with HAART therapy.

Table 17.3 Prevention strategies for intravenous drug users

- Education/awareness
  - Refrain from sharing needles/paraphernalia
  - Promote consistent condom use
  - Reduce other risky sexual behavior
- Treatment of concomitant psychiatric issues
- Needle and syringe exchange programs (NEP)
- Substance abuse treatment
- Opioid agonist therapy (OAT)

Substance Abuse Treatment

Ideally, all persons who use illicit drugs would be referred to a substance abuse treatment program and successfully complete the program and remain drug-free. Unfortunately, nearly 50% of patients decline substance abuse treatment (SAT) at the time of recommendation [43]. Women and persons with a history of injection drug use are more likely to participate in SAT. To be most successful, SATs must be combined with evaluation and treatment of psychiatric illness, specifically depression and anxiety. Furthermore, an assessment of complicating factors such as housing, transportation, medication acquisition, and other needs can further facilitate a successful SAT.

Given that many persons will refuse SAT, other risk reduction strategies are necessary, specifically for injection drug use. Intravenous injection provides the strongest drug effect and is also the most cost-effective for most drug users. Unfortunately, intravenous injection is also the most efficient means to transmit blood-borne pathogens such as HBV, HCV, and HIV. While the high rates of transmission are often reduced to blaming the risky individual, we must recognize that many factors contribute to transmission. These include but are not limited to the following: a lack of knowledge and awareness of the risk associated with injection drug use, lack of access to sterile injection drug equipment, the use of "shooter's galleries" in which a drug dealer lends needles and syringes to multiple persons [44]. It is, therefore, incumbent on providers to identify persons at risk and educate them about risk reduction strategies.

Opioid Replacement Therapy

While some persons can successfully abstain from recurrence of use of illicit drugs through abstinence-based programs such as Narcotics Anonymous or other programs, opioid agonist therapy (OAT) with maintenance methadone or buprenorphine have proven very successful in the outpatient setting [45]. Numerous studies of methadone maintenance therapy have yielded successful results reducing the use of heroin and significantly reducing the transmission of HIV and hepatitis [46–48]. While there has been recent increased concern about methadone toxicity and attributable mortality, numerous studies have illustrated a 40–70% reduction in mortality with methadone maintenance compared to time periods before the institution of methadone programs [49, 50]. Given the concern for cardiac toxicity with methadone, many providers are using buprenorphine, a partial opioid agonist to reduce heroin use [51, 52]. Head-to-head comparisons showed that long-term adherence was better with methadone but greater reduction of opioid consumption was reported with buprenorphine [53]. There is significant literature supporting both agents and providers are encouraged to refer patients for routine focused counseling when buprenorphine is given in the office-based setting. Unfortunately, for persons using amphetamines or cocaine, there are currently no effective pharmaceutical agents for replacement therapy. There are even fewer resources for those with prescription drug addiction.

Needle Exchange Programs

HBV and HCV have been demonstrated to remain viable in syringes stored at room temperature up to 8 months after inoculation and HIV may be recoverable up to 30 days (but generally 1–2 days) after inoculation [54, 55]. While disinfecting equipment using bleach can inactivate these viruses, trials have shown mixed results regarding reduction in HIV transmission [56]. Alternatively, needle [and syringe] exchange programs (NEP) can facilitate the use of sterile equipment for persons who continue to use injection drugs. The first NEPs were met with skepticism in Amsterdam in the mid-1980s but have since proven successful in both developed and developing countries [57, 58]. Ideally, NEP allow for the dissemination of education materials and other risk reduction strategies such as condom distribution, vaccination, access to SATs, and other health services [38]. Numerous studies have illustrated the effectiveness of NEP and a recent cost-effectiveness analysis illustrated that widespread NEPs in the USA would prevent 12,350 incident cases of HIV with a savings of 1.3 billion dollars in treatment costs for HIV alone [59]. Despite the widespread recognition of the success of NEPs, the restrictive legal apparatus of many countries has made the widespread uptake of this intervention difficult in many settings [60]. An alternative approach is to utilize pharmacies as a resource for sterile needles and syringes although the benefits of other risk reduction efforts may be less emphasized and there is concern that some patients do not like this approach due to stigmatization or cost issues [61]. Some hospital- and community-based harm reduction programs prefer to distribute syringes/needles directly rather than exchange and also provide opioid overdose prevention supplies including naloxone.

Overview of Vaccination

The administration of preventive vaccines remains an important preventive measure in the care of persons living with HIV. Current guidelines recommend all HBV seronegative HIV-infected persons receive HBV vaccination shortly after their initial visit [9, 33, 34, 62]. HAV vaccination is routinely recommended for all nonimmune HCV-coinfected patients, because of their increased risk of fulminant HAV, and for persons in high-risk groups, although some clinicians routinely vaccinate all HIV-infected persons regardless of HCV status [33, 62]. For the asymptomatic patient with a high CD4 cell count, these vaccinations are administered before initiating antiretroviral therapy (ART). Questions remain about the appropriate timing of vaccine administration with regard to current CD4 count, nadir CD4 count, level of HIV viremia, and administration of potent ART. If clinicians wait until the plasma HIV RNA levels are undetectable or for CD4 counts to increase for persons presenting late to care, many patients may be at risk for infection with these preventable pathogens. The issue is complicated by the fact that HIV-infected persons respond poorly to vaccinations, with seroprotection rates ranging from 18 to 56% for HBV and 52 to 94% for HAV vaccine compared with greater than 95% in HIV-seronegative adults [63]. This section reviews recent literature regarding hepatitis vaccine responses, the role of immune reconstitution and HIV virologic suppression on these responses, and the use of hepatitis vaccines by practitioners.

Hepatitis A Vaccination

Although the most recent Advisory Committee on Immunization Practices (ACIP) adult immunization schedule recommends HAV vaccination for persons with chronic liver disease, those requiring clotting factors, certain occupational risk groups, travelers to endemic areas, and persons with specific behavioral risk factors (e.g., MSM and injection drug users), it does not specifically recommend vaccination for all persons with HIV infection [64]. Nevertheless, many providers offer HAV vaccination to their HAV-seronegative patients regardless of risk factors because of the possible complications of acute HAV and given the prevalence of HAV seropositivity in HIV-infected populations (more than 20%) [65, 66]. Two recent articles specifically evaluated the poor response rates in adult HIV-infected populations in the current ART era, and a third attempted to evaluate the role of immune reconstitution for HAV vaccine response [66–68].

In the first study, 334 HIV-infected, HAV antibody seronegative subjects received HAV vaccination [66]. Of those vaccinated, 133 subjects (50%) developed protective antibody after vaccination. Two thirds of the cohort was receiving ART at the time of vaccination. Although there was no difference among different CD4 cell count strata, responders had significantly lower HIV viral loads than nonresponders. By multivariate analysis, both low HIV viral load at time of vaccination and male gender were associated with a protective vaccine response. The second study evaluated HAV vaccine responses in 214 HIV-infected subjects with a seroconversion rate of 61% [67]. By univariate analysis, vaccine response correlated with the level of HIV viremia and current and nadir CD4 cell counts. By multivariate analysis, only higher current CD4 was associated with a response to vaccine.

Taken together, these studies suggest that response to HAV vaccine is less than optimal in HIV-infected persons and that immune status mediates the response, whether because of absolute number of CD4 cells or the level of HIV viremia. Clearly, the patient's immune status should be considered when vaccinating against HAV. Another study, from the Pediatric AIDS Clinical Trials Group, attempted to address this very question [68]. This study included 152 HAV-seronegative HIV-infected youth with a median age of 9.2 years (range, 2–21 years) who were on stable ART with a baseline median CD4 count of 830 cells/mm^3 (median, 32%). After two vaccine doses, 97% of the subjects seroconverted, although only 53% were considered to have developed a high antibody titer (>250 mIU/mL). A significantly higher proportion of subjects with high antibody response also had undetectable HIV viral loads. Of note, although seroconversion rates approached those of uninfected youth, the titers were lower in the HIV-infected subjects by a magnitude of approximately two. Because of this lower peak antibody production, titers waned to below the level of protection in 10% of HIV-infected children by 12 months after vaccination. Overall, this study suggests that control of viremia improves humoral responses to HAV vaccine. Whether the direct mechanism is mediated through absolute CD4 cell count, improved B-cell function, or reduction in viral loads remains to be fully elucidated. However, these studies suggest that in persons with low CD4 cell counts, HAV vaccination should be deferred until immune reconstitution has occurred with CD4 cell count increases above 200 cells/mm^3.

Hepatitis B Vaccination

Numerous studies have demonstrated that HIV-infected persons do not respond optimally to HBV vaccination. Ungulkraiwit et al. [69] enrolled 65 HIV-infected subjects in a series of three injections with a double dose of HBV vaccine. At first vaccination, the mean CD4 cell count was 354 cells/mm^3; 88% of the cohort was receiving HAART, with 75% having an undetectable HIV viral load. Unfortunately, only 46% of the vaccines responded. Response rates correlated with younger age and higher CD4 counts. There was also a trend toward lower HIV viral loads in responders. Another recent study evaluated responses in 55 subjects observed at a single site in Brazil using a higher dose of HBV vaccine [70]. Overall, 59% of the subjects responded, and response correlated with higher CD4 cell counts and lower HIV viral loads. The third study compared standard (10 mcg) vs. high (40 mcg) doses of HBV vaccine in 79 HIV-infected individuals observed at a single site in Mexico [71]. Overall, 61% of the subjects responded with no difference between the two arms. Mean CD4 counts were 225 and 245 cells/mm^3, respectively, and only 19% had HIV viral loads below the limits of quantification at time of vaccination.

Given that these studies confirm that our current approaches yield poor responses, researchers have looked for alternative strategies. A small study from Canada evaluated the use of four intradermal injections in 12 HIV-infected subjects who failed to respond to six doses of standard intramuscular vaccine [72]. By improving antigen presentation mediated through the Langerhans cells in the dermis, this strategy has yielded protection in non-responding health care workers and dialysis patients. Unfortunately, only 6 of the 12 HIV-infected subjects responded, with one individual maintaining protective immunity at 12 months. Therefore, this intradermal route of administration does not appear to be an effective strategy.

Use of higher dose HBV vaccine (40 mcg dose) is another alternative given the ACIP recommendations regarding dialysis patients and other immunocompromised individuals [64]. Fonseca et al. [73] randomized 210 HIV-infected persons to standard (20 mcg dose) vs. double dose (40 mcg dose) and reported a better seroconversion with the higher dose (47 vs. 34%, $p=0.07$) [74]. This improvement was most noticeable for those with CD4+ T-cell counts ≥ 350 c/mm^3 (64 vs. 39%) and HIV viral loads <10,000 cp/mL (58 vs. 37%). However, another trial comparing 10 vs. 40 mcg dosing of HBV vaccine reported no differences in seroconversion rates between the two strategies (61 and 62%, respectively) [71]. Still, more subjects who received the 40 mcg dose developed HBsAb titers >100 mIU/mL. Sasaki et al. reported a seroconversion rate of 66% in 80 HIV-infected age 18–35 years with CD4+ T-count >350 c/mm^3 who received the 40 mcg dose of vaccine [74]. Similarly, Overton et al. recently reported a 59% seroconversion rate with a 40 mcg dose of HBV vaccine [75]. While there is a trend to better responses with these higher vaccine doses, they remain below what is reported in immunocompetent individuals.

A second alternative strategy that has been pursued to improve antibody responses is the use of adjuvants. The formulations of hepatitis vaccines that are currently approved by the Food and Drug Administration (FDA) are precipitated with alum (potassium aluminum sulfate) to form bulk vaccine adjuvanted with amorphous aluminum hydroxyphosphate sulfate or adsorbed onto the alum [76]. It is believed that the effective adjuvanticity of alum is a function of the degree of adsorption of antigen on the adjuvant, and this in turn is the basis of the depot theory. The aluminum adjuvants allow the slow release of antigen at the site of vaccine injection, prolonging the interaction between antigen and APCs and lymphocytes. Unfortunately, as noted above, HIV-infected persons do not respond adequately to the currently available alum-adsorbed vaccines. Therefore, other adjuvants are being evaluated.

One adjuvant that has shown promise in HIV-infected patients is CpG adjuvant, an oligodeoxynucleotide-containing immunostimulatory motif that directly activates B cells and plasmacytoid dendritic cells via toll-like receptors.

Cooper et al. have recently published data from a randomized controlled trial of 36 HIV-infected subjects receiving 40 mcg of HBV vaccine with or without this adjuvant [77]. Response was significantly greater in those receiving the novel adjuvant (85 vs. 40%) at 60 months after vaccination. These data were particularly intriguing given that the rate of response was similar to that in historical controls. Confirmatory results are expected from larger studies.

Other possible adjuvants have been evaluated. Two meta-analyses have compiled data regarding the role of granulocyte-macrophage colony-stimulating factor (GM-CSF) on immune responses to HBV vaccine. The first meta-analysis identified 187 patients with end-stage renal disease from seven different prospective trials. The odds ratio of having a protective response rate was 4.63 (95% CI, 1.42–15.14) for those receiving adjuvant GM-CSF [78]. Cruciani et al. [79] identified 734 subjects from 13 studies and also reported a benefit for GM-CSF, particularly in generating protection after the first dose of HBV vaccine.

This strategy has also been evaluated in HIV-infected subjects with mixed results. Sasaki et al. [74] evaluated the efficacy of a single 20 mcg dose of GM-CSF to augment response to double-dose HBV vaccine in 80 HIV-infected persons with CD4 cell counts greater than 350 cells/mm^3 90% of who were on HAART. A significant increase in the development of hepatitis B surface antibody (HBsAb) was noted in the GM-CSF group (62%) vs. the placebo group (30%) after the second vaccine dose ($p<0.0074$). One month after vaccination, 72% of the patients in the GM-CSF group and 60% in the placebo group developed protective titers that were significantly higher in the GM-CSF group (645 vs. 375 IU/L; $p<0.01$). These results suggest promise for the role of cytokines in augmenting immune response to vaccination in HIV-infected persons. However, a recent study from the AIDS Clinical Trials Group evaluating the use of higher-dose GM-CSF (250 mcg) with 40 mcg HBV vaccine administered at weeks 0, 4, and 12 weeks yielded differing results [75]. The overall response rate was 59% 1 month after completion of the vaccine series with no differences between the study arm who received GM-CSF and the vaccine only arm. Additional research is needed to clarify if there is a dose threshold for the use of GM-CSF as an adjuvant for HBV vaccination.

Issues with Isolated Hepatitis B Core Positivity

Screening for hepatitis serologies has become the standard of care for HIV care providers. As noted earlier, evidence of active or past coinfection with HBV is very prevalent in HIV-infected patients. The pattern of HBV surface antigen negative-HBV core antibody (HBcAb) positive is also more often found in HIV-infected individuals. The question arises as to whether this reflects cleared infection in the distant past, occult HBV infection, or a false-positive HBcAb assay. For a patient who is currently receiving HAART with HBV activity, it may be difficult to discern the actual meaning of isolated HBcAb, although the presence of HBV e antibody (HBeAb) can confirm past infection; however, this test is not 100% reliable as the HBeAb may wane and disappear over time. Several studies evaluated this issue and assessed the utility of HBV vaccination for HIV-infected subjects with isolated HBcAb.

The University of Pennsylvania's Center for AIDS Research evaluated the prevalence of isolated HBcAb serology in their database and identified 699 (59%) of 1,193 HIV-infected subjects with this pattern [80]. To assess for occult HBV infection, 179 subjects were randomly selected to have stored serum sent for HBV DNA and 17 subjects (10%) were identified with occult infection. This number may actually underestimate the prevalence of occult HBV as 61% of HBV DNA-negative subjects were receiving more than one active agent against HBV. Detectable HIV viremia was associated with occult HBV, and the authors suggest that immune dysfunction may contribute to persistent low-level HBV replication. Of note, persons coinfected with HCV were less likely to have occult HBV, raising questions of either a false-positive result or the possible dominance of HCV over concomitant HBV infection.

Two additional studies also looked at the prevalence of this serologic pattern and its impact on HBV vaccination. Gandhi et al. [81] evaluated vaccine responses in 69 subjects, 29 with isolated HBcAb and 40 with negative HBcAb. Isolated HBcAb serology was associated with HCV antibody positivity, male gender, white race, and elevated transaminases but not level of HIV viremia or CD4 cell count. An anamnestic response to a single booster dose of HBV vaccine occurred in only 16% of subjects overall; this result did not differ between the groups. Interestingly, the 50% of subjects who were HBcAb positive–HBeAb positive had a significantly higher anamnestic response than did isolated HBcAb-positive subjects (43 vs. 7%, respectively). The authors suggested that the former pattern likely represents past infection and thereby enhanced the vaccine response. A second study from Thailand found 28 of 140 patients (20%) with isolated HBcAb [82]. Risk factors for this pattern again included HCV antibody positivity and history of intravenous drug use. Only 2 of the 28 subjects (7%) had an anamnestic response to HBV vaccination.

Another study evaluated the perception of this serologic pattern among 40 HIV practitioners at a Chicago clinic with more than 4,500 HIV-infected patients [83]. Of 3,810 patients with complete HBV serology, 698 (18%) were found to have isolated HBcAb. Once again this pattern was more common in HCV antibody-positive than in HIV-monoinfected patients (36 vs. 13%). The majority of providers (77.5%) believed this pattern to reflect past infection with resulting immunity while the remaining providers (22.5%) believed that this represented occult HBV disease. Only six providers (15%) reported routinely vaccinating patients with this serologic pattern.

The authors of the two vaccine studies recommended additional research to evaluate the appropriate vaccine strategy for this common serologic pattern. One approach at present is to check quantitative HBsAb 2–4 weeks after a single dose of HBV vaccine and if an anamnestic response has not occurred, complete the three-dose series [62]. Alternatively, one could vaccinate these patients with the three-dose series and then check the HBsAb titer. The latter approach may be more practical as the anamnestic response was very poor in both studies and the additional vaccine doses will serve to boost immunity and yield higher protective HBsAb titers. Furthermore, having patients return for the 2- to 4-week visit may be impractical in the clinical setting.

Perceptions About Hepatitis Vaccination

As noted above, while providers are aware of risk factors for hepatitis coinfection, many still fail to adequately screen their patients for serologic evidence of hepatitis coinfection. In the current era of potent ART, providers must recognize the appropriate prevention measures for HIV-infected patients, whether those are age-appropriate cancer screenings, behavioral modification, or disease-preventing vaccines. Several recent studies evaluated the perceptions of patients and providers of hepatitis vaccination and provider utilization of hepatitis vaccines and illustrated that we need appropriate medical education regarding vaccine-preventable diseases.

Ho et al. [84] interviewed 144 HIV-infected subjects at a single site in Brazil regarding receipt of several recommended vaccines, including hepatitis B, influenza, pneumococcal, and diphtheria/tetanus. Brazil's National Immunization Program offers free vaccinations to all HIV-infected persons, thus removing any financial burden related to vaccine administration. Overall, the cohort had a mean CD4 count of 443 cells/mm^3 and 87% of the subjects were receiving ART, indicating that they were engaged in care. The subjects reported vaccine coverage as follows: 77% HBV vaccine, 55% pneumococcal vaccine, 36% diphtheria/tetanus vaccine, and 24% influenza vaccine in the past 3 years. Only 17% of the entire sample had received all appropriate vaccines.

A second study from the French Aquitaine cohort specifically evaluated patient and provider perceptions regarding HBV vaccination [5]. Almost all the physicians (93%) reported being vaccinated against HBV, whereas only 113 of 512 HIV-infected patients (22%) reported HBV vaccination.

One of four physicians reported that they did not routinely perform HBV serologic testing, and only 23% reported that they evaluated patients with post-vaccination serologic testing. Physicians reported the following reasons for failure to vaccinate: forgetting (78%), difficulty in identifying at-risk patients (44%), and concern regarding post-vaccination complications (32%). Notably, a large majority of the HIV-infected patients (82%) reported risk factors for HBV infection. Overall, vaccination coverage was suboptimal in this at-risk population, and the authors recommended developing educational campaigns for both patients and providers.

These reports on vaccination practices by HIV providers indicate that we are missing an opportunity to prevent viral hepatitis. These issues are important not only for the individual patient but also from the public health perspective; universal vaccination could improve population immunity and assist in our progress toward elimination of hepatitis infections. Data from the CDC confirm that the incidence of acute HBV declined 94% among US children and adolescents from 1990 to 2004, coinciding with the integration of HBV vaccine into routine childhood vaccinations [85, 86]. Two recent studies of intravenous drug user (IVDU) populations in the USA and the UK illustrate that vigilant HBV immunization programs are needed to reduce HBV in those high-risk populations as well. In a cohort of 831 IVDUs in San Francisco, only 22% of subjects had evidence of vaccine-induced immunity whereas 56% were naïve for all HBV markers and 21% had evidence of past or chronic infection [87].

The UK study evaluated trends regarding HBV infection among 31,913 IVDUs from 1992, when universal HBV vaccination was recommended by the World Health Organization, through 2004 [88]. Rates of HBV infection were cut in half from 1992, when 50% of IVDUs tested were HBcAb positive, to 1999, when only 25% of those tested were HBcAb positive. Unfortunately, the rates subsequently increased slightly, particularly among young IVDUs. Although these data illustrate that the current UK vaccination program focusing on intravenous drug use as a risk factor has had a tremendous impact, there is still progress to be made in terms of education and promotion of hepatitis vaccination.

Summary

In the current ART era, we expect the life span of HIV-infected persons to approach that of those without HIV infection. Given this fact, addressing prevention issues is critical, whether we focus on cardiovascular risk factors or vaccine-preventable diseases. In the Data Collection on Adverse Events of Anti-HIV Drugs (D:A:D) study, liver disease was the most common cause of mortality for HIV-infected persons other than AIDS-related deaths [3]. Surprisingly, at CD4 cell counts above 200 cells/mm^3, liver-related mortality was the single most important cause of death in this large cohort. Both HBV and HCV were significantly associated with increased mortality. These findings serve as a clear reminder of the importance of hepatitis prevention.

We recommend that all HIV-infected patients undergo hepatitis serology testing (HAV antibody total, HBV core antibody total, HBV surface antibody, HBV surface antigen, and HCV antibody) at baseline and then annually (if susceptible) to monitor for incident infection. Given the concern for liver toxicity, we recommend vaccination against both HAV and HBV for patients who are seronegative for these viruses, even for those who do not fall into traditional risk groups for HAV. Persons with isolated HBcAb without occult HBV infection should also be offered HBV vaccination as outlined previously.

The current ACIP guidelines recommend the use of higher-dose (40 mcg) HBV vaccine for dialysis patients and other immunocompromised patients [64]. The revised US Public Health Service guidelines for opportunistic infections explicitly urge providers to vaccinate patients who have CD4 cell counts above 350 cells/mm^3 as early as possible [62]. For patients with more advanced disease, ART should be optimized to suppress HIV replication and increase CD4 cell counts to generate a better vaccine response.

To improve the likelihood of seroconversion, we recommend the current two-dose series of HAV vaccine and a three-dose series of HBV vaccine using the higher, 40-mcg dosing used in dialysis patients. Care providers should evaluate HBsAb and HAV antibody status after vaccination and perform annual quantitative HBV surface antibody assays. Patients who fail to develop protective antibody after completing the vaccine series may be offered a second vaccination series, although development of protection remains low and current strategies for these patients are inadequate. For a person whose titer wanes to below 10 IU/L, one should consider administering a booster vaccine, as recommended for dialysis patients [64]. The role of adjuvants and other immunomodulating agents to improve vaccine responses are currently under study and hopefully will enhance this preventive strategy.

Finally, frank discussion with patients about risk reduction strategies to avoid infection with viral hepatitis is also needed. With the recognition of high morbidity and mortality associated with liver-related diseases, it is imperative to counsel patients on avoidance of these life-threatening comorbidities.

References

1. Palella Jr FJ, Delaney KM, Moorman AC, et al. Declining morbidity and mortality among patients with advanced human immunodeficiency virus infection. HIV Outpatient Study Investigators. N Engl J Med. 1998;338:853–60.

2. Vellozzi C, Brooks JT, Bush TJ, et al. The study to understand the natural history of HIV and AIDS in the Era of effective therapy (SUN study). Am J Epidemiol. 2009;169:642–52.
3. Weber R, Sabin CA, Friis-Møller N, et al. Liver-related deaths in persons infected with the human immunodeficiency virus: the D:A:D study. Arch Intern Med. 2006;166:1632–41.
4. Antiretroviral Therapy Cohort Collaboration. Causes of death in HIV-1-infected patients treated with antiretroviral therapy, 1996–2006: collaborative analysis of 13 HIV cohort studies. Clin Infect Dis. 2010;50:1387–96.
5. Winnock M, Neau D, Castera L, et al. Hepatitis B vaccination in HIV-infected patients: a survey of physicians and patients participating in the Aquitaine cohort. Gastroenterol Clin Biol. 2006;30:189–95.
6. Shehab TM, Sonnad SS, Lok AS. Management of hepatitis C patients by primary care physicians in the USA: results of a national survey. J Viral Hepat. 2001;8:377–83.
7. Daniels D, Grytdal S. Centers for disease control and prevention (CDC). Surveillance for acute viral hepatitis – United States, 2007. MMWR Surveill Summ. 2009;58:1–27.
8. Diamond C, Thiede H, Perdue T, et al. Viral hepatitis among young men who have sex with men: prevalence of infection, risk behaviors, and vaccination. Sex Transm Dis. 2003;30:425–32.
9. New York State Department of Health Institute. HIV Clinical Resource. http://www.hivguidelines.org. Accessed 27 May 2010.
10. Lutwick LI. Clinical interactions between human immunodeficiency virus and the human hepatitis viruses. Infect Dis Clin Prac. 1999;8:9–20.
11. Ida S, Tachikawa N, Nakajima A, et al. Influence of human immunodeficiency virus type 1 infection on acute hepatitis A virus infection. Clin Infect Dis. 2002;34:379–85.
12. Alter M. Epidemiology of viral hepatitis and HIV co-infection. J Hepatol. 2006;44:6–9.
13. Soriano V, Puoti M, Peters M, et al. Care of HIV patients with chronic hepatitis B: updated recommendations from the HIV-Hepatitis B Virus International Panel. AIDS. 2008;22:1399–410.
14. Lee WM, Hepatitis B. Virus infection. N Engl J Med. 1997;337:1733–45.
15. Weinbaum CM, Williams I, Mast EE, et al. Recommendations for identification and public health management of persons with chronic hepatitis B virus infection. MMWR Recomm Rep. 2008;57:1–20.
16. Vong S, Bell BP. Chronic liver disease mortality in the United States, 1990–1998. Hepatology. 2004;39:476–83.
17. Kellerman SE, Hanson DL, McNaghten AD, Fleming PL. Prevalence of chronic hepatitis B and incidence of acute hepatitis B infection in human immunodeficiency virus-infected subjects. J Infect Dis. 2003;188:571–7.
18. Tien PC, Kovacs A, Bacchetti P, et al. Association between syphilis, antibodies to herpes simplex virus type 2, and recreational drug use and hepatitis B virus infection in the Women's Interagency HIV Study. Clin Infect Dis. 2004;39:1363–70.
19. Bodsworth N, Cooper D, Donovan B. The influence of human immunodeficiency virus type 1 infection on the development of the hepatitis B virus carrier state. J Infect Dis. 1991;163:1138–40.
20. Gilson RJ, Hawkins AE, Beecham MR, et al. Interactions between HIV and hepatitis B in homosexual men: effects on the natural history of infection. AIDS. 1997;11:597–606.
21. Thio CL, Seaberg EC, Skolasdy Jr R, et al. HIV-1, hepatitis B, and risk of liver-related mortality in the Multicenter AIDS Cohort Study (MACS). Lancet. 2002;360:1921–6.
22. Eskild A, Magnus P, Petersen G, et al. Hepatitis B antibodies in HIV-infected homosexual men are associated with more rapid progression to AIDS. AIDS. 1992;6:571–4.
23. Solomon RE, Van Raden M, Kaslow RA, et al. Association of hepatitis B surface antigen and core antibody with acquisition and manifestations of HIV-1 infection. Am J Public Health. 1990;80:1475–8.
24. Alter MJ. Epidemiology of hepatitis C. Hepatology. 1997;26:62S–5.
25. Wasley A, Grytdal S. Centers for disease control and prevention (CDC). Surveillance for acute viral hepatitis – United States, 2006. MMWR Surveill Summ. 2008;57:1–24.
26. Kim WR. The burden of hepatitis C in the United States. Hepatology. 2002;36:S30–4.
27. Alter MJ. Epidemiology of hepatitis C virus infection. World J Gastroenterol. 2007;13:2436–41.
28. Khalsa JH, Elkashef A. Interventions for HIV and hepatitis C virus infections in recreational drug users. Clin Infect Dis. 2010;50:1505–11.
29. Gotz HM, van Doornum G, Niesters HG, et al. A cluster of acute hepatitis C virus infection among men who have sex with men – results from contact tracing and public health implications. AIDS. 2005;19:969–74.
30. Richardson D, Fisher M, Sabin CA. Sexual transmission of hepatitis C in MSM may not be confined to those with HIV infection. J Infect Dis. 2008;197:1213–4.
31. Wang CC, Krantz E, Klarquist J, et al. Acute hepatitis C in a contemporary US cohort: modes of acquisition and factors influencing viral clearance. J Infect Dis. 2007;196:1474–82.
32. Mast EE, Hwang LY, Seto DS, et al. Risk factors for perinatal transmission of hepatitis C virus (HCV) and the natural history of HCV infection acquired in infancy. J Infect Dis. 2005;192:1880–9.
33. Aberg JA, Kaplan JE, Libman H, et al. Primary care guidelines for the management of persons infected with human immunodeficiency virus: 2009 update by the HIV medicine Association of the Infectious Diseases Society of America. Clin Infect Dis. 2009;49:651–81.
34. European AIDS Clinical Society. Guidelines: Clinical Management and Treatment of HIV Infected Adults in Europe. http://www.europeanaidsclinicalsociety.org. Accessed 27 May 2010.
35. Chamie G, Bonacini M, Bangsberg DR, et al. Factors associated with seronegative chronic hepatitis C virus infection in HIV-infection. Clin Infect Dis. 2007;44:577–83.
36. Centers for Disease Control and Prevention (CDC), Health Resources and Services Administration, National Institutes of Health, HIV Medicine Association of the Infectious Diseases Society of America. Incorporating HIV prevention into the medical care of persons living with HIV. Recommendations of CDC, the Health Resources and Services Administration, the National Institutes of Health, and the HIV Medicine Association of the Infectious Diseases Society of America. MMWR Recomm Rep. 2003;52:1–24.
37. U S Department of Health and Human Services. The HIV/AIDS Program: HAB Performance Measures. http://hab.hrsa.gov. Accessed 10 Apr 2010.
38. Vlahov D, Robertson AM, Strathdee SA. Prevention of HIV infection among injection drug users in resource-limited settings. Clin Infect Dis. 2010;50:S114–21.
39. Galvan FH, Bing EG, Fleishman JA, et al. The prevalence of alcohol consumption and heavy drinking among people with HIV in the United States: results from the HIV Cost and Services Utilization Study. J Stud Alcohol. 2002;63:179–86.
40. McNeely J, Silvera R, Torres K, Bernstein K, et al. Current Substance Misuse and HIV Risk Behavior Among Highly Sexually Active Men Who Have Sex with Men (MSM) Attending Commercial Sex Venues, Events and Parties (CSVEP) in New York City. Society of General Internal Medicine (SGIM) 33rd Annual Meeting, April 28–May 1, 2010, Minneapolis MN. Abstract #198149.
41. Valle M, Levy J. Weighing the consequences: self-disclosure of HIV-positive status among African American injection drug users. Health Educ Behav. 2009;36:155–66.

42. Gorbach PM, Galea JT, Amani B, et al. Don't ask, don't tell: patterns of HIV disclosure among HIV positive men who have sex with men with recent STI practising high risk behavior in Los Angeles and Seattle. Sex Transm Infect. 2004;80:512–7.
43. Pisu M, Cloud G, Austin S, et al. Substance abuse treatment in an urban HIV clinic: who enrolls and what are the benefits? AIDS Care. 2010;22:348–54.
44. Des Jarlais DC, Semaan S. HIV prevention for injecting drug users: the first 25 years and counting. Psychosom Med. 2008;70:606–11.
45. Krantz MJ, Mehler PS. Treating opioid dependence. Growing implications for primary care. Arch Intern Med. 2004;164:277–88.
46. Sees KL, Delucchi KL, Masson C, et al. Methadone maintenance vs. 180-day psychosocially enriched detoxification for treatment of opioid dependence: a randomized controlled trial. JAMA. 2000;283:1303–10.
47. Novick DM, Joseph H, Croxson TS, et al. Absence of antibody to human immunodeficiency virus in long-term, socially rehabilitated methadone maintenance patients. Arch Intern Med. 1990;150:97–9.
48. Gowing LR, Farrell M, Bornemann R, Sullivan LE, Ali RL. Methadone treatment of injecting opioid users for prevention of HIV infection. J Gen Intern Med. 2006;21:193–5.
49. Bell J, Zador D. A risk-benefit analysis of methadone maintenance treatment. Drug Saf. 2000;22:179–90.
50. Clausen T, Anchersen K, Waal H. Mortality prior to, during and after opioid maintenance treatment (OMT): a national prospective cross-registry study. Drug Alcohol Depend. 2008;94:151–7.
51. Krantz MJ, Martin J, Stimmel B, Mehta D, Haigney MC. QTc interval screening in methadone treatment. Ann Intern Med. 2009;150:387–95.
52. Johnson RE, Chutuape MA, Strain EC, et al. A comparison of levomethadyl acetate, buprenorphine, and methadone for opioid dependence. N Engl J Med. 2000;343:1290–7.
53. Fischer G, Gombas W, Eder H, et al. Buprenorphine versus methadone maintenance for the treatment of opioid dependence. Addiction. 1999;94:1337–47.
54. Heimer R, Khoshnood K, Jariwala-Freeman B, Duncan B, Harima Y. Hepatitis in used syringes: the limits of sensitivity of techniques to detect hepatitis B virus (HBV) DNA, hepatitis C virus (HCV) RNA, and antibodies to HBV core and HCV antigens. J Infect Dis. 1996;173:997–1000.
55. Abdala N, Stephens PC, Griffith BP, Heimer R. Survival of HIV-1 in syringes. J Acquir Immune Defic Syndr Hum Retrovirol. 1999;20:73–80.
56. Gleghorn AA, Doherty MC, Vlahov D, Celentano DD, Jones TS. Inadequate bleach contact times during syringe cleaning among injection drug users. J Acquir Immune Defic Syndr. 1994;7:767–72.
57. Institute of Medicine. Preventing HIV infection among injecting drug users in high risk countries: an assessment of the evidence. http://www.iom.edu/CMS/3783/30188/37071.aspx. Accessed 27 May 2010.
58. World Health Organization. Effectiveness of sterile needle and syringe programming in reducing HIV/AIDS among injecting drug users. http://www.who.int/hiv/pub/prev_care/effectivenesssterileneedle.pdf. Accessed 27 May 2010.
59. Holtgrave DR, Pinkerton SD, Jones TS, Lurie P, Vlahov D. Cost and cost-effectiveness of increasing access to sterile syringes and needles as an HIV prevention intervention in the United States. J Acquir Immune Defic Syndr Hum Retrovirol. 1998;18:S133–8.
60. International Harm Reduction Association and Human Rights Watch. Building consensus: a reference guide to human rights and drug policy. http://www.ihra.net/BookofAuthorities. Accessed 27 May 2010.
61. Ramos R, Ferreira-Pinto JB, Brouwer KC, et al. A tale of two cities: social and environmental influences shaping risk factors and protective behaviors in two Mexico-US border cities. Health Place. 2009;15:999–1005.
62. Kaplan JE, Benson C, Holmes KH, et al. Guidelines for prevention and treatment of opportunistic infections in HIV-infected adults and adolescents: recommendations from CDC, the National Institutes of Health, and the HIV Medicine Association of the Infectious Diseases Society of America. MMWR Recomm Rep. 2009;58:1–207.
63. Overton ET, Aberg JA. Hepatitis A and B immunization in persons infected with HIV. The Year in Hepat Vaccin. 2008;2:31–7.
64. Advisory Committee on Immunization Practices. Recommended adult immunization schedule: United States, 2010. Ann Intern Med. 2010;152:36–9.
65. Overton ET, Nurutdinova D, Sungkanuparph S, et al. Predictors of immunity after hepatitis A vaccination in HIV-infected persons. J Viral Hepat. 2007;14:189–93.
66. Tedaldi EM, Baker RK, Moorman AC, et al. Hepatitis A and B vaccination practices for ambulatory patients infected with HIV. Clin Infect Dis. 2004;38:1478–84.
67. Rimland D, Guest JL. Response to hepatitis A vaccine in HIV patients in the HAART era. AIDS. 2005;19:1702–4.
68. Weinberg A, Gona P, Nachman SA, et al. Antibody responses to hepatitis A virus vaccine in HIV-infected children with evidence of immunologic reconstitution while receiving highly active antiretroviral therapy. J Infect Dis. 2006;193:302–11.
69. Ungulkraiwit P, Jongjirawisan Y, Atamasirikul K, Sungkanuparph S. Factors for predicting successful immune response to hepatitis B vaccination in HIV-1 infected patients. Southeast Asian J Trop Med Public Health. 2007;38:680–5.
70. Veiga AP, Casseb J, Duarte AJ. Humoral response to hepatitis B vaccination and its relationship with T CD45RA+ (naïve) and CD45RO+ (memory) subsets in HIV-1-infected subjects. Vaccine. 2006;24:7124–8.
71. Cornejo-Juarez P, Volkow-Fernandez P, Escobedo-Lopez K. Randomized controlled trial of hepatitis B virus vaccine in HIV-1-infected patients comparing two different doses. AIDS Res Ther. 2006;6:3–9.
72. Shafran SD, Mashinter LD, Lindemulder A, et al. Poor efficacy of intradermal administration of recombinant hepatitis B virus immunization in HIV-infected individuals who fail to respond to intramuscular administration of hepatitis B virus vaccine. HIV Med. 2007;8:295–9.
73. Fonseca MO, Pang LW, de Paula Cavalheiro N, Barone AA, Heloisa Lopes M. Randomized trial of recombinant hepatitis B vaccine in HIV-infected adult patients comparing a standard dose to a double dose. Vaccine. 2005;23:2902–8.
74. Sasaki M, Foccacia R, deMessias-Reason IJ. Efficacy of granulocyte-macrophage colony-stimulating factor (GM-CSF) as a vaccine adjuvant for hepatitis B virus in patients with HIV infection. Vaccine. 2003;21:4545–9.
75. Overton ET, Kang M, Peters MG, et al. Immune Response to Hepatitis B Vaccine in HIV-Infected Subjects Using Granulocyte-Macrophage Colony-Stimulating Factor (GM-CSF) as a Vaccine Adjuvant: ACTG Study 5220. Vaccine. Accepted for publication June 8, 2010.
76. Baylor NW, Egan W, Richman P. Aluminum salts in vaccines – US perspective. Vaccine. 2002;20:S18–23.
77. Cooper CL, Angel JB, Seguin I, Davis HL, Cameron DW. CPG 7909 adjuvant plus hepatitis B virus vaccination in HIV-infected adults achieves long-term seroprotection for up to 5 years. Clin Infect Dis. 2008;46(8):1310–4.
78. Fabrizi F, Ganeshan SV, Dixit V, Martin P. Meta-analysis: the adjuvant role of granulocyte macrophage-colony stimulating factor on immunological response to hepatitis B virus vaccine in end-stage renal disease. Aliment Pharmacol Ther. 2006;24:789–96.
79. Cruciani M, Mengoli C, Serpelloni G, et al. Granulocyte macrophage colony-stimulating factor as an adjuvant for hepatitis B vaccination: a meta-analysis. Vaccine. 2007;25:709–18.

80. Re 3rd VL, Frank I, Gross R, et al. Prevalence, risk factors, and outcomes for occult hepatitis B virus infection among HIV-infected patients. J Acquir Immune Defic Syndr. 2007;44:315–20.
81. Gandhi RT, Wurcel A, Lee H, et al. Response to hepatitis B vaccine in HIV-1-positive subjects who test positive for isolated antibody to hepatitis B core antigen: implications for hepatitis B vaccine strategies. J Infect Dis. 2005;191:1435–41.
82. Jongjirawisan Y, Ungulkraiwit P, Sungkanuparph S. Isolated antibody to hepatitis B core antigen in HIV-1 infected patients and a pilot study of vaccination to determine the anamnestic response. J Med Assoc Thai. 2006;89:2028–34.
83. Thomas-Gosain N, Adeyemi OM. Perceived significance of isolated HBcAb in patients with HIV: a survey of practitioners. AIDS Patient Care STDS. 2007;21:385–9.
84. Ho YL, Enohata T, Lopes MH, De Sousa Dos Santos S. Vaccination in Brazilian HIV-infected adults: a cross-sectional study. AIDS Patient Care STDS. 2008;22:65–70.
85. Mast EE, Margolis HS, Fiore AE, et al. A comprehensive immunization strategy to eliminate transmission of hepatitis B virus infection in the United States: recommendations of the Advisory Committee on Immunization Practices (ACIP) Part 1: immunization of infants, children, and adolescents. MMWR Recomm Rep. 2005;54:1–31.
86. Mast EE, Weinbaum CM, Fiore AE, et al. A comprehensive immunization strategy to eliminate transmission of hepatitis B virus infection in the United States: recommendations of the Advisory Committee on Immunization Practices (ACIP) Part II: immunization of adults. MMWR Recomm Rep. 2006;55:1–33.
87. Lum PJ, Hahn JA, Shafer KP, et al. Hepatitis B virus infection and immunization status in a new generation of injection drug users in San Francisco. J Viral Hepat. 2008;15:229–36.
88. Judd A, Hickman M, Hope VD, et al. Twenty years of selective hepatitis B vaccination: is hepatitis B declining among injecting drug users in England and Wales? J Viral Hepat. 2007;14:584–91.

Antiretroviral Therapy and Hepatotoxicity

18

Norah J. Shire

Introduction

The advent of antiretroviral therapy (ART) for treatment of HIV has significantly delayed HIV-related disease progression, allowing those infected to live longer without opportunistic infections. To some extent, HIV has become a chronic disease requiring long-term treatment with multidrug regimens. A probability model of the survival benefit of AIDS therapy in the USA demonstrated that the projected per-person survival after a diagnosis of AIDS increased 13.3 years from 19 months with no available treatment to 14.9 years in 2003 [1]. However, risks associated with ART pose challenges to patient care. Of particular concern is the potential for hepatotoxicity, especially in HIV-infected patients who may be at increased risk from liver injury due to underlying liver disease from causes such as viral hepatitis. Flares in aminotransferases, often interpreted as hepatotoxicity in those on ART, may cause treatment discontinuation, appropriately in some cases but unnecessarily in others.

This chapter discusses the definition, mechanisms, diagnosis, and frequency of hepatotoxicity attributable to ART and reviews the added impact of viral coinfection.

Defining Hepatotoxicity

Hepatotoxicity is typically diagnosed when there are liver enzyme elevations in the absence of other causes of elevation, such as viral hepatitis, alcohol or drug abuse, immune reconstitution syndrome, or biliary tract disorders. Updated reference ranges for the upper limit of "normal" alanine aminotransferase (ALT) have been suggested: 30 U/L for men, and 19 U/L for women [2], corresponding to the 95th percentiles of ALT levels in a cohort of nearly 4,000 first-time blood donors at low risk for liver disease. Although ALT is certainly one marker of liver injury, it is not sufficiently sensitive or specific to define or categorize hepatotoxicity, as it is found in tissues other than the liver [3]. A commonly used grading scheme for hepatotoxicity in HIV was derived from the Adult AIDS Clinical Trials Group (AACTG) (Table 18.1) [4]. However, this scale implies a "normal" baseline value against which to assess transaminase abnormalities. In many patients with HIV, baseline values are above normal limits, often due to viral hepatitis coinfection. Thus, a modification to this scale was developed to measure fold-change from baseline, and it defines severe hepatotoxicity as grade 3 or 4 change in aspartate aminotransferase (AST) or ALT levels during treatment (only one enzyme elevation is needed to meet the hepatotoxicity definition) (Table 18.1) [5].

More recently, the US Food and Drug Administration (FDA) released guidance for the pharmaceutical industry on evaluating drug-induced liver injury (DILI) in the post-licensure context [6]. In this guidance, the FDA suggests that the most critical evaluation of potential for severe hepatotoxicity is "Hy's Law," the moniker given to an algorithm that combines assessment of liver injury with altered liver function. Hy's Law, derived from Hy Zimmerman's observation that patients with ALT/AST elevations with concomitant jaundice had a poor prognosis [7], is met by the following criteria:

1. ALT or AST >3× ULN,
2. Total bilirubin >2× ULN, and
3. There is no other cause for these enzyme elevations.

In the context of drug trials, it is also important to consider the frequency of ALT/AST elevations compared to the placebo or control group, and whether there are even higher elevations (e.g., >5× or 10× ULN or change from baseline) seen in the treatment group versus the control group.

N.J. Shire (✉)
Experimental Medicine, Infections Diseases, Merck, Sharp, and Dohme Corp., 351 Sumneytown Pike, North Wales, PA 19454, USA
e-mail: norah_shire@merck.com

Table 18.1 ALT and AST elevations and hepatoxicity grading

Grade	Description	AACTG ALT or AST elevation	Modified ALT or AST elevation
0			<1.5× baseline
1	Mild	1.25–2.5× ULN	1.25–2.5× baseline
2	Moderate	2.51–5× ULN	2.6–3.5× baseline
3	Severe	5.1–10.0× ULN	3.6–5× baseline
4	Potentially life-threatening	>10.0× ULN	>5× baseline

AACTG Adult AIDS Clinical Trials Group, *ALT* alanine aminotransferase, *AST* aspartate aminotransferase, *ULN* upper limit of normal

Mechanisms of ART-Associated Hepatoxicity

Mitochondrial Toxicity

Hepatotoxicity and lactic acidosis in patients treated with nonnucleoside polymerase inhibitors (NRTIs) have been observed for nearly two decades, both preclinically [8–11] and clinically [12, 13]. NRTIs inhibit HIV replication by incorporating into viral genetic material and acting as chain terminators. However, NRTIs are also able to inhibit human DNA polymerase γ (pol-γ), which is responsible for mitochondrial DNA (mtDNA) replication. This inhibition leads to mitochondrial dysfunction due to DNA depletion, along with the potential for mtDNA mutations, microvesicular steatosis, and oxidative stress [14, 15]. Evaluations of various NRTI compounds in HepG2 cells have demonstrated differing effects of various compounds on mitochondrial function. Walker et al. [12] analyzed effects of zalcitibine (ddC), didanosine (ddI), stavudine (d4T), lamivudine (3TC), and zidovudine (ZDV) and found that ddC, ddI, and d4T, in this order, had the greatest depletion on mtDNA, whereas 3TC had no effect. Similarly, when put in combination, 3TC–ZDV and ddC–d4T had the greatest effect. A separate study yielded comparable results: ddC, ddI, d4T, ZDV, and 3TC/abacavir (ABC)/tenofovir (TDF) decreased mtDNA levels in this order [16].

Recently, reports of mitochondrial toxicity manifested by pancreatitis, lactic acidosis and hepatic failure in patients coinfected with HIV and HCV receiving ddI plus ribavirin (RBV) or ddI/d4T and RBV, generated a review by the US FDA [17]. The Adverse Event Reporting System was analyzed for adverse events associated with both RBV and with approved NRTIs. Results demonstrated a significantly elevated risk of mitochondrial toxicity in those taking RBV and ddI (OR, 12.4; 95% CI, 3.8–40.8) or RBV and ddI/d4T (OR, 8.0; 95% CI, 2.9–21.9) compared with patients on RBV and other NRTIs. Fleischer et al. [17] hypothesized that the ability of RBV to facilitate phosphorylation of ddI to its active metabolite may at least partially explain this synergistic effect. These data led to a contraindication for RBV added to the ddI label in 2009 [18].

It should be noted that this toxicity may also affect newborns of HIV-infected mothers. Deleterious NRTI effects on placental mitochondria have been described [19]. However, it has also been suggested that the risks of mitochondrial toxicity remain small compared to the risks of mother-to-child transmission, and the balance falls in favor of the benefits of effective therapy at preventing horizontal transmission [20].

Direct Hepatotoxicity

Like many drugs and other chemicals, ART can induce direct liver toxicity. This may occur when polymorphisms in cytochrome metabolic pathways are present and alter drug metabolism and exposure. For example, efavirenz (EFV) is metabolized by cytochrome P450 2B6 (CYP2B6), and various polymorphisms have been associated with very high plasma levels of the agent [21–23]. In the double nonnucleoside (2NN) study of 1216 HIV-infected patients randomized to EFV or nevirapine (NVP) plus a double NRTI backbone, induction plasma concentrations of EFV appeared to be related to risk of liver enzyme elevations in the first 6 weeks of treatment [24]. Hepatocyte toxicity can also occur through activity of Fas ligand and tumor necrosis factor α (TNF-α), which trigger hepatocyte apoptosis and necrosis [25]. Proinflammatory cytokine expression and signaling may be increased in the context of HIV and HCV coinfection [26] and it has also been demonstrated that HIV may increase hepatocyte susceptibility to TRAIL-mediated apoptosis [27]. Although data linking specific ART agents or regimens to altered cytokine expression and resulting hepatotoxicity are sparse, assessing expression of genes regulating hepatocellular apoptosis may help in early screening for potential hepatotoxicity.

Hypersensitivity Reactions

Hypersensitivity reactions are unpredictable immunological responses to drugs or other foreign agents and may or may not be mediated by dosage, route of administration, and duration of treatment [26, 28]. There are several ART agents that have known propensity to trigger hypersensitivity reactions in the liver. NVP, for example, may result in rare but potentially fatal hepatic hypersensitivity reaction. Martin et al. reported that the interaction of haplotype HLA-DRB1*0101 and higher CD4 cell count renders individuals susceptible to immune-mediated hypersensitivity reactions [29]. This is consistent with results from Shenton et al. [30] that suggest a CD4-mediated immune response to NVP, and also suggest that tolerance at low doses is due to hepatic metabolic tolerance rather than immune tolerance. Recently, SNPs in cytochrome genes CYP2B6 and CYP3A5 and the transporter gene ABCB1 have been implicated in the potential for NVP hepatotoxicity [31]. In ACTG 5095, NVP was substituted for EFV when an EFV-related adverse event occurred unless administration of NVP was contraindicated [32]. Grade 3/4 hepatotoxicity occurred in 14% of patients who switched compared to 6% in patients who did not switch; however, only three patients discontinued NVP because of hepatotoxicity. The incidence of hypersensitivity reactions leading to NVP discontinuation in the 3,752-patient AIDS Therapy Evaluation in The Netherlands (ATHENA) cohort was 6%; this manifested as hepatotoxicity in 1.5%, rash in 4.9%, and both in 0.2 [33]. Importantly, significant risk factors for hypersensitivity included prior treatment with high CD4 counts, Asian race, female sex, and detectable HIV viral load at the start of treatment. Race and sex differences may stem from variability of haplotypes or metabolic/transporter gene SNPs in the study population.

The NRTI abacavir (ABC) may also cause a hypersensitivity reaction that is characterized by rapid onset of rash, fever, gastrointestinal symptoms, and less frequently respiratory complaints. This reaction is known to be associated with the haplotype HLA-B*5701, with positive and negative predictive values of 100 and 97%, respectively [34, 35]. A recent, large, and prospective epidemiological analysis reported that HLA-B*5701 prevalence in Europe was approximately 5%, with the highest proportions in Caucasians and the lowest in those of Black race [36], consistent with the racial variability in reaction incidence observed in clinical studies. The complex hepatic metabolism of ABC gives rise to several metabolites which, in the setting of the identified haplotype, may provoke a strong T-cell response. It is not often that ABC causes reactions in the absence of the offending haplotype, but cases of HCV-negative, HBV-negative patients with severe hepatotoxicity after ABC initiation have been described [37].

Steatohepatitis

Hepatic steatosis refers to accumulation of lipids within hepatocytes and is termed "nonalcoholic fatty liver disease (NAFLD)" in the absence of other identifiable etiologies such as excessive alcohol use, viral infections, drug or other toxicities, and autoimmune disease. Over 5% of hepatocytes must have evidence of fatty infiltration for NAFLD to be diagnosed [38]. Nearly 40% of patients with NAFLD will progress to nonalcoholic steatohepatitis, or NASH, which is characterized by inflammation and/or fibrosis and may result in end-stage liver disease, hepatocellular carcinoma, and death in 10–15% [39, 40]. As described above, antiretroviral-related inhibition of mitochondrial DNA synthesis by NRTIs may lead to hepatic steatosis and lactic acidosis, which in some cases may be fatal [41]. Steatohepatitis can also occur with use of protease inhibitors, which may lead to dyslipidemia and insulin resistance that results in triglyceride accumulation in the liver [42, 43]. Both mechanisms of steatosis development may be facilitated by concomitant HCV infection, especially genotype 3 [44–46]. It is important to note that although viral hepatitis and alcohol use may be predisposing factors, their absence does not preclude development of NAFLD or NASH, or even rapid progression to cirrhosis [47]. In a report of 225 HIV-monoinfected patients without a history of alcohol abuse, the prevalence of NAFLD was 37% [48]. Multivariable analysis of these results suggested that longer NRTI exposure was significantly associated with NAFLD, along with male sex, waist circumference, and high serum ALT/AST ratio. Other studies [49], though not all [46, 50] have reported similar trends.

Immune Reconstitution/Inflammatory Syndrome

An additional mechanism for ART-related hepatotoxicity is immune reconstitution/inflammatory syndrome, which typically occurs with viral hepatitis coinfection. The immune response that follows successful ART initiation may be directed at viral antigens in the liver, resulting in cell death and release of aminotransferases. Several studies have demonstrated a correlation between an increase in CD4+ count after ART initiation and ALT/AST flares [5, 51–53], and some of these studies demonstrated a concomitant increase in HCV viral load as well [52, 54]. Similarly, HBV-active ART initiation in those with HBV coinfection may result in ALT/AST flares mediated by proinflammatory cytokines [5, 55]. Conversely, withdrawal of HBV-active ART such as 3TC or tenofovir (TDF)/emtricitibine (FTC) can result in HBV viral load rebound and severe transaminase flares [56, 57].

The challenge for patient management is to determine when a transaminase flare is truly reflective of hepatic injury, and when it is transient and clinically insignificant. In the case of HBV coinfection, treatment interruptions appear to exacerbate flares caused by immune reconstitution and may lead to increased HBV treatment resistance; thus, treatment should be maintained if the flare is not severe [57]. When concomitant HCV is present, transaminase flares should be evaluated for severity and in the context of increasing or decreasing HCV viral load. Many flares are mild-to-moderate and transient and do not require treatment modification. However, persistent HCV viral load increases may be suggestive of immune pressure facilitating HCV quasispecies evolution and mutations that could adversely affect future HCV treatment response.

Hyperbilirubinemia

Some ART agents, especially protease inhibitors, may cause unconjugated hyperbilirubinemia. It has been demonstrated that indinavir (IDV) competitively inhibits bilirubin UDP-glucuronosyltransferase (UGT) activity, leading to increases in serum levels of unconjugated bilirubin [58]. The same mechanism has been observed for atazanavir (ATV) [59]. Presence of the Gilbert's polymorphism in the UGT1 gene increases the risk of this event. Generally, this phenomenon is reversible upon withdrawal of the offending agent, and is not associated with hepatocellular injury or concomitant transaminase elevations. Grade IV hyperbilirubinemia is rare compared to lower elevations [60] and is typically associated with UGT1A1 polymorphisms [61]. A recent analysis of prospectively collected data from a cohort of more than 2,400 patients suggested that higher baseline CD4+ counts, abnormal bilirubin levels at baseline, and concomitant RTV use increase risk of grade 3/4 hyperbilirubinemia, while female sex and NNRTI use are protective [60]. Interestingly, HCV antibody positivity was not a predictive factor for hyperbilirubinemia in multivariable analysis in this study.

Incidence and Predictors of Hepatotoxicity

Incidence of hepatotoxicity varies significantly by therapeutic regimen and patient population, but including newer agents such as entry and integrase inhibitors, generally ranges between 2 and 26% for grade 3/4 transaminase elevations [52, 62–68]. Steatosis incidence is difficult to assess due to a paucity of liver biopsy data from HIV trials but prevalence of steatosis is highly variable, ranging from 13 to 69% [44, 49, 69].

Therapeutic classes, agents, and hepatoxocity mechanisms and frequency are summarized in Table 18.2. Although the potential for hepatotoxicity is associated with every class of ART, novel FDA-approved agents such as the integrase and entry inhibitors appear to have relatively low hepatotoxic

Table 18.2 FDA-approved therapeutic agents for HIV and hepatic toxicity incidence

Drug class/agent	Typical toxicity mechanisms	Incidence/prevalence
Nucleoside reverse-transcriptase inhibitors (NRTIs) Abacavir (ABC) Didanosine (ddI) Emtricitibine (FTC) Lamivudine (3TC) Stavudine (D4T) Tenofovir (TDF) Zidovudine (ZDV)	Mitochondrial toxicity (especially ddC, ddI, and d4T, and especially ddI/D4T when combined with ribavirin) Steatohepatitis (HCV is an important cofactor) Hypersensitivity reaction (ABC)	Mitochondrial toxicity: Incidence, 5–8.5% [45, 71, 72] Steatohepatitis: Incidence, 20.9/1000 PY [73]; Prevalence of severe steatosis, 13% [49]; Prevalence of any steatosis, 67–69% [44, 69] Hypersensitivity reaction: Incidence, 5–6% [35]
Nonnucleoside reverse-transcriptase inhibitors (NNRTIs) Delavirdine (DLV) Efavirenz (EFV) Etravirine (ETV) Nevirapine (NVP)	Direct hepatotoxicity (NVP, EFV; viral hepatitis is a significant cofactor) Hypersensitivity (NVP)	Direct hepatotoxicity incidence: 8–16% [68]; 1.26–2.63/100 PY [74]; 3.6–7.6/100 PY [75]; 1.3–2.1% [76]; 18.5/100 PY–44.4/100 PY [77] Hepatic hypersensitivity: 1.5% [33]
Protease inhibitors (Pis) Amprenavir (APV) Atazanavir (ATV) Darunavir (DRV) Indinavir (IDV) Lopinavir (LPV) Nelfinavir (NFV) Ritonavir (RTV) Saquinavir (SQV) Tipranavir (TPV)	Steatohepatitis Immune reconstitution/inflammatory syndrome Viral hepatitis exacerbation Hyperbilirubinemia (ATV, IDV)	Overall grade 3/4 transaminase elevations: 9–17% [68]; 19–26% [66]; 18% [67]; 7–19.5% [52] Hyperbilirubinemia: ~50% [60]; 30–38% [66]; 25% [78]. Grade 3/4 jaundice, 37% [61]
Integrase inhibitors Raltegravir (RAL)	Liver enzyme elevations (LEE)	Any liver enzyme elevation: 7.9% [70] 2.8–3/100PY [65] Grade 3/4 LEE: 2–4.2% [63, 79]
Entry inhibitors Enfurvitide (ENF) Maraviroc (MVC)	Liver enzyme elevations (LEE)	Grade 3/4 LEE: 6.5%, or 5.9/100PY (ENF in combination with TPV/RTV) [64] 3–5% (MVC in triple-class resistant patients) [62]

propensity. Maraviroc and raltegravir both demonstrated transaminase elevations at rates comparable to placebo in clinical trials [62, 63, 65]. In a prospective observational analysis of 126 HIV-monoinfected and 92 HIV–HCV coinfected patients initiating raltegravir, 1.4% experienced grade 3 or 4 ALT or AST flares [70]. The only independent predictor of such elevations was HCV coinfection and no flares could be attributed to raltegravir.

It was recently demonstrated that coadministration of TPV/RTV with the fusion inhibitor enfuvirtide (ENF) increased plasma trough levels of both TPV and RTV [80]. This interaction was cited as the etiology for grade 4 transaminase elevations (including AST, ALT, and gamma-glutamyltransferase) in an HBV-coinfected patient with low HBV viral load and no evidence of cirrhosis or history of excessive alcohol use [81]. The authors posited that the hepatotoxicity was induced by increased TPV/RTV serum levels and recommended monitoring of TPV levels, TPV dose adjustment if necessary, and adjustment or discontinuation of RTV if TPV is coadministered with ENF. However, a subsequent subanalysis of the Randomized Evaluation of Strategic Intervention in multidrug resiStant patients with Tipranavir (RESIST) 1 and 2 studies, in which 22% of patients administered TPV/RTV and 18% of those receiving RTV-boosted comparator PI were on concomitant ENF, showed that grade 3/4 ALT flares were lower in the TPV/RTV plus ENF arm compared to the TPV/RTV arm without EVF (6.5 and 12.9%, respectively, $p<0.05$) [64]. The same trend was true for the comparator PI arm. The rate of clinically reported hepatic events was also lower in the TPV/RTV + ENF arm was lower than the TPV/RTV arm without ENF (5.9 vs. 9.3 events/100PY), although rates were slightly higher in the RTV/PI arm with versus without ENF (3.9 vs. 2.9/100PY). Thus, while increases in TPV (and other PI) plasma concentrations may occur with concomitant ENF and RTV, this does not translate into increased risk of hepatotoxicity.

Several studies have examined predictors and risk factors for severe hepatotoxicity. A retrospective analysis of 16 AACTG trials, comprising nearly 9,000 HIV-positive patients treated between 1990 and 1999, assessed predictors of severe hepatotoxicity and mortality from hepatic-related causes [82]. Subjects from each study were categorized by baseline treatment: single NRTI, multiple NNRTs, NRTI(s) plus NNRTI(s), and NRTI(s) plus PI(s). Overall, 9.3% developed severe hepatotoxicity in the first year of treatment, although this decreased to 8.7% if IDV-related hyperbilirubinemia was excluded. Liver-related deaths occurred in 0.9% of patients. Factors that were associated with risk of severe hepatotoxicity for all regimens included elevated transaminases at baseline (NRTIs and NNTRIs), thrombocytopenia (single NRTI), concomitant medications with potential for hepatotoxicity (NRTIs), and renal insufficiency (multiple NRTIs). For those on IDV (PI), risk factors included elevated baseline transaminases and bilirubin, concomitant d4T, other hepatotoxic medications, injection drug use, and abnormal baseline bilirubin. Hepatitis C infection was a strong predictor, but HBV infection failed to reach statistical significance, possibly due to small patient numbers. Conversely, in the HIV-Netherlands Australia Thailand Research Collaboration (HIV-NAT) trials, nearly 700 patients were treated with two NRTIs and subsets were treated with a PI ($n=135$) or NNRTI ($n=215$) [77]. Both HCV and HBV coinfection (9 and 7% of the study participants, respectively) and NNRTI use as independent predictors of severe hepatotoxicity

As elevated baseline transaminases are common in those with viral hepatitis coinfection, these were adjusted for in a 400-subject study, of whom 15% were HCV+ and 8% were HBV+ [67]. After adjustment, viral hepatitis remained associated with an increased risk of hepatotoxicity with relative risks of 2.78 (95% CI, 1.50–5.16) and 2.46 (95% CI, 1.43–4.24) for HBV and HCV infection, respectively.

Although treatment for HCV is generally initiated only when HIV is controlled with ART, it is important to note that sustained viral response to HCV treatment may decrease hepatoxicity risk with ART for HIV. In one study, the annual incidence of hepatic events was statistically significantly reduced in patients who achieved SVR compared to those who did not (3.1 vs. 12.9%, respectively) [83]. Other factors associated with risk of hepatotoxicity included NRTI use (increased risk) and PI use (decreased risk).

Summary

Hepatotoxicity in the context of ART is complex and multicausal. Although some hepatic events are class effects, others are agent-specific, rendering study comparisons difficult. In many cases, mechanisms underlying elevated transaminases are best identified by liver biopsy, which can be costly and difficult. Although novel agents appear to be relatively safe for the liver, patients with other forms of liver disease may be at increased risk and should be monitored for signs of hepatotoxicity. Even in these patients, early ALT/AST elevations may resolve without clinical implications. New pharmacogenomic methods may help identify patients at increased risk for hepatotoxicity, and may also help in identifying the safest new agents and optimal combinations of agents. Until then, the clear quality-of-life and survival benefits conferred by ART continue to outweigh risks for most patients.

References

1. Walensky RP, Paltiel AD, Losina E, Mercincavage LM, Schackman BR, Sax PE, et al. The survival benefits of AIDS treatment in the United States. J Infect Dis. 2006;194(1):11–9.
2. Prati D, Taioli E, Zanella A, Della TE, Butelli S, Del Vecchio E, et al. Updated definitions of healthy ranges for serum alanine aminotransferase levels. Ann Intern Med. 2002;137(1):1–10.
3. Green RM, Flamm S. AGA technical review on the evaluation of liver chemistry tests. Gastroenterology. 2002;123(4):1367–84.

4. Table of grading severity of adult adverse experiences. Rockville, MD: Division of AIDS, National Institute of Allergy and Infectious Diseases; 1996.
5. Sulkowski MS, Thomas DL, Chaisson RE, Moore RD. Hepatotoxicity associated with antiretroviral therapy in adults infected with human immunodeficiency virus and the role of hepatitis C or B virus infection. JAMA. 2000;283(1):74–80.
6. Food and Drug Administration. Guidance for industry drug-induced liver injury: premarketing clinical evaluation. 2009.
7. Zimmerman HJ. Drug-induced liver disease. Drugs. 1978;16(1): 25–45.
8. Chen CH, Vazquez-Padua M, Cheng YC. Effect of anti-human immunodeficiency virus nucleoside analogs on mitochondrial DNA and its implication for delayed toxicity. Mol Pharmacol. 1991;39(5):625–8.
9. Gerschenson M, Nguyen VT, St Claire MC, Harbaugh SW, Harbaugh JW, Proia LA, et al. Chronic stavudine exposure induces hepatic mitochondrial toxicity in adult Erythrocebus patas monkeys. J Hum Virol. 2001;4(6):335–42.
10. Mansuri MM, Hitchcock MJ, Buroker RA, Bregman CL, Ghazzouli I, Desiderio JV, et al. Comparison of in vitro biological properties and mouse toxicities of three thymidine analogs active against human immunodeficiency virus. Antimicrob Agents Chemother. 1990;34(4):637–41.
11. Wu Y, Li N, Zhang T, Wu H, Huang C, Chen D. Mitochondrial DNA base excision repair and mitochondrial DNA mutation in human hepatic HuH-7 cells exposed to stavudine. Mutat Res. 2009;664(1–2):28–38.
12. Walker UA, Bickel M, Lutke Volksbeck SI, Ketelsen UP, Schofer H, Setzer B, et al. Evidence of nucleoside analogue reverse transcriptase inhibitor–associated genetic and structural defects of mitochondria in adipose tissue of HIV-infected patients. J Acquir Immune Defic Syndr. 2002;29(2):117–21.
13. Bissuel F, Bruneel F, Habersetzer F, Chassard D, Cotte L, Chevallier M, et al. Fulminant hepatitis with severe lactate acidosis in HIV-infected patients on didanosine therapy. J Intern Med. 1994;235(4): 367–71.
14. Lewis W, Day BJ, Copeland WC. Mitochondrial toxicity of NRTI antiviral drugs: an integrated cellular perspective. Nat Rev Drug Discov. 2003;2(10):812–22.
15. Walker UA. Antiretroviral therapy-induced liver alterations. Curr Opin HIV AIDS. 2007;2(4):293–8.
16. Birkus G, Hitchcock MJ, Cihlar T. Assessment of mitochondrial toxicity in human cells treated with tenofovir: comparison with other nucleoside reverse transcriptase inhibitors. Antimicrob Agents Chemother. 2002;46(3):716–23.
17. Fleischer R, Boxwell D, Sherman KE. Nucleoside analogues and mitochondrial toxicity. Clin Infect Dis. 2004;38(8):e79–80.
18. Videx [package insert]. Princeton, NJ: Bristol-Myers Squibb; 2010.
19. Gingelmaier A, Grubert TA, Kost BP, Setzer B, Lebrecht D, Mylonas I, et al. Mitochondrial toxicity in HIV type-1-exposed pregnancies in the era of highly active antiretroviral therapy. Antivir Ther. 2009;14(3):331–8.
20. Ciaranello AL, Seage III GR, Freedberg KA, Weinstein MC, Lockman S, Walensky RP. Antiretroviral drugs for preventing mother-to-child transmission of HIV in sub-Saharan Africa: balancing efficacy and infant toxicity. AIDS. 2008;22(17):2359–69.
21. Ribaudo HJ, Haas DW, Tierney C, Kim RB, Wilkinson GR, Gulick RM, et al. Pharmacogenetics of plasma efavirenz exposure after treatment discontinuation: an Adult AIDS Clinical Trials Group Study. Clin Infect Dis. 2006;42(3):401–7.
22. Rodriguez-Novoa S, Barreiro P, Rendon A, Jimenez-Nacher I, Gonzalez-Lahoz J, Soriano V. Influence of 516 G>T polymorphisms at the gene encoding the CYP450-2B6 isoenzyme on efavirenz plasma concentrations in HIV-infected subjects. Clin Infect Dis. 2005;40(9):1358–61.
23. Rotger M, Colombo S, Furrer H, Bleiber G, Buclin T, Lee BL, et al. Influence of CYP2B6 polymorphism on plasma and intracellular concentrations and toxicity of efavirenz and nevirapine in HIV-infected patients. Pharmacogenet Genomics. 2005; 15(1):1–5.
24. Kappelhoff BS, van Leth F, Robinson PA, MacGregor TR, Baraldi E, Montella F, et al. Are adverse events of nevirapine and efavirenz related to plasma concentrations? Antivir Ther. 2005; 10(4):489–98.
25. Leist M, Gantner F, Kunstle G, Wendel A. Cytokine-mediated hepatic apoptosis. Rev Physiol Biochem Pharmacol. 1998;133: 109–55.
26. Blackard JT, Kang M, St Clair JB, Lin W, Kamegaya Y, Sherman KE, et al. Viral factors associated with cytokine expression during HCV/HIV co-infection. J Interferon Cytokine Res. 2007;27(4): 263–9.
27. Babu CK, Suwansrinon K, Bren GD, Badley AD, Rizza SA. HIV induces TRAIL sensitivity in hepatocytes. PLoS One. 2009; 4(2):e4623.
28. Burns-Naas LA, Meade BJ, Munson AL. Toxic responses of the immune system. In: Klaassen CD, editor. Toxicology. USA: McGraw-Hill; 2001. p. 419–70.
29. Martin AM, Nolan D, James I, Cameron P, Keller J, Moore C, et al. Predisposition to nevirapine hypersensitivity associated with HLA-DRB1*0101 and abrogated by low CD4 T-cell counts. AIDS. 2005;19(1):97–9.
30. Shenton JM, Popovic M, Chen J, Masson MJ, Uetrecht JP. Evidence of an immune-mediated mechanism for an idiosyncratic nevirapine-induced reaction in the female Brown Norway rat. Chem Res Toxicol. 2005;18(12):1799–813.
31. Ciccacci C, Borgiani P, Ceffa S, Sirianni E, Marazzi MC, Altan AM, et al. Nevirapine-induced hepatotoxicity and pharmacogenetics: a retrospective study in a population from Mozambique. Pharmacogenomics. 2010;11(1):23–31.
32. Schouten JT, Krambrink A, Ribaudo HJ, Kmack A, Webb N, Shikuma C, et al. Substitution of nevirapine because of efavirenz toxicity in AIDS clinical trials group A5095. Clin Infect Dis. 2010;50(5):787–91.
33. Wit FW, Kesselring AM, Gras L, Richter C, van der Ende ME, Brinkman K, et al. Discontinuation of nevirapine because of hypersensitivity reactions in patients with prior treatment experience, compared with treatment-naive patients: the ATHENA cohort study. Clin Infect Dis. 2008;46(6):933–40.
34. Hetherington S, Hughes AR, Mosteller M, Shortino D, Baker KL, Spreen W, et al. Genetic variations in HLA-B region and hypersensitivity reactions to abacavir. Lancet. 2002;359(9312):1121–2.
35. Mallal S, Nolan D, Witt C, Masel G, Martin AM, Moore C, et al. Association between presence of HLA-B*5701, HLA-DR7, and HLA-DQ3 and hypersensitivity to HIV-1 reverse-transcriptase inhibitor abacavir. Lancet. 2002;359(9308):727–32.
36. Orkin C, Wang J, Bergin C, Molina JM, Lazzarin A, Cavassini M, et al. An epidemiologic study to determine the prevalence of the HLA-B*5701 allele among HIV-positive patients in Europe. Pharmacogenet Genomics. 2010;20(5):307–14.
37. Soni S, Churchill DR, Gilleece Y. Abacavir-induced hepatotoxicity: a report of two cases. AIDS. 2008;22(18):2557–8.
38. Neuschwander-Tetri BA, Caldwell SH. Nonalcoholic steatohepatitis: summary of an AASLD Single Topic Conference. Hepatology. 2003;37(5):1202–19.
39. Adams LA, Lymp JF, St Sauver J, Sanderson SO, Lindor KD, Feldstein A, et al. The natural history of nonalcoholic fatty liver disease: a population-based cohort study. Gastroenterology. 2005;129(1):113–21.
40. Adams LA, Sanderson S, Lindor KD, Angulo P. The histological course of nonalcoholic fatty liver disease: a longitudinal study of 103 patients with sequential liver biopsies. J Hepatol. 2005; 42(1):132–8.

41. Fortgang IS, Belitsos PC, Chaisson RE, Moore RD. Hepatomegaly and steatosis in HIV-infected patients receiving nucleoside analog antiretroviral therapy. Am J Gastroenterol. 1995;90(9):1433–6.
42. Carr A, Miller J, Law M, Cooper DA. A syndrome of lipoatrophy, lactic acidaemia and liver dysfunction associated with HIV nucleoside analogue therapy: contribution to protease inhibitor-related lipodystrophy syndrome. AIDS. 2000;14(3):F25–32.
43. Ingiliz P, Valantin MA, Duvivier C, Medja F, Dominguez S, Charlotte F, et al. Liver damage underlying unexplained transaminase elevation in human immunodeficiency virus-1 mono-infected patients on antiretroviral therapy. Hepatology. 2009;49(2):436–42.
44. McGovern BH, Ditelberg JS, Taylor LE, Gandhi RT, Christopoulos KA, Chapman S, et al. Hepatic steatosis is associated with fibrosis, nucleoside analogue use, and hepatitis C virus genotype 3 infection in HIV-seropositive patients. Clin Infect Dis. 2006;43(3):365–72.
45. Sulkowski MS, Mehta SH, Torbenson M, Afdhal NH, Mirel L, Moore RD, et al. Hepatic steatosis and antiretroviral drug use among adults coinfected with HIV and hepatitis C virus. AIDS. 2005;19(6):585–92.
46. Lonardo A, Adinolfi LE, Loria P, Carulli N, Ruggiero G, Day CP. Steatosis and hepatitis C virus: mechanisms and significance for hepatic and extrahepatic disease. Gastroenterology. 2004;126(2):586–97.
47. Loulergue P, Callard P, Bonnard P, Pialoux G. Hepatic steatosis as an emerging cause of cirrhosis in HIV-infected patients. J Acquir Immune Defic Syndr. 2007;45(3):365.
48. Guaraldi G, Squillace N, Stentarelli C, Orlando G, D'Amico R, Ligabue G, et al. Nonalcoholic fatty liver disease in HIV-infected patients referred to a metabolic clinic: prevalence, characteristics, and predictors. Clin Infect Dis. 2008;47(2):250–7.
49. Ryan P, Blanco F, Garcia-Gasco P, Garcia-Merchan J, Vispo E, Barreiro P, et al. Predictors of severe hepatic steatosis using abdominal ultrasound in HIV-infected patients. HIV Med. 2009;10(1):53–9.
50. Crum-Cianflone N, Dilay A, Collins G, Asher D, Campin R, Medina S, et al. Nonalcoholic fatty liver disease among HIV-infected persons. J Acquir Immune Defic Syndr. 2009;50(5):464–73.
51. Puoti M, Torti C, Ripamonti D, Castelli F, Zaltron S, Zanini B, et al. Severe hepatotoxicity during combination antiretroviral treatment: incidence, liver histology, and outcome. J Acquir Immune Defic Syndr. 2003;32(3):259–67.
52. Sherman KE, Shire NJ, Cernohous P, Rouster SD, Omachi JH, Brun S, et al. Liver injury and changes in hepatitis C Virus (HCV) RNA load associated with protease inhibitor-based antiretroviral therapy for treatment-naive HCV-HIV-coinfected patients: lopinavir-ritonavir versus nelfinavir. Clin Infect Dis. 2005;41(8):1186–95.
53. Chung RT, Evans SR, Yang Y, Theodore D, Valdez H, Clark R, et al. Immune recovery is associated with persistent rise in hepatitis C virus RNA, infrequent liver test flares, and is not impaired by hepatitis C virus in co-infected subjects. AIDS. 2002;16(14):1915–23.
54. Vento S, Garofano T, Renzini C, Casali F, Ferraro T, Concia E. Enhancement of hepatitis C virus replication and liver damage in HIV-coinfected patients on antiretroviral combination therapy. AIDS. 1998;12(1):116–7.
55. Crane M, Oliver B, Matthews G, Avihingsanon A, Ubolyam S, Markovska V, et al. Immunopathogenesis of hepatic flare in HIV/hepatitis B virus (HBV)-coinfected individuals after the initiation of HBV-active antiretroviral therapy. J Infect Dis. 2009;199(7):974–81.
56. Bellini C, Keiser O, Chave JP, Evison J, Fehr J, Kaiser L, et al. Liver enzyme elevation after lamivudine withdrawal in HIV-hepatitis B virus co-infected patients: the Swiss HIV Cohort Study. HIV Med. 2009;10(1):12–8.
57. Nuesch R, Ananworanich J, Srasuebkul P, Chetchotisakd P, Prasithsirikul W, Klinbuayam W, et al. Interruptions of tenofovir/emtricitabine-based antiretroviral therapy in patients with HIV/hepatitis B virus co-infection. AIDS. 2008;22(1):152–4.
58. Zucker SD, Qin X, Rouster SD, Yu F, Green RM, Keshavan P, et al. Mechanism of indinavir-induced hyperbilirubinemia. Proc Natl Acad Sci USA. 2001;98(22):12671–6.
59. Zhang D, Chando TJ, Everett DW, Patten CJ, Dehal SS, Humphreys WG. In vitro inhibition of UDP glucuronosyltransferases by atazanavir and other HIV protease inhibitors and the relationship of this property to in vivo bilirubin glucuronidation. Drug Metab Dispos. 2005;33(11):1729–39.
60. Torti C, Lapadula G, Antinori A, Quirino T, Maserati R, Castelnuovo F, et al. Hyperbilirubinemia during atazanavir treatment in 2,404 patients in the Italian atazanavir expanded access program and MASTER Cohorts. Infection. 2009;37(3):244–9.
61. Lankisch TO, Moebius U, Wehmeier M, Behrens G, Manns MP, Schmidt RE, et al. Gilbert's disease and atazanavir: from phenotype to UDP-glucuronosyltransferase haplotype. Hepatology. 2006;44(5):1324–32.
62. Gulick RM, Lalezari J, Goodrich J, Clumeck N, Dejesus E, Horban A, et al. Maraviroc for previously treated patients with R5 HIV-1 infection. N Engl J Med. 2008;359(14):1429–41.
63. Lennox JL, Dejesus E, Lazzarin A, Pollard RB, Madruga JV, Berger DS, et al. Safety and efficacy of raltegravir-based versus efavirenz-based combination therapy in treatment-naive patients with HIV-1 infection: a multicentre, double-blind randomised controlled trial. Lancet. 2009;374(9692):796–806.
64. Raffi F, Battegay M, Rusconi S, Opravil M, Blick G, Steigbigel RT, et al. Combined tipranavir and enfuvirtide use associated with higher plasma tipranavir concentrations but not with increased hepatotoxicity: sub-analysis from RESIST. AIDS. 2007;22(13):1977–80.
65. Steigbigel RT, Cooper DA, Teppler H, Eron JJ, Gatell JM, Kumar PN, et al. Long-term efficacy and safety of Raltegravir combined with optimized background therapy in treatment-experienced patients with drug-resistant HIV infection: week 96 results of the BENCHMRK 1 and 2 Phase III trials. Clin Infect Dis. 2010;50(4):605–12.
66. Cooper CL, Parbhakar MA, Angel JB. Hepatotoxicity associated with antiretroviral therapy containing dual versus single protease inhibitors in individuals coinfected with hepatitis C virus and human immunodeficiency virus. Clin Infect Dis. 2002;34(9):1259–63.
67. den Brinker M, Wit FW, Wertheim-van Dillen PM, Jurriaans S, Weel J, van Leeuwen R, et al. Hepatitis B and C virus co-infection and the risk for hepatotoxicity of highly active antiretroviral therapy in HIV-1 infection. AIDS. 2000;14(18):2895–902.
68. Sulkowski MS, Thomas DL, Mehta SH, Chaisson RE, Moore RD. Hepatotoxicity associated with nevirapine or efavirenz containing antiretroviral therapy: role of hepatitis C and B infections. Hepatology. 2002;35(1):182–9.
69. Neau D, Winnock M, Castera L, Bail BL, Loko MA, Geraut L, et al. Prevalence of and factors associated with hepatic steatosis in patients coinfected with hepatitis C virus and HIV: Agence Nationale pour la Recherche contre le SIDA et les hepatites virales CO₃ Aquitaine Cohort. J Acquir Immune Defic Syndr. 2007;45(2):168–73.
70. Vispo E, Mena A, Maida I, Blanco F, Cordoba M, Labarga P, et al. Hepatic safety profile of raltegravir in HIV-infected patients with chronic hepatitis C. J Antimicrob Chemother. 2010;65(3):543–7.
71. Saves M, Vandentorren S, Daucourt V, Marimoutou C, Dupon M, Couzigou P, et al. Severe hepatic cytolysis: incidence and risk factors in patients treated by antiretroviral combinations. Aquitaine Cohort, France, 1996–1998. Groupe dEpidemiologie Clinique de Sida en Aquitaine (GECSA). AIDS. 1999;13(17):F115–21.
72. Verucchi G, Calza L, Manfredi R, Chiodo F. Incidence of liver toxicity in HIV-infected patients receiving isolated dual nucleoside

analogue antiretroviral therapy. J Acquir Immune Defic Syndr. 2003;33(4):546–8.
73. Lonergan JT, Behling C, Pfander H, Hassanein TI, Mathews WC. Hyperlactatemia and hepatic abnormalities in 10 human immunodeficiency virus-infected patients receiving nucleoside analogue combination regimens. Clin Infect Dis. 2000;31(1):162–6.
74. Antela A, Ocampo A, Gomez R, Lopez MJ, Marino A, Losada E, et al. Liver toxicity after switching or simplifying to nevirapine-based therapy is not related to CD4 cell counts: results of the TOSCANA Study. HIV Clin Trials. 2010;11(1):11–7.
75. Chu KM, Boulle AM, Ford N, Goemaere E, Asselman V, Van Cutsem G. Nevirapine-associated early hepatotoxicity: incidence, risk factors, and associated mortality in a primary care ART programme in South Africa. PLoS One. 2010;5(2):e9183.
76. Bruck S, Witte S, Brust J, Schuster D, Mosthaf F, Procaccianti M, et al. Hepatotoxicity in patients prescribed efavirenz or nevirapine. Eur J Med Res. 2008;13(7):343–8.
77. Law WP, Dore GJ, Duncombe CJ, Mahanontharit A, Boyd MA, Ruxrungtham K, et al. Risk of severe hepatotoxicity associated with antiretroviral therapy in the HIV-NAT Cohort, Thailand, 1996–2001. AIDS. 2003;17(15):2191–9.
78. McMahon DK, Dinubile MJ, Meibohm AR, Marino DR, Robertson MN. Efficacy, safety, and tolerability of long-term combination antiretroviral therapy in asymptomatic treatment-naive adults with early HIV infection. HIV Clin Trials. 2007;8(5):269–81.
79. Steigbigel RT, Cooper DA, Kumar PN, Eron JE, Schechter M, Markowitz M, et al. Raltegravir with optimized background therapy for resistant HIV-1 infection. N Engl J Med. 2008;359(4):339–54.
80. González de Requena D, Calcagno A, Bonora S, Ladetto L, D'Avolio A, Sciandra M, et al. Unexpected drug–drug interaction between tipranavir/ritonavir and enfuvirtide. AIDS. 2006;20(15):1977–9.
81. Julg B, Bogner JR, Goebel FD. Severe hepatotoxicity associated with the combination of enfuvirtide and tipranavir/ritonavir: case report. AIDS. 2006;20(11):1563.
82. Servoss JC, Kitch DW, Andersen JW, Reisler RB, Chung RT, Robbins GK. Predictors of antiretroviral-related hepatotoxicity in the adult AIDS Clinical Trial Group (1989–1999). J Acquir Immune Defic Syndr. 2006;43(3):320–3.
83. Labarga P, Soriano V, Vispo ME, Pinilla J, Martin-Carbonero L, Castellares C, et al. Hepatotoxicity of antiretroviral drugs is reduced after successful treatment of chronic hepatitis C in HIV-infected patients. J Infect Dis. 2007;196(5):670–6.

Management of End-Stage Liver Disease and the Role of Liver Transplantation in HIV-Infected Patients

Marion G. Peters and Peter G. Stock

Cirrhosis in HIV Patients

Liver disease is the second most frequent cause of death in HIV patients after AIDS, accounting for a greater proportion of deaths than cardiovascular disease or non-AIDS-related cancers [1]. The major contributor to end-stage liver disease (ESLD) in HIV-infected patients is the high rate of coinfection with hepatitis C virus (HCV) or hepatitis B virus (HBV), estimated at 30% and 10%, respectively [2]. Rates of both coinfections vary in the population depending upon the route and timing of transmission. Because individuals with HIV are living longer without AIDS and progression to cirrhosis is more rapid in patients with liver disease and HIV, ESLD is now common in HIV patients. Cirrhosis may be present in up to 15% of patients without any clinical findings, so called "silent cirrhosis" [3]. Serum ALT is not a good marker of ongoing liver disease and normal ALT has been shown to be associated with significant fibrosis in 25–40% of HIV–HCV coinfected patients [4]. On the positive side, introduction of highly active antiretroviral therapy (HAART) has reduced the risk of developing ESLD in those HIV patients with HCV coinfection [5] and therapy for HCV or HBV may halt or reverse progression of liver disease.

Cirrhosis and its complications in HIV patients should be managed as it is in HIV-seronegative patients (Table 19.1). All patients with cirrhosis should undergo upper endoscopy to evaluate for varices and should undergo routine screening for hepatocellular carcinoma (HCC). If Grade 2 or greater varices are found, primary prophylaxis with a nonselective beta blocker (propranolol or nadolol) should be initiated to decrease the heart rate by 10%. Lower doses of beta blockers are required to decrease splanchnic pressure than are used to decrease systemic blood pressure (e.g., propranolol 10–20 mg twice or thrice daily). If beta blockers cannot be tolerated, then band ligation is recommended.

HCC risk appears to be increased in HIV patients with cirrhosis [6, 7]. All patients with cirrhosis should be monitored for HCC. Ultrasonography is recommended every 6 months to 12 months (every 6 months in patients on the transplant waiting list), with quadruple-phase computed tomography (CT) used to confirm and further delineate abnormalities. The risk of HCC in cirrhotics is 1–4% per year and the doubling time of HCC tumors is estimated to be 136 days. Alfa-fetoprotein (AFP) testing should be confirmed with liver imaging studies because of poor specificity and sensitivity. The utility of serum AFP for HCC screening in persons with HIV is unknown. Patients with HCC should be offered all conventional therapies including chemoembolization and transplantation.

Decompensated Cirrhosis

Cirrhosis from any cause can progress to decompensated liver disease with the development of varices, ascites, hepatic encephalopathy, or synthetic dysfunction [low albumin, increased international normalized ratio (INR) and jaundice]. It is estimated that 5–7% of patients with cirrhosis without HIV decompensate per year [8]. It is difficult to predict clinically which cirrhotic patients will progress, although an elevated hepatic venous pressure gradient (HVPG) of greater than 10 mmHg has been shown to be the best predictor of decompensation [8]. This evaluation requires catheterization of the hepatic vein with wedge pressure measurement and is not routinely performed in the clinical setting.

Funding: Peter Stock and Marion Peters were supported in part by the Solid Organ Transplantation in HIV: Multi-Site Study (A1052748) and Women's Interagency HIV Study (U02 AI034989), respectively, both funded by the National Institute of Allergy and Infectious Diseases.

M.G. Peters (✉)
Department of Medicine, University of California-San Francisco, 513 Parnassus Ave S357, San Francisco, CA 94143-0538, USA
e-mail: marion.peters@ucsf.edu

Table 19.1 Monitoring of patients with cirrhosis and HIV

Test	Outcome	Treatment
Upper endoscopy	Varices	Nonselective beta blocker
	No varices	Repeat in 2 years
HCC surveillance: liver imaging every 6 months	HCC	Treat as for non-HIV patients
Ascites	All patients require paracentesis	Check ascitic albumin, protein
		White cell count and differential
		Place fluid in blood culture bottles
Check serum to ascites albumin gradient (SAAG)	>1.1	Antibiotic prophylaxis
Spontaneous bacterial peritonitis	PMN > 250 or positive culture	Antibiotics for SBP
	Ascitic protein < 1 MELD > 9	Primary SBP prophylaxis antibiotics see text
	After one episode of SBP	Secondary SBP prophylaxis
Hepatic encephaolopathy	Search for precipitating cause	• Nonabsorbable disaccharides
		• Nonabsorbable antibiotics
Liver decompensation	Evaluate for transplantation	

HCC hepatocellular carcinoma, *PMN* polymorphonuclear cells, *MELD* model for end-stage liver disease, *SBP* spontaneous bacterial peritonitis

Table 19.2 Child–Pugh–Turcotte score

Points	1	2	3
Hepatic encephalopathy*	None	1–2	3–4
Ascites	Absent	Slight or diuretic controlled	Moderate (despite diuretics) or severe
Bilirubin (mg/dL)	<2	2–3	>3
Albumin (g/dL)	>3.5	2.8–3.5	<2.8
Prothrombin time	<4 s prolonged	4–6 s	>6 s
Or INR	<1.7	1.7–2.3	>2.3

Child class: A: 5–6, B: 7–9, C: >9
INR international normalized ratio
* see table 19.3 for Hepatic encephalopathy staging
Note: If there is elevated bilirubin, check direct and indirect bilirubin. If only indirect bilirubin levels are elevated, use direct value for the CPT score. If both the direct and indirect bilirubin levels are elevated, use the total bilirubin level for the CPT score

The clinical severity of cirrhosis predicts mortality: stage 1 is compensated cirrhosis with absence of varices; stage 2 compensated cirrhosis with varices; stage 3 decompensated cirrhosis with ascites but without hemorrhage; and stage 4 decompensated cirrhosis and variceal hemorrhage with or without ascites. One year mortality in a large cohort of untreated patients was 1% in patients with stage 1 disease; increasing to 3%, 20% and 57% in those with stage 2, 3, and 4, respectively [9]. The presence of varices on CT scan or upper endoscopy provides evidence of portal hypertension, as does a low platelet count with splenomegaly.

There have been a number of studies showing that time to cirrhosis and liver decompensation is shortened in HIV patients with liver disease. After the first evidence of liver decompensation in a group of patients with HIV–HCV coinfection, 54% survived 1 year, compared to 74% of those with HCV alone [10]. This increased rate of decompensation continued over time in HCV/HIV patients, with 40% and 25% surviving 2 and 5 years, compared to 61% and 44% survival in those with HCV monoinfection alone. Death due to ESLD is increased in those HIV patients with concomitant viral coinfection: 44% of those HIV patients with HBV and HCV coinfection died a liver related death; compared to 31% of those with HCV coinfection; 22% of those with HBV coinfection; and 1.2% of HIV patients without viral coinfection [11].

Tools used to assess disease severity and predict death in cirrhosis include the Child-Pugh-Turcotte (CPT) score and Model for End-Stage Liver Disease (MELD) score. The CPT score was developed in the 1970s to assess risk of death in cirrhotic patients, mainly in patients who received portacaval shunting. CPT utilizes both clinical assessment and laboratory values: grading of encephalopathy and ascites, serum albumin level, bilirubin level, and prothrombin time or INR (Table 19.2) [12]. Class A (CPT score 5–6) indicates well-compensated cirrhotic disease, with Class B indicating milder decompensation (CPT score 7–9) and Class C indicating the most severe decompensation (CPT score > 9). If there is elevated serum bilirubin in patients on HAART, direct and indirect bilirubin should be evaluated as hyperbilirubinemia can be due to atazanavir or indinivir. If only indirect bilirubin levels are elevated, then the direct value for the CPT score is used. If both the direct and indirect bilirubin levels are elevated, then the total bilirubin level for the CPT score should be used. This scoring system was initially used for determining severity of liver disease for liver transplant recipients. However, it is has been replaced by the MELD scoring system, which is less subjective and ulitizes only serum bilirubin level, INR, and creatinine level [13]. MELD was shown to predict 3-month mortality after transjugular intrahepatic portosystemic shunting (TIPS), and subsequent studies showed it to be a better predictor of survival of patients on the liver transplant waiting list than was the CPT score [14]. Since 2002, MELD score has been used to determine severity of disease on the liver transplantation waiting list. There is no correction for MELD in patients with unconjugated hyperbilirubinemia.

Ascites

An increase in intrahepatic resistance in cirrhotic patients leads to portal hypertension, splanchnic and systemic vasodilation, a reduction in effective arterial blood volume, activation of neurohumoral systems, and sodium retention with the development of ascites. All patients with ascites require a diagnostic paracentesis for analysis to evaluate for portal hypertension and to exclude spontaneous bacterial peritonitis (SBP) [15, 16]. Portal hypertension is determined by measuring the serum to ascites albumin gradient (SAAG); SAAG ≥ 1.1 mg/dL suggests that the ascites is secondary to portal hypertension. Lower values should precipitate a search for other etiologies including peritoneal tuberculosis and carcinomatosis.

Management of ascites includes sodium restriction (<2 g/day) to alleviate fluid retention and diuretics [8]. Sodium intake can be checked by measuring sodium levels in the urine. If a patient reports no response to diuretics but has significant sodium in the urine, he/she is likely not adhering to a low-salt diet. The recommended starting diuretic regimen is spironolactone alone or in combination with furosemide (ratio of 40 mg furosemide: 100 mg spironolactone). Spironolactone increases serum potassium and furosemide reduces it, so the two drugs need to be used in balance to maintain normal serum potassium levels. The doses of spironolactone can be increased up to 300–400 mg as needed with concomitant increases in furosemide (60–80 mg twice daily) adjusting for serum potassium.

If these measures are ineffective, other interventions include large-volume paracentesis with albumin replacement and TIPS. With progressive decompensation, ascites may become refractory to diuretic. Treatment of refractory ascites usually requires large-volume paracentesis. For every liter of ascites removed, 50 cc of 25% sal-poor albumin must be given intravenously. Albumin or peritoneovenous shunting increases the effective arterial blood volume but peritoneovenous shunting is rarely used now because it has a high failure rate and complications. While TIPS leads to prompt drop in portal pressure, ascites may not reverse for 4–6 weeks. Thus, while portal hypertension is clearly important in the generation of ascites, reduction of portal pressure alone is rarely sufficient to induce prompt reversal of ascites, showing the importance of neurohumoral factors. Although TIPS is associated with greater transplant-free survival than large volume paracentesis, it also has a much higher rate of hepatic encephalopathy [17]. The risk of hepatic encephalopathy reflects the shunting of blood away from the liver to the systemic circulation permitting toxins and other substances from the gut that would ordinarily be metabolized by the liver to act as neurotoxins.

Spontaneous Bacterial Peritonitis

Spontaneous bacterial peritonitis (SBP) is the most common type of bacterial infection in hospitalized liver patients, with *Escherichia coli* being the most common pathogen [16]. Clinical suspicion is raised by unexplained encephalopathy, jaundice, or worsening renal failure. In less than 50% of cases, there is fever, abdominal pain or leukocytosis. The diagnosis of SBP requires paracentesis. A diagnostic paracentesis removes 20–30 cc of ascitic fluid and places fluid in blood culture bottles and a CBC tube to measure the percent of polymorphonuclear cells (PMN) and to culture the ascites. Gram stain is not of value and fluid is more likely to produce a positive culture if placed in blood culture bottles [16]. The recommended initial treatment is cephalosporins, with adjustment based on results of ascitic fluid culture sensitivities. In SBP, renal dysfunction is a major cause of death. Administration of intravenous albumin has been shown to prevent hepatorenal dysfunction and subsequent death in patients who have a serum bilirubin level greater than 4 mg/dL, serum creatinine level greater than 1 g/dL, or blood urea nitrogen level greater than 30 mg/dL [18]. Recurrence of SBP can be decreased by prophylactic treatment with antibiotics: ciprofloxacin, trimethoprim-sulfamethoxazole, or norfloxacin. Primary prophylaxis against SBP should be given in those patients with an ascitic protein level <1 g/dL, with oral antibiotics such as weekly ciprofloxacin (750 mg), daily TMP-SMX or norfloxacin (400 mg). Secondary antibiotic prophylaxis is recommended for all persons with a history of SBP and is advisable in any HIV patient with a MELD score > 9.

Esophagogastric Varices

Esophagogastroduodenoscopy (EGD) should be performed in all persons with cirrhosis at the time of diagnosis, particularly those with thrombocytopenia and who have evidence of portal hypertension. If no gastroesophageal varices are noted,

EGD should be repeated every 2 years. For persons with grade 2 or higher varices, nonselective beta blockers (e.g., nadolol or propranolol) are used to decrease splanchnic pressure. Effectiveness is assessed by decreasing the heart rate by 10%. Nonselective beta blockers are the mainstay of both primary and secondary prevention of variceal hemorrhage. However, esophageal variceal ligation (EVL) or banding is another preventive option, particularly for persons who cannot tolerate beta blockers.

Treatment of variceal hemorrhage includes antibiotics (which improve survival) and resuscitation aimed at achieving a hemoglobin level of 9 g/dL [8]. Factors associated with increased risk of death in the first 6 weeks after variceal bleeding include a MELD score of 18 or greater, the use of four or more units of packed red blood cells in the first 24 h, and active bleeding at endoscopy. Specific therapies for acute variceal hemorrhage include intravenous vasoconstrictors (e.g., somatostatin, terlipressin, octreotide) given for 2–5 days in an intensive care unit, though large randomized clinical trials have reported conflicting results in terms of improved survival. Endoscopic EVL to obliterate varices is the preferred treatment over sclerotherapy, which is associated with a higher risk of esophageal stricture. If these measures fail TIPS may be performed. TIPS has largely replaced surgical treatments such as selective splenorenal shunting. For prevention of variceal recurrence, the combination of a nonselective beta-blocker (e.g., propranolol) and EVL is superior to EVL alone, with a rebleeding rate of 12% observed with the combination versus 38% with EVL alone in one study [19]. Vasoconstrictors reduce splanchnic flow and splanchnic pressure disproportionately to their reduction of systemic blood pressure. The goal of TIPS or another shunting procedure is to reduce portal pressure to <12 mmHg.

Hepatorenal Syndrome

Hepatorenal syndrome (HRS) results from renal vasoconstriction which is characterized by decreased cortical flow and increased medullary flow in the kidney, leading to a marked reduction in effective arterial blood volume. Acute renal failure occurs in 14–25% of hospitalized patients with cirrhosis [8] with HRS the primary form of prerenal failure accounting for 60–80% of cases. To exclude a prerenal state, all patients should receive 48 h of fluid challenge (usually albumin) before the diagnosis of HRS can be made. Acute tubular necrosis accounts for the remaining 20–40% of cases of renal failure. There are two forms of HRS: a rapidly progressive type 1 which produces acute renal failure within 2 weeks and is associated with a doubling of serum creatinine level or halving of creatinine clearance to <20 mL/min. Type I HRS is more common in those patients with refractory ascites, hyponatremia, or both, and carries a <50% survival at 1 month. Type 2 HRS is a more slowly progressing form characterized by an increase in serum creatinine level to greater than 1.5 mg/dL, creatinine clearance <40 mL/min, and urine sodium level of less than 10 mEq. Type 2 HRS is often precipitated by excessive diuresis of patients who are diuretic resistant. It carries a median survival of 6 months. Treatment for Type I HRS consists of liver transplantation. In type 2 HRS associated some small studies have shown benefit with midodrine and octreotide in reversing vasodilation and albumin to increase intravascular volume [20]. However, no controlled trials have demonstrated that this improves survival. In those patients with hyponatremia, treatment consists of fluid restriction and vasopressin-2 receptor antagonists or midodrine. Hypertonic saline should not be used: patients with hyponatremia have normal levels of total body sodium with massive fluid overload, and hypertonic sodium exacerbates the problem. Dialysis may be performed in patients with type 1 HRS who are on the transplant waiting list. However, most patients require continuous venovenous hemodialysis in an intensive care unit because they usually have systemic hypotension and cannot tolerate intermittent hemodialysis.

Hepatic Encephalopathy

Hepatic encephalopathy results from a combination of portosystemic shunting and failure to metabolize neurotoxic substances. The nature of these false neurotransmitters absorbed from the gut in the setting of liver dysfunction remains unclear after decades of research. Ammonia levels actually correlate poorly with stage of encephalopathy in cirrhosis. Early stage 1 encephalopathy may have subtle findings such as euphoria, fluctuating mild confusion, slowness of mentation, slurred speech, sleep–wake disturbance, and loss of second language. The stages of encephalopathy are depicted in Table 19.3.

Hepatic encephalopathy can be precipitated by infection (e.g., urinary tract or SBP), gastrointestinal bleeding (with an increased protein load in the gut), electrolyte imbalance, portal vein thrombosis, worsening liver disease, or shunting of blood away from the liver (as seen after TIPS). Treatment is aimed at reducing production of ammonia (and other toxins) from the colon through use of nonabsorbable disaccharides (e.g., lactulose, lactitol, lactose) and nonabsorbable antibiotics such as neomycin and rifamixin; data indicate that rifamixin is less absorbable than neomycin [21]. Patients with HIV may not tolerate lactulose because of already present diarrhea and benefit from therapy with zinc and rifaximin. Protein restriction is no longer recommended as it promotes protein degradation, may worsen nutritional status, and decrease muscle mass when maintained for long periods. A 40 g protein diet is recommended.

Table 19.3 Hepatic encephalopathy staging

Stage	Mental state	Tremor	EEG
I	Euphoria, occasionally depression, fluctuant mild confusion, slowness of mentation, untidy, slurred speech, sleep–wake disturbance	Slight Increased reflexes	
II	Accentuation of stage I, drowsiness, inappropriate behavior	Present, easily elicited	Abnormal, generalized slowing
III	Most of the time but can be aroused by vocal stimuli speech is incoherent and confusion is marked	Present if subject is cooperative	Abnormal
IV, early	Cannot be aroused by vocal stimuli but reactive to noxious stimuli	None	Abnormal
IV, late	Cannot be aroused by vocal stimuli and uncoordinated reactivity to noxious stimuli	None	Abnormal

EEG electroencephalogram

Liver Transplantation

HIV Transplant Candidacy

The management of HIV patients who are undergoing liver transplantation requires close collaboration of hepatologist, surgeon, and infectious disease specialists because of the complexity of diagnosis, management, and drug–drug interactions. All HIV-infected persons with decompensated liver disease and/or early HCC are potential candidates for orthotopic liver transplantation. This is because HIV infection is no longer a contraindication to organ transplantation with the use of effective HAART [22, 23]. Development of decompensation such as ascites, variceal hemorrhage, or hepatic encephalopathy is associated with a median survival of 1.5 years. Eligibility for transplantation is based on MELD score. Those patients with CPT score ≥7 and/or MELD score >10 should be referred for evaluation for liver transplantation. However, MELD underestimates the need for transplantation in patient with chronic encephalopathy, hepatic hydrothorax, hepatopulmonary syndrome, and portopulmonary hypertension and HIV patients may deteriorate at a lower MELD than non-HIV patients. For these patients, other options that should be considered include "higher risk" donors and living donors.

All HIV candidates for transplantation must fulfill standard requirements for non-HIV patients including absence of life-threatening extrahepatic disease and ability to adhere to post-transplantation care (Table 19.4). In addition, there are certain specific HIV exclusions which include progressive multifocal leukoencephalopathy (PML), chronic cryptosporidiosis, drug resistant fungal infections and visceral Kaposi's sarcoma (KS). For listing for liver transplantation, CD4 counts are required to be at least 100/mm^3. This is lower than required for renal transplantation because CD4 counts may be lower due to common occurrence of portal hypertension and hypersplenism. Patients who are unable to tolerate posttransplantation antiretroviral therapy (ART) medication have poorer outcomes and those patients with multidrug resistant HIV may not be candidates [23]. Determining posttransplantation HIV control is particularly difficult with the many patients coinfected with HIV–HCV who may be unable to tolerate HAART pre transplant. In these patients, careful assessment by an infectious disease specialist is required, including HIV resistance testing to predict whether the patient will respond to HAART post transplantation. Significant wasting and/or malnutrition are additional relative contraindications to transplantation.

Posttransplantation Management

A summary of posttransplantation management in HIV patients is outlined in Table 19.5.

Immunosuppressive Strategies

The immunosuppressive regimens used following liver transplantation in HIV infected recipients were originally chosen as a result of their antiretroviral qualities. The majority of the maintenance immunosuppressive regimens include a calcineurin inhibitor [(CNI): Cyclosprin A (CSA)] and tacrolimus, mycophenolate mofetil, and steroids. The early utilization of lymphocyte depleting agents, most notably thymoglobulin, has been avoided in liver transplant recipients based on a rapid septic death in a HIV-positive liver transplant recipient following treatment with thymoglobulin [23]. It is speculated that lymphodepletion associated with thymoglobulin may exacerbate the compromised immune state associated with a recovering liver, and overwhelm the immune system in an HIV+ recipient. Since early control of rejection can be achieved in liver transplant recipients without lymphodepleting induction therapy, induction therapy is not recommended.

Table 19.4 Candidacy for liver transplantation in HIV patients with end-stage liver disease

Indications	Standard criteria as for non-HIV patients
	CD4 ≥ 100/mm³
	Deemed able to tolerate HAART post transplantation
	Stable HIV disease
	HIV expertise in primary medical provider
	HIV undetectable is ideal. If patient off HAART, HIV must be predicted to be controlled post transplantation
	Compliance with HAART and transplant regimens
Contraindications	Progressive multifocal leukoencephalopathy
	Chronic cryptosporidiosis
	Drug-resistant fungal infections
	Visceral Kaposi's sarcoma
	Multidrug-resistant HIV
	Substance use per transplant program policy
	Malnutrition and wasting

HAART highly active antiretroviral therapy

Table 19.5 Posttransplant management of HIV patients

HBV coinfection	• Hepatitis B immune globulin and nucleoside analogs as with non-HIV patients
	• Start/stop all HBV drugs and HAART simultaneously
HCV coinfection	• As for HCV monoinfected patients
HAART	• Start/stop all medications at the same time
	• Usually start with pre transplant HAART regimen
	• Usually started at day 4–7 post transplantation
Immunosuppression	• NNRTIs lower CNI levels
	• PIs increase CNI levels
	• Avoid lymphodepletion therapies
Immunization	• Require pre OLT vaccination against Pneumococcus, Hepatitis A and B
	• Varicella vaccine should NOT be given, instead IgG postexposure
	• Avoid live attenuated vaccines (oral polio, smallpox) to household contacts
Prophylaxis	• CMV, fungal infections, *Pneumocystis carinii*
	• MAC if CD4 <75 mm³
Malignancy screening	• Increased risk of standard tumors in HIV patients
	• Papanicolaou test smears of the cervix and/or anal canal annually

CNI calcineurin inhibitors, *PI* protease inhibitors, *MAC Mycobacterium avium* complex, *HAART* highly active antiretroviral therapy, *HCV* hepatitis C virus, *CMV* cytomegalovirus, *HBV* hepatitis B virus, *NNRTI* nonnucleoside reverse-transcriptase inhibitors, *OLT* orthotopic liver transplantation

Both CSA and tacrolimus have a significant role in most immunosuppressive regimens in HIV-negative recipients and also have well-documented antiretroviral qualities. Despite their efficacy, both of these agents are nephrogenic and diabetogenic. These detrimental side effects can be exacerbated by antiretroviral regimens which include protease inhibitors (PI). PIs are diabetogenic, and may increase the risks of diabetes associated with both tacrolimus and CSA. Most liver transplant centers in the USA favor tacrolimus over CSA as the CNI of choice in the majority of liver transplant recipients. Unfortunately, the diabetogenicity of tacrolimus is probably greater than CSA, and CSA may be chosen in recipients that are at a high risk for developing diabetes. Perhaps the greatest problem is the inhibition of the cytochrome p450 3A4 (CYP3A4) system in HIV-positive recipients that are on HAART regimens that include PIs. Owing to this inhibition, patients on PI and CSA required only 20% of the dose given to recipients that do not have a PI as part of the HAART regimen. For subjects on tacrolimus or sirolimus, the dose was markedly decreased and the dosing interval was increased up to fivefold [24]. There is no question that recipients on HAART regimens which require HAART require close monitoring. Despite the recognition that HIV infected transplanted recipients require significantly lower doses of CNI if their regimen includes a PI, a significant number of patients have developed toxic CNI levels, which in turn have been associated with nephrotoxicity [23]. For all these reasons, there is some consideration to switching antiretroviral regimens if they include a PI, to HAART regimens which avoid PIs (see Section "HAART Strategies" below).

Another immunosuppressive agent which may have a special place in regimens used in HIV+recipients is sirolimus, a target of rapamycin (TOR) inhibitor and antiproliferative agent [25]. This drug has less nephrotoxicity than CNI, and is less diabetogenic than CNIs. Since sirolimus also downregulates the CCR5 receptor on lymphocytes, the entry port for HIV, it may prevent the virus from entering the cell [26]. Finally, sirolimus inhibits vascular endothelial growth factor and is effective in the treatment of KS, which is an HHV-8 derived opportunistic neoplasm and can be problematic in people infected with HIV [27]. For all these reasons, sirolimus is utilized in several HIV-infected recipients in the absence of any CNI.

HAART Strategies

In the early trials of transplantation in HIV+recipients, immunosuppression did not cause progression of HIV to AIDS [28]. Since HIV+ patients in all clinical trials have had well controlled HIV on a stable HAART regimen, clinicians have been reluctant to change the stable antiretroviral regimen which was controlling progression of HIV. Nonetheless, based on the problems obtaining safe and adequate levels of CNI inhibitors in people on HAART regimens which include PIs, there has been a debate about switching HAART regimens pretransplant and provide PI-free regimens. Some centers have been using HAART regimens that use the new integrase inhibitors and exclude PIs [29]. In fact, these centers are reporting lower rejection rates in HIV-positive transplant recipients, which in turn may be related to more stable CNI drug levels in patients which have been switched off of the PI based regimens. The debate to switch to PI free regimens pretransplant remains controversial, although many transplant centers appear to be leaning in the direction of switching to PI free HAART regimens pretransplant.

During the posttransplantation period, the HIV-positive liver transplant recipient may develop several of the toxicities associated with HAART, including hepatotoxicity and neuropathies. If the HAART regimen is suspected to be involved with the toxicity, it is imperative that all drugs of the HAART regimen be discontinued temporarily without risk and to avoid the development of HIV drug-resistance. Following resolution of the toxicity, a new antiretroviral regimen can be initiated based on recommendations from the HIV provider.

HBV and HCV Management Post Transplantation

HBV–HIV coinfected patients have similar patient and graft survival to with HBV mono-infection [30]. This success can be attributed to the ability to control the HBV coinfection post transplantation with combination nucleoside analogs and HBV immune globulin. The fact the both patient and graft survival in liver transplants performed in HBV–HIV coinfected recipients is comparable to HBV monoinfected recipients is really the proof that liver transplantation can be performed safely in people infected with HIV, as long as the viral hepatitis can be controlled post transplantation.

Unfortunately, the same success observed in the HBV–HIV coinfected liver transplant recipients has not been seen in the HCV–HIV coinfected transplant recipients [23, 31]. Rapid recurrence of HCV has been problematic in all patients transplanted for HCV, but there is no question that recipients with HIV–HCV coinfection have a higher morbidity and mortality than those with HCV monoinfection. Nonetheless, there have been some HCV–HIV coinfected patients who have done extremely well and cleared HCV with interferon therapy post transplantation. In addition, a few HCV–HIV coinfected patients have cleared HCV spontaneously. It is possible that some of the antiretroviral drugs may impact HCV. Some transplant centers prefer the use of CSA in maintenance regimens over tacrolimus, in that CSA has both anti-HCV and anti-HIV properties [32]. As with monoinfected HCV liver transplant recipients, bolus steroids should be avoided in the treatment of rejection in light of the exacerbation of HCV which has previously been reported [33]. The future for newer agents to control HCV post transplantation is very promising, and hopefully the HIV–HCV liver coinfected liver transplant recipients will enjoy the same degree of success as the HIV–HBV coinfected recipients.

Opportunistic Infections and Malignancies Post Transplantation

Transplant recipients infected with HIV are susceptible to cancers specific to HIV as well as cancers associated with immunosuppression [23]. As is done in HIV-uninfected liver transplant recipients, HIV-positive recipients should receive prophylaxis for cytomegalovirus, fungal infections, and *Pneumocytys carinii* pneumonia. If CD4 counts drop below 75 cell/μl, HIV+recipients should also receive prophylaxis for *Mycobacterium avium* complex. KS and non-Hodgkin's lymphoma have been associated with AIDS, but fortunately have not been seen with a high frequency in the early studies. Although de novo cutaneous KS has been seen in a couple of posttransplantation HIV-infected transplant recipients, it has been very effectively treated with rapamycin [27] (see Section "Immunsuppressive Strategies", above). Unfortunately, the human papillomavirus (HPV) and associated anal and cervical cancers may be problematic in HIV-positive transplant recipients. Patients with low-grade cellular abnormalities have progressed to anal cancer following liver transplantation and immunosuppression. The University of

California–San Francisco (UCSF) screening guidelines recommends that these patients should be screened with PAP smears of the cervix and anal canal on an annual basis.

Summary

HIV-positive patients with cirrhosis should receive the same management and prophylaxis as cirrhotic patients without HIV. This usually requires comanagement by HIV provider and hepatologist. Early referral for liver transplantation is critical to allow HIV patients to be evaluated for optimal timing of liver transplant. HBV–HIV coinfected patients have similar posttransplantation survival to those with HBV alone as recurrent HBV infection is generally well controlled with combination nucleoside analogs and HBV immune globulin. Recurrent HCV infection remains a difficult problem in all patients transplanted for HCV, but those with HIV–HCV coinfection have a higher morbidity and mortality than those with HCV monoinfection. Some successes are noted and there is hope with newer direct acting antivirals will achieve higher clearance rates of HCV infection before and post transplantation. Immunosuppressive treatment for transplantation in HIV patients is complicated with the use of multiple drugs, especially HAART, provided by many physicians. For this reason, close collaboration between HIV physicians and transplant physicians is necessary to avoid drug interactions that pose especial risks for organ rejection and calcineurin toxicity.

References

1. Weber R, Sabin CA, Friis-Moller N, Reiss P, El Sadr WM, Kirk O, et al. Liver-related deaths in persons infected with the human immunodeficiency virus: the D:A:D study. Arch Intern Med. 2006;166(15):1632–41.
2. Koziel MJ, Peters MG. Viral hepatitis in HIV infection. N Engl J Med. 2007;356(14):1445–54.
3. Sterling RK, Contos MJ, Sanyal AJ, Luketic VA, Stravitz RT, Wilson MS, et al. The clinical spectrum of hepatitis C virus in HIV coinfection. J Acquir Immune Defic Syndr. 2003;32(1):30–7.
4. Martin-Carbonero L, Benhamou Y, Puoti M, Berenguer J, Mallolas J, Quereda C, et al. Incidence and predictors of severe liver fibrosis in human immunodeficiency virus-infected patients with chronic hepatitis C: a European collaborative study. Clin Infect Dis. 2004;38(1):128–33.
5. Qurishi N, Kreuzberg C, Luchters G, Effenberger W, Kupfer B, Sauerbruch T, et al. Effect of antiretroviral therapy on liver-related mortality in patients with HIV and hepatitis C virus coinfection. Lancet. 2003;362(9397):1708–13.
6. Garcia-Samaniego J, Rodriguez M, Berenguer J, Rodriguez-Rosado R, Carbo J, Asensi V, et al. Hepatocellular carcinoma in HIV-infected patients with chronic hepatitis C. Am J Gastroenterol. 2001;96(1):179–83.
7. Brau N, Fox RK, Xiao P, Marks K, Naqvi Z, Taylor LE, et al. Presentation and outcome of hepatocellular carcinoma in HIV-infected patients: a U.S.-Canadian multicenter study. J Hepatol. 2007;47(4):527–37.
8. Garcia-Tsao G, Lim JK. Management and treatment of patients with cirrhosis and portal hypertension: recommendations from the Department of Veterans Affairs Hepatitis C Resource Center Program and the National Hepatitis C Program. Am J Gastroenterol. 2009;104(7):1802–29.
9. D'Amico G, Morabito A, Pagliaro L, Marubini E. Survival and prognostic indicators in compensated and decompensated cirrhosis. Dig Dis Sci. 1986;31(5):468–75.
10. Pineda JA, Garcia-Garcia JA, Aguilar-Guisado M, Rios-Villegas MJ, Ruiz-Morales J, Rivero A, et al. Clinical progression of hepatitis C virus-related chronic liver disease in human immunodeficiency virus-infected patients undergoing highly active antiretroviral therapy. Hepatology. 2007;46(3):622–30.
11. Salmon-Ceron D, Lewden C, Morlat P, Bevilacqua S, Jougla E, Bonnet F, et al. Liver disease as a major cause of death among HIV infected patients: role of hepatitis C and B viruses and alcohol. J Hepatol. 2005;42(6):799–805.
12. Pugh RN. Pugh's grading in the classification of liver decompensation. Gut. 1992;33(11):1583.
13. Kamath PS, Kim WR. The model for end-stage liver disease (MELD). Hepatology. 2007;45(3):797–805.
14. Wiesner RH, McDiarmid SV, Kamath PS, Edwards EB, Malinchoc M, Kremers WK, et al. MELD and PELD: application of survival models to liver allocation. Liver Transpl. 2001;7(7):567–80.
15. Runyon BA, Antillon MR, Akriviadis EA, McHutchison JG. Bedside inoculation of blood culture bottles with ascitic fluid is superior to delayed inoculation in the detection of spontaneous bacterial peritonitis. J Clin Microbiol. 1990;28:2811–2.
16. Runyon BA. Management of adult patients with ascites due to cirrhosis: an update. Hepatology. 2009;49(6):2087–107.
17. Gines P, Uriz J, Calahorra B, Garcia-Tsao G, Kamath PS, Del Arbol LR, et al. Transjugular intrahepatic portosystemic shunting versus paracentesis plus albumin for refractory ascites in cirrhosis. Gastroenterology. 2002;123(6):1839–47.
18. Fernandez J, Navasa M, Garcia-Pagan JC, Garcia-Pagan JC, G-Abraldes J, Jimenez W, et al. Effect of intravenous albumin on systemic and hepatic hemodynamics and vasoactive neurohormonal systems in patients with cirrhosis and spontaneous bacterial peritonitis. J Hepatol. 2004;41(3):384–90.
19. de la Pena J, Brullet E, Sanchez-Hernandez E, Rivero M, Vergara M, Martin-Lorente JL, et al. Variceal ligation plus nadolol compared with ligation for prophylaxis of variceal rebleeding: a multicenter trial. Hepatology. 2005;41(3):572–8.
20. Skagen C, Einstein M, Lucey MR, Said A. Combination treatment with octreotide, midodrine, and albumin improves survival in patients with type 1 and type 2 hepatorenal syndrome. J Clin Gastroenterol. 2009;43(7):680–5.
21. Bass NM, Mullen KD, Sanyal A, Poordad F, Neff G, Leevy CB, et al. Rifaximin treatment in hepatic encephalopathy. N Engl J Med. 2010;362(12):1071–81.
22. Miro JM, Torre-Cisnero J, Moreno A, Tuset M, Quereda C, Laguno M, et al. GESIDA/GESITRA-SEIMC, PNS and ONT consensus document on solid organ transplant (SOT) in HIV-infected patients in Spain (March, 2005). Enferm Infecc Microbiol Clin. 2005;23(6):353–62.
23. Tan-Tam CC, Frassetto LA, Stock PG. Liver and kidney transplantation in HIV-infected patients. AIDS Rev. 2009;11(4):190–204.
24. Frassetto LA, Browne M, Cheng A, Wolfe AR, Roland ME, Stock PG, et al. Immunosuppressant pharmacokinetics and dosing modifications in HIV-1 infected liver and kidney transplant recipients. Am J Transplant. 2007;7(12):2816–20.
25. Sehgal SN. Sirolimus: its discovery, biological properties, and mechanism of action. Transplant Proc. 2003;35(3 Suppl):7S–14S.

26. Heredia A, Amoroso A, Davis C, Le N, Reardon E, Dominique JK, et al. Rapamycin causes down-regulation of CCR5 and accumulation of anti-HIV beta-chemokines: an approach to suppress R5 strains of HIV-1. Proc Natl Acad Sci USA. 2003;100(18): 10411–6.
27. Stallone G, Schena A, Infante B, Di Paolo S, Loverre A, Maggio G, et al. Sirolimus for Kaposi's sarcoma in renal-transplant recipients. N Engl J Med. 2005;352(13):1317–23.
28. Stock PG, Roland ME. Evolving clinical strategies for transplantation in the HIV-positive recipient. Transplantation. 2007;84(5):563–71.
29. Moreno A, Perez-Elias MJ, Casado JL, Fortun J, Barcena R, Quereda C, et al. Raltegravir-based highly active antiretroviral therapy has beneficial effects on the renal function of human immunodeficiency virus-infected patients after solid organ transplantation. Liver Transpl. 2010;16(4):530–2.
30. Coffin CS, Stock PG, Dove LM, Berg CL, Nissen NN, Curry MP, et al. Virologic and clinical outcomes of hepatitis B virus infection in HIV-HBV coinfected transplant recipients. Am J Transplant. 2010;10(5):1268–75.
31. Roland ME, Barin B, Carlson L, Frassetto LA, Terrault NA, Hirose R, et al. HIV-infected liver and kidney transplant recipients: 1- and 3-year outcomes. Am J Transplant. 2008;8(2):355–65.
32. Ishii N, Watashi K, Hishiki T, Goto K, Inoue D, Hijikata M, et al. Diverse effects of cyclosporine on hepatitis C virus strain replication. J Virol. 2006;80(9):4510–20.
33. Berenguer M, Aguilera V, Prieto M, San Juan F, Rayon JM, Benlloch S, et al. Significant improvement in the outcome of HCV-infected transplant recipients by avoiding rapid steroid tapering and potent induction immunosuppression. J Hepatol. 2006;44(4): 717–22.

Assessment and Treatment of Alcohol- and Substance-Use Disorders in Patients with HIV Infection

Ashley D. Bone and Andrew F. Angelino

Introduction

Throughout the world, alcohol and substance use can be described as vectors of HIV infection. Transmission of HIV related to alcohol and substance use may be direct or indirect. Direct transmission of HIV comes through the sharing of needles or other "works" among injection drug users (IDUs), or through exposure to blood by other means, such as sharing a contaminated straw used for intranasal inhalation of cocaine. Indirect transmission occurs when substance users, often while under the influence of the substance, become vulnerable to unsafe practices, such as trading sex for drugs or money to get drugs, failure to use condoms or safer sex practices, or failure to maintain stable relationships, thus increasing the number of sexual partners, about whom they may know very little.

Furthermore, alcohol and substance use and their sequelae are significant factors reducing adherence to treatment [1, 2]. Patients who are actively using may be vulnerable to fail to come for appointments, to not remember to take medicine, to beliefs about not wanting to take medicine while under the influence and thus having erratic dosing, and to adherence lapses due to experiencing other negative consequences of use, such as arrest or intermittent homelessness. The Healthy Living Trial Group found almost a third of their sample to be intermittently homeless over a 37-month period [3]. It is imperative that providers working with patients with substance-use disorders understand the larger picture of the patients' lives and how substance use has figured into the equation.

Among patients with HIV infection, alcohol- and substance-use disorders of all kinds are found in high prevalence. In a point prevalence study at the Johns Hopkins University HIV (Moore) Clinic, substance-use problems were identified in 74% of patients presenting for initial HIV treatment [4]. In a more recent study performed by the National Institute of Mental Health (NIMH) investigating acute/early HIV infection, 85% of participants had a history of alcohol or substance-use disorder [5]. Hearing this prevalence may lead some to make various assumptions about the population of patients with HIV infection ("they all use drugs, share needles, smoke crack," etc.), the overall drug problem in major cities, or the rationale of use ("if I had that infection, I'd use too," etc.). The point of this statement is to entreat the practitioner to overcome the urge to make assumptions, and to rather ask the question "What kinds of people and problems went into making up those high point prevalences, and how can I assess my patients to see if they have similar issues for which I might intervene?"

Definitions of Alcohol and Substance-Use Disorders

For the purpose of discussion, it is useful to begin with definitions of the various types of substance-use problems and disorders with which patients may present. First among these is substance *misuse*. Misuse occurs when a patient uses a psychoactive substance for a purpose other than its intended purpose. An example of this is the use of leftover narcotic prescription tablets to attempt to alleviate insomnia on some occasion. This type of problem is of unknown prevalence, but suspected to be very high. It may be the topic of discussion for providers and patients, generally in the form of admonitions against self-assessment and treatment, but for the purposes of this chapter, it is outside the scope of further discussion.

A.D. Bone (✉)
Department of Psychiatry and Behavioral Sciences,
Johns Hopkins University School of Medicine,
4940 Easten Ave A4C-456, Baltimore, MD 21224, USA
e-mail: abone2@jhmi.edu

The second type of disorder is *substance abuse*. This term may be somewhat confusing, since it is improperly used in a general way to describe any and all substance problems, most often by the media, legislators, administrators, but even on occasion by experts in the field. However, substance abuse relates specifically to continued use of a substance despite the experience of adverse consequences. An example is continuing to drink alcohol to excess despite arrests for driving under the influence, loss of job, and damage to a relationship. Individuals with substance abuse may or may not be using every day, and may also have substance dependence.

Third, *substance dependence* is a disorder that requires either the development of tolerance to a substance, or the development of a physical withdrawal syndrome when the substance use is stopped, or the steady increase in devotion of life of the individual to the thinking about the substance, planning for its use, obtaining funding for the substance, obtaining the substance, using the substance, being under the influence of the substance, withdrawing from the substance, and starting the cycle over. While the first two criteria may not be easily demonstrable for all substances (tolerance to cocaine is less clear than for opiates, for example, and some argue there is no physical withdrawal syndrome for cocaine), the third criterion really describes the process of selective behavior shaping by a series of positive and negative reinforcements, and thus describes a patient with a narrowly proscribed set of behaviors that incrementally preclude the healthy expression of a wider variety of behaviors.

Last among the definitions for this discussion is *addiction*. Politically charged, and with good reason, addiction describes those individuals who have become enslaved to the substance to the point of utter devastation of life. While much of the present literature is either moving away from using the term or applying it to a wider range of behaviors (such as sex, eating, video games, or work) which may be diluting the impact of the term, it is a powerful word that is well known to those who suffer from it. Addicts will describe to providers, when asked and as part of a trusting, committed provider-patient relationship, behaviors that seem overwhelmingly irrational, such as injecting water from the toilet based on the belief that some cocaine powder was spilled into the toilet while using in a restroom stall. The above clinical terms simply lack the emotional power to describe this, and while the provider may document the above as part of a substance dependence diagnosis, the therapy will center on the addiction. The proper use of this word, however, requires a level of professionalism and education that will endeavor to stigmatize the behavior and not the patient, helping the patient to recognize his or her loss of identity to the enslaving substance so that the patient can increase his or her power to choose other behaviors and, ultimately, outcomes.

Assessment of Patients for Alcohol and Substance-Use Disorders

Probably the most important factor in the assessment of patients for alcohol- and substance-use disorders is a high index of suspicion on the part of the clinician. While it is not suggested that the clinician automatically assume all patients are actively using and/or lying about use, it is useful for clinicians to begin thinking about each patient as if she/he may be using so that an assessment may be undertaken and therapeutic decisions based on fact, rather than assumption. Many clinics choose to administer screening tools to all patients. Among these are the CAGE questionnaire [6] (tried to *C*ut back, *A*nnoyed by questions about use, *G*uilt over use, needing an *E*ye-opener in the morning) for alcohol use and the 28-item Drug Abuse Screening Tool (DAST) [7] for other substances (see Table 20.1). Once a patient "screens positive," a full assessment is recommended to the patient. Another approach is administering the Addiction Severity Index (ASI) to all patients [8]. This may be useful, as the ASI can be readministered as indicated to track change over time. Screening tools used in the recovery community to help a patient identify if they have alcohol or substance addiction include pamphlets such as "Is AA for you?" from Alcoholics Anonymous (see Table 20.2) and "Am I an addict?" from Narcotics Anonymous (see Table 20.3).

This difficulty with assessment for substance-use disorders stems from the willingness of the patient to acknowledge the problem and begin the process of change. The stages of change model, first described by Prochaska and DiClemente [9] is a useful theoretical construct for understanding how people move through the process of changing behavior. In this model, individuals begin in the precontemplative stage, in which there is no recognition of the problem, no desire to change and no activity in the direction of change, except by chance. The next stage is the contemplative stage, in which individuals are recognizing a problem or potential to change, beginning to think about the steps of changing, and, as they progress, trying out new behaviors in line with the proposed plan of changing. From this stage, people move to the active stage, where the individual is practicing new behaviors in a concerted effort, finally moving to a "whatever it takes" attitude. These stages of course are not static and concrete, but rather represent a continuum over which people move generally in the direction of change, but perhaps in a halting, erratic, meandering or "three-steps-forward-and-two-back" way.

Understanding this theoretical process is useful to the clinician, as it helps to explain why patients may or may not be forthcoming about details of alcohol or substance use. As a tool to help patients move forward on the process of change while gathering necessary information, a technique called Motivational Interviewing was described by Miller and colleagues [10, 11].

Table 20.1 DAST items [7]

1. Have you used drugs other than those required for medical reasons?
2. Have you abused prescription drugs?
3. Do you abuse more than one drug at a time?
4. Can you get through the week without using drugs (other than those required for medical reasons)?
5. Are you always able to stop using drugs when you want to?
6. Do you abuse drugs on a continuous basis?
7. Do you try to limit your drug use to certain situations?
8. Have you had "blackouts" or "flashbacks" as a result of drug use?
9. Do you ever feel bad about your drug abuse?
10. Does your spouse (or parents) ever complain about your involvement with drugs?
11. Do your friends or relatives know or suspect you abuse drugs?
12. Has drug abuse ever created problems between you and your spouse?
13. Has any family member ever sought help for problems related to your drug;se?
14. Have you ever lost friends because of your use of drugs?
15. Have you ever neglected your family or missed work because of your use of drugs?
16. Have you ever been in trouble at work because of drug abuse?
17. Have you ever lost a job because of drug abuse?
18. Have you gotten into fights when under the influence of drugs?
19. Have you ever been arrested because of unusual behavior while under the influence of drugs?
20. Have you ever been arrested for driving while under the influence of drugs?
21. Have you engaged in illegal activities in order to obtain drugs?
22. Have you ever been arrested for possession of illegal drugs?
23. Have you ever experienced withdrawal symptoms as a result of heavy drug intake?
24. Have you had medical problems as a result of your drug use (e.g., memory loss, hepatitis, convulsions, bleeding, etc.)?
25. Have you ever gone to anyone for help for a drug problem?
26. Have you ever been in hospital for medical problems related to your drug use?
27. Have you ever been involved in a treatment program specifically related to drug use?
28. Have you been treated as an out-patient for problems related to drug abuse?

Scoring and interpretation: A score of "1" is given for each YES response, except for items 4, 5, and 7, for which a NO response is given a score of "1." Based on data from a heterogeneous psychiatric patient population, cutoff scores of 6 through 11 are considered to be optimal for screening for substance-use disorders. Using a cutoff score of 6 has been found to provide excellent sensitivity for identifying patients with substance-use disorders as well as satisfactory specificity (i.e., identification of patients who do not have substance-use disorders). Using a cutoff score of <11 somewhat reduces the sensitivity for identifying patients with substance-use disorders, but more accurately identifies the patients who do not have a substance-use disorders. Over 12 is definitely a substance abuse problem. In a heterogeneous psychiatric patient population, most items have been shown to correlate at least moderately well with the total scale scores. The items that correlate poorly with the total scale scores appear to be items 4, 7, 16, 20, and 22

Table 20.2 The 12 questions have been excerpted from the pamphlet "Is A.A. for you?"

1. Have you ever decided to stop drinking for a week or so, but only lasted for a couple of days?
2. Do you wish people would mind their own business about your drinking – stop telling you what to do?
3. Have you ever switched from one kind of drink to another in the hope that this would keep you from getting drunk?
4. Have you had to have an eye-opener upon awakening during the past year?
5. Do you envy people who can drink without getting into trouble?
6. Have you had problems connected with drinking during the past year?
7. Has your drinking caused trouble at home?
8. Do you ever try to get "extra" drinks at a party because you do not get enough?
9. Do you tell yourself you can stop drinking any time you want to, even though you keep getting drunk when you don't mean to?
10. Have you missed days of work or school because of drinking?
11. Do you have "blackouts"?
12. Have you ever felt that your life would be better if you did not drink?

If individuals answered four or more questions YES, then they were considered to have a problem with their drinking. Reprinted with permission by AA World Services, Inc. All rights reserved

In this technique, the clinician lends emotional reward to the patient's responses to questions, leading the patient to see the benefits of change. Part assessment, part therapy, this approach is often generally adopted by substance-use disorder treatment counselors of all types, even if adherence to the formal "rules" of the technique is minimal. Through the process, the provider hopes to help the patient with the process of conversion – moving forward on the states of change continuum.

A full assessment of substance-use history is a detailed interview and may take 30 min or more to complete, depending on the patient's comfort level. The history will describe the age of first exposure and initial experiences, early influences in use (e.g., parents, peers), which substances are used, how much and how often of each type, patterns of use and associated stimuli that trigger use, consequences of use and their effect on the individual and the substance use, periods of abstinence and prior attempts at recovery, and current motivation and support for recovery.

In addition to this evaluation, providers should obtain a medical history with attention to those illnesses that often result from substance use. Of course, information about HIV and hepatitis infections should be obtained, but in addition, the review should cover other illnesses such as cellulitis, abscesses (integumentary as well as intramuscular, intracranial, epidural, and pulmonary), osteomyelitis, endocarditis,

Table 20.3 The 29 questions have been excerpted from the pamphlet "Am I an Addict?"

1. Do you ever use alone?
2. Have you ever substituted one drug for another, thinking that one particular drug was the problem?
3. Have you ever manipulated or lied to a doctor to obtain prescription drugs?
4. Have you ever stolen drugs or stolen to obtain drugs?
5. Do you regularly use a drug when you wake up or when you go to bed?
6. Have you ever taken one drug to overcome the effects of another?
7. Do you avoid people or places that do not approve of you using drugs?
8. Have you ever used a drug without knowing what it was or what it would do to you?
9. Has your job or school performance ever suffered from the effects of your drug use?
10. Have you ever been arrested as a result of using drugs?
11. Have you ever lied about what or how much you use?
12. Do you put the purchase of drugs ahead of your financial responsibilities?
13. Have you ever tried to stop or control your using?
14. Have you ever been in a jail, hospital, or drug rehabilitation center because of your using?
15. Does using interfere with your sleeping or eating?
16. Does the thought of running out of drugs terrify you?
17. Do you feel it is impossible for you to live without drugs?
18. Do you ever question your own sanity?
19. Is your drug use making life at home unhappy?
20. Have you ever thought you couldn't fit in or have a good time without drugs?
21. Have you ever felt defensive, guilty, or ashamed about your using?
22. Do you think a lot about drugs?
23. Have you had irrational or indefinable fears?
24. Has using affected your sexual relationships?
25. Have you ever taken drugs you didn't prefer?
26. Have you ever used drugs because of emotional pain or stress?
27. Have you ever overdosed on any drugs?
28. Do you continue to use despite negative consequences?
29. Do you think you might have a drug problem?

The NA World Services pamphlet notes that addicts all answered different numbers of these questions "yes." They specifically state that actual number of "yes" responses was not as important as *how individuals felt inside* and *how addiction had affected their lives*. Reprinted with permission by NA World Services, Inc. All rights reserved

Chronic Obstructive Pulmonary Disease (COPD), nephropathies, cirrhosis, neuropathies and ataxia, nasal septum erosions, heart disease (cardiomyopathies, myocardial infarction, congestive heart failure), malnutrition, frostbite and hypothermia (dependent on geography), and tuberculosis.

Finally, it cannot be stressed strongly enough that patients with substance-use disorders must be evaluated for comorbid mental illnesses. It is well established that there is a high degree of comorbidity of mental disorders with substance-use disorders [12]. Most commonly seen are major depression, adjustment disorders, anxiety disorders of all types (including panic, generalized anxiety, and posttraumatic stress disorder), bipolar disorders, and personality disorders. In the NIMH multisite acute HIV infection study, 53% of participants had a history of an affective disorder [5]. The full assessment and treatment of these disorders is outside the scope of this chapter, but it should be noted that if the patient reports severe, potentially life-threatening psychiatric symptoms such as suicidal thinking, they should be referred for expert psychiatric evaluation and treatment as soon as possible.

The Motivated Behavior Concept and Its Use as a Framework for Designing Treatment

In *The Perspectives of Psychiatry*, McHugh and Slavney [15] describe a model for understanding reinforced behaviors and the role of drive in the continuance of certain behaviors (see Fig. 20.1). In short, it is understood that behaviors that are rewarded are generally repeated, and behaviors that result in adverse consequences are generally extinguished [13, 14]. However, some behaviors are continued despite negative consequences because of a programmed drive in the brain. Examples of such types of drives are hunger, thirst, and sex drive. Even if an individual has severe food poisoning and she/he has developed repulsion to the particular kind of food that caused the illness, hunger will eventually return and lead to resumption of eating. This feature is self-preservative – it ensures that a behavior necessary for life (and in the case of sex drive, the survival of the species) will continue. The issue for these behaviors, however, is that positive feedback loops that reinforce behavior are dangerous in biologic systems and can lead to illness. Therefore, for these types of normal behaviors, the brain also has a feedback system that turns off the behavior – the ability to achieve satiety. After eating a full meal, there is little interest in reviewing the menu of entrees again – it holds little salience because the reward systems for food stimuli have been dampened. These two features, drive and satiety, are highly important to the regulation of motivated behaviors (eating, drinking, sleep, sex), and are precisely the features that are corrupted in the development of reinforced behaviors of substance use.

When substances have the ability to short-circuit the cycle because of a short half-life or abrupt termination of action, as in the case of short-acting benzodiazepines, intravenous or smoked cocaine, or intravenous amphetamine, the satiety brake on the cycle is disabled and the cycle can spin out of control for the duration of the episode of use. The cycle becomes smoke crack, feel high for a period (an hour or less), feel an intense dysphoria as the cocaine wears off and dopamine reuptake begins again abruptly, find a way to obtain more crack quickly (pay, perform sexual act, etc.), use more crack, feel high for a short time, feel intense dysphoria, and on and on until the individual is no longer able to continue.

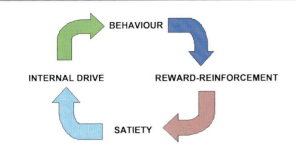

Fig. 20.1 The motivated behavior model. *From: McHugh PR, Slavney PR. The Perspectives of Psychiatry, 2nd edition. Baltimore: Johns Hopkins University Press, 1998* [13]

This binge pattern is a commonly described one and is often a critical factor in the documentation of a diagnosis of substance abuse, and sometimes, substance dependence (if there is an increasing preoccupation with returning to this cycle of use). Clearly, therapies designed to address this type of problem for a patient will focus strongly on never using the first time, since once the use is begun the patient is "off to the races" and becomes swept up in the spinning cycle until it burns itself out.

In contrast to this type of pattern, individuals who use substances that lead to the development of a new drive, such as heroin, prescription narcotics, alcohol, intranasal cocaine and amphetamine, and longer-acting benzodiazepines, may eventually settle into a more ordered cycle of behavior. The quintessential example of this is heroin use, where patients initially feel high for some time from the heroin, but with repeated use, develop tolerance, and then develop withdrawal symptoms when they do not get the heroin regularly. By this time, the patient will be using heroin fairly regularly – often three to four times a day with a regimented periodicity – simply to maintain a withdrawal-free existence. This type of pattern is easily documented to support the diagnosis of substance dependence. In such cases, the therapy often has an initial focus on detoxification and overcoming craving, and then a focus on relapse prevention, since once withdrawal is gone, the patient is drawn again to the intoxicating effects of the drug.

Treatment of Alcohol- and Substance-Use Disorders

First and foremost, the treatment of any substance-use disorder cannot begin until the goal and path of treatment has been established. While it would be easiest to say that the goal of treatment is complete abstinence in every case, this is more of a dogmatic approach, and thus, less individualized. It will be clear from the patient's history if there are circumstances during which alcohol use, for example, is handled responsibly and does not lead to adverse outcomes. For such individuals, a moderation approach may be appropriate [15], but extreme caution should be exercised in recommending this path, as there are significant risks associated with failure. For illicit drug users or patients abusing prescription drugs, abstinence may be the only plausible ultimate goal, although the path to the abstinent state may require an intermediate step of agonist substitution.

In particular, opioid-dependent patients need careful guidance when deciding between an agonist-based or abstinence-based recovery. For patients who have failed several attempts at abstinence, who have significant psychiatric and/or medical, especially chronic pain, comorbidities, or who have few supports and little structure to their lives, agonist-based therapies, such as buprenorphine or methadone maintenance treatment, are the standard of care. Patients who have less severe opioid problems, have stable, more structured lives with social supports, and who have no significant comorbidities may benefit from an abstinence-based approach from the beginning. Ultimately, one might envision that the agonist-based patients will improve in stability and structure to the point where they can slowly move toward complete abstinence.

The universal beginning of therapy, however, is the process of role induction for the patient. This is best accomplished in a reasonably focused patient, and so it may require that the patient have a brief detoxification period so as to eliminate effects of intoxication or acute withdrawal on attention and judgment. During the role induction, the provider outlines for the patient what the jobs of the treatment team members will be, what the patient's responsibilities are, and how the relationship will proceed. General ideas to be covered are that substance use is a behavior with many steps and the process will involve the patient's hard work to identify and enhance points of control in the behavior and even harder work to exercise that control and choose different, albeit less established, more difficult behaviors. Further, the concept of prescribed behaviors, such as attendance at meetings, should be discussed, with an emphasis on establishing a set of normalizing behaviors to replace the routines of substance-use behaviors. Last, the patient should learn the part that providers and medications will play in the recovery, and understand the need for adherence to all aspects of treatment.

Nonpharmacologic treatment of substance-use disorders is essential in every case, but may take more or less structured forms. Some patients may benefit from a locked residential setting with restricted visitors, while some may function well enough with a "recovery house", where individuals in recovery live together and support each other, but there is little to no structured oversight and residents are encouraged to go out to work or school during the day. All patients benefit from developing a support network, be it made up of friends or family or both, to be available in times of crisis and promote maintenance of normal behaviors.

Table 20.4 The 12 steps of alcoholics anonymous

1. We admitted we were powerless over alcohol – that our lives had become unmanageable
2. Came to believe that a Power greater than ourselves could restore us to sanity
3. Made a decision to turn our will and our lives over to the care of God as we understood Him
4. Made a searching and fearless moral inventory of ourselves
5. Admitted to God, to ourselves, and to another human being the exact nature of our wrongs
6. Were entirely ready to have God remove all these defects of character
7. Humbly asked Him to remove our shortcomings
8. Made a list of all persons we had harmed, and became willing to make amends to them all
9. Made direct amends to such people wherever possible, except when to do so would injure them or others
10. Continued to take personal inventory and when we were wrong promptly admitted it
11. Sought through prayer and meditation to improve our conscious contact with God, *as we understood Him*, praying only for knowledge of His will for us and the power to carry that out
12. Having had a spiritual awakening as the result of these Steps, we tried to carry this message to alcoholics, and to practice these principles in all our affairs

Reprinted with permission of A.A. World Services, Inc. Permission to reprint this material by A.A. World Services, Inc means that AAWS has not reviewed and/or endorses this publication. A.A. is a program of recovery for alcoholism only- use of A.A. material in any non-A.A. context does not imply otherwise

Table 20.5 The 12 steps of narcotics anonymous

1. We admitted that we were powerless over our addiction, that our lives had become unmanageable
2. We came to believe that a Power greater than ourselves could restore us to sanity
3. We made a decision to turn our will and our lives over to the care of God as we understood Him
4. We made a searching and fearless moral inventory of ourselves
5. We admitted to God, to ourselves, and to another human being the exact nature of our wrongs
6. We were entirely ready to have God remove all these defects of character
7. We humbly asked Him to remove our shortcomings
8. We made a list of all persons we had harmed, and became willing to make amends to them all
9. We made direct amends to such people wherever possible, except when to do so would injure them or others
10. We continued to take personal inventory and when we were wrong promptly admitted it
11. We sought through prayer and meditation to improve our conscious contact with God as we understood Him, praying only for knowledge of His will for us and the power to carry that out
12. Having had a spiritual awakening as a result of these steps, we tried to carry this message to addicts, and to practice these principles in all our affairs

Reprinted with permission of N.A. World Services, Inc.

A mainstay of therapy for substance-use disorders is group therapy. Substance-use disorder programs rely heavily on the group process to reinforce cognitive and behavior change. Substance-use patterns are identified and sustaining factors reinforcing use can be explored and addressed. Through the group process, patients challenge each other to identify "triggers" – stimuli that have become associated with substance use – and to "change people, places and things" so as to break habits and find new responses to cravings. The knowledge shared by more experienced patients helps those newer to recovery, and the networking of patients allows for a support system that extends beyond the group meeting for when unanticipated challenges arise.

A widely accepted framework for the therapeutic process that meshes well with the group method is the 12-step framework. The foundation of the 12-step model is built upon an individual's admission of the disorder and recognition for the need for help. Emphasis is placed on the individual having a spiritual transformation to overcome his/her addiction. Individuals examine and admit past indiscretions, and, where necessary, they attempt to mend their relationships. Finally, the process culminates in individuals rebuilding their lives without use and helping others that suffer from similar addictions through shared experiences. Members of 12 step programs often utilize sponsors (experienced members) to take them through this process. The 12-steps are published throughout the world and are recognized as an effective program to recovery. There are well over 200 kinds of 12-step programs addressing various kinds of addictions. The two most popular are Alcoholics Anonymous and Narcotics Anonymous (Tables 20.4 and 20.5, respectively, outline the original 12 original steps of each program).

Individual therapy for substance-use disorders is of use for many patients, but there are potential pitfalls. The isolated nature of individual therapy allows for a separation of the therapeutic setting from the "real world," thus leading to a sense that the discussions are either theoretical and not specifically applicable to daily challenges, or that discussions are after-the-fact analyses of events, and do not generalize. Further, individual therapy typically occurs once to twice weekly, and may not allow for the daily support and networking available from group meetings, which can be attended several times per day. Therefore, it is generally recommended that individual therapy not be the sole mode of nonpharmacologic intervention for substance-use disorders.

Pharmacologic Interventions for Substance-Use Disorders

Certain pharmacologic interventions have been shown to be of some benefit for patients with alcohol or opioid use disorders. While these medications are not a substitute for the cognitive and behavior changes brought about by psychotherapy and group meetings, they provide powerful adjuncts that may support patients through the process of recovery. The mechanisms of action of these agents differ, so each requires a discussion with the patient as to the proper use and expected outcomes. Most importantly, however, the majority of these medicines require daily administration, and so their effectiveness is limited to patients who maintain adherence.

There are three medications used in the treatment of alcohol use disorders. The first of these is disulfiram. Disulfiram blocks the action of acetaldehyde dehydrogenase, which causes a buildup of acetaldehyde when an individual ingests alcohol. Since acetaldehyde is toxic, the individual will experience a degree of acetaldehyde poisoning, with symptoms of flushing, headache, nausea and vomiting. Disulfiram works for 1–3 days after ingestion, so it is usually prescribed daily. In principle, the use of disulfiram reinforces the commitment the patient makes to sobriety, acting like a promise made not to drink, the knowledge of which deters drinking if a significant craving should occur. Before prescribing disulfiram, patients should be checked for elevations of liver transaminases, as disulfiram can cause a chemical hepatitis.

Naltrexone can be used for patients with binge drinking problems, as it has been shown to reduce the amounts or alcohol during relapse. The mechanism of action is believed to be that blockade of opioid reward lessens the reward triggered by alcohol ingestion. Again, patients should be tested for abnormalities of liver transaminases prior to prescribing naltrexone. Patients occasionally report that other rewarding sensations are reduced while taking naltrexone, thus limiting adherence sometimes. Since binges occur sporadically, patients often have difficulty taking medicine daily when there are no daily effects. However, patients who have the idea that naltrexone reduces alcohol craving may have improved confidence in their ability to resist or limit use.

Acamprosate is a medicine used for patients with alcohol dependence. The proposed mechanism of action is a reduction of anxiety symptoms that accompany the withdrawal and craving states. The medication takes about 1 week to begin working. Patients must be free of alcohol for several days before starting and should have liver transaminases checked before prescription. Studies have reported positive outcomes in some settings, specifically where the medication is coupled with some form of group therapy.

There are three medications prescribed for opioid-dependent patients. Methadone is a full opioid receptor agonist with a half-life that supports once daily dosing. It is used to occupy opioid receptors and thus, remove a patient's need to use shorter-acting agents repeatedly throughout the day. By satisfying withdrawal-induced craving, methadone maintenance provides a biological stability that can be a platform for building psychosocial stability and structure, which ultimately may support an abstinent lifestyle.

Buprenorphine is a partial agonist at the opioid receptor, binding tightly, but only stimulating weakly. The effect is again a reduced withdrawal-driven craving, which provides the same support to the patient. In one preparation, it is coformulated with naloxone, an opioid antagonist, in a sublingual tablet. Since buprenorphine is well absorbed sublingually while naloxone is not, tablets administered by this route provide full buprenorphine activity but no antagonist activity of naloxone. However, if the tablet is crushed, suspended and injected, the effect will be all naloxone, and thus unpleasant for an opioid-dependent person. The coformulation, therefore, decreases diversion of the medication to street use, which was a factor in the Food and Drug Administration (FDA)'s decision to permit office-based prescription. Further, since buprenorphine is a partial agonist, competitive inhibition of metabolic enzymes that affects its serum concentration has less impact on clinical effect than seen with the full agonist methadone. This renders buprenorphine a good choice for use in HIV-infected patients on antiretrovirals such as efavirenz and ritonavir, which inhibit cytochrome P450 3A4, the major metabolic pathway for both methadone and buprenorphine (see Table 20.6) [16].

Finally, naltrexone has been used to help patients with opioid dependence. Available in a depot preparation, it blocks the opioid receptor for up to 4 weeks. Since typical opioid use will result in no stimulation of the receptor, this knowledge can strengthen patients' resolve to not use. Of risk though, is that when a patient does relapse, she/he may try to override the naltrexone blockade of the receptor, to dire outcome, as overdosage will lead to respiratory suppression prior to the intoxicating effects.

Table 20.6 Drug interactions

	No. or insignificant interaction	Clinical relevant interaction
Methadone	Abacavir	Didanosine
	Emtricitabine	Stavudine
	Lamivudine	Zidovudine
	Tenofovir	Delavirdine
	Etravirine	Efavirenz
	Amprenavir	Nevirapine
	Atazanavir	Lopinavir/Ritonavir
	Darunavir	Nelfinavir
	Fosamprenavir	Ritonavir
	Indinavir	
	Saquinavir	
	Tipranivir	
	Enfurvitide	
	Maraviroc	
	Raltegravir	
Buprenorphine	Abacavir	Delavirdine
	Didanosine	Efavirenz
	Emtricitabine	
	Stavudine	
	Lamivudine	
	Zidovudine	
	Tenofovir	
	Etravirine	
	Nevirapine	
	Amprenavir	
	Atazanavir	
	Darunavir	
	Fosamprenavir	
	Indinavir	
	Lopinavir/Ritonavir	
	Nelfinavir	
	Ritonavir	
	Saquinavir	
	Tipranivir	
	Enfurvitide	
	Maraviroc	
	Raltegravir	

Reprinted with permission from: Batkis MF, Treisman GJ, and Angelino AF. Integrating Opioid Use Disorder and HIV Treatment: Rationale, Clinical Guidelines for Addiction Treatment, and Review of Interactions of Antiretroviral Agents and Opioid Agonist Therapist 2010;24 (1): 115–22 [17]

Summary

Substance-use disorders are important vectors of HIV transmission and are highly prevalent among patients with HIV infection. Further, substance-use disorders are often comorbid with other mental illnesses and can lead to impaired adherence and poorer HIV outcomes. Providers should be familiar with substance-use disorders, their assessment and underlying mechanisms, and with available psychotherapeutic and pharmacologic treatment options. Aggressive treatment of substance-use disorders improves patients' lives and may improve HIV outcomes.

References

1. Singh N, Squier C, Sivek C, Wagener M, Nguyen MH, Yu VL. Determinants of compliance with antiretroviral therapy in patients with human immunodeficiency virus: prospective assessment with implications for enhancing compliance. AIDS Care. 1996;8:261–9.
2. Bouhnik A-D, Chesney M, Carrieri P, Gallais H, Moreau J, Moatti JP, Obadia Y, Spire B; the MANIF 2000 Study Group. Nonadherence among HIV-infected injecting drug users: the impact of social instability. J Acquir Immune Defic Syndr. 2002;31 Suppl 3:S149–53.
3. Rotheram-Borus MJ, Desmond K, Comulada WS, Arnold EM, Johnson M, the Healthy Living Group. Reducing risky sexual behavior and substance us among currently and formerly homeless adults living with HIV. Research and Practice. 2009;99(6):1100–7.
4. Lyketsos CG, Hanson A, Fishman M, McHugh PR, Treisman GJ. Screening for psychiatric morbidity in a medical outpatient clinic for HIV infection: the need for a psychiatric presence. Int J Psychiatry Med. 1994;24:103–13.
5. Atkinson JH, Higgins JA, Vigil O, Dubrow R, Remien RH, Steward WT, et al. Psychiatric context of acute/early HIV infection. The NIMH multisite acute HIV infection study: IV. AIDS Behav. 2009;13:1061–7.
6. Mayfield D, McLeod G, Hall P. The CAGE questionnaire: a validation of a new alcoholism screening instrument. Am J Psychiatry. 1974;131:1121–3.
7. Skinner HA. The drug abuse screening test. Addict Behav. 1982;7:363–71.
8. McLellan AT, Luborsky L, Woody GE, Obrien CP. An improved diagnostic evaluation instrument for substance abuse patients, the Addiction Severity Index. J Nerv Ment Dis. 1980;168:26–33.
9. Prochaska JO, DiClemente CC, Norcross JC. In search of how people change. Applications to addictive behaviors. Am Psychol. 1992;47:1102–14.
10. Miller WR, Rollnick S. Motivational interviewing: preparing people to change addictive behavior. New York: Guilford; 1991.
11. Miller WR, Benefield G, Tonigan JS. Enhancing motivation for change in problem drinking: a controlled comparison of two therapist styles. J Consult Clin Psychol. 1993;61:455–61.
12. Regier DA, Farmer ME, Rae DS, Locke BZ, Keith SJ, Judd LL, et al. Comorbidity of mental disorders with alcohol and other drug abuse: results from the Epidemiologic Catchment Area (ECA) Study. JAMA. 1990;264:2511–8.
13. McHugh PR, Slavney PR. The Perspectives of Psychiatry. 2nd ed. Baltimore: Johns Hopkins University Press; 1998.
14. Thorndike E. Educational psychology: the psychology of learning. New York: Teacher's College Press; 1921. p. 172.
15. Ferster CB, Skinner BF. Schedules of reinforcement. Acton, MA: Copley; 1957.
16. Levy MS. Take control of your drinking…and you may not need to quit. Baltimore: Johns Hopkins; 2007.
17. Batkis MF, Treisman GJ, Angelino AF. Integrated opioid use disorder and HIV treatment: rationale, clinical guidelines for addiction treatment, and review of interactions of antiretroviral agents and opioid agonist therapies. AIDS Patient Care STDS. 2010;24: 15–22.

Racial Disparities in HIV and Liver Disease

Nyingi M. Kemmer

Introduction

Based on the recent Center of Disease Control (CDC) report, an estimated 1.1 million persons in the USA are infected with the human immunodeficiency virus (HIV). Several US-based population studies have consistently shown a significant ethnic variation in HIV prevalence, with ethnic minorities accounting for about 70% of those living with HIV. In 1997, for the purposes of federal statistics reporting, the Office of Management and Budget revised the classification of individuals by race and ethnicity. The revision identified five racial and two ethnic groups. The racial categories are as follows: (1) White, (2) Black or African American, (3) Asian, (4) Native Hawaiian or other Pacific Islander, and (5) American Indian or Alaskan Native; the ethnic categories are as follows: (1) Hispanic or Latino and (2) non-Hispanic/Latino. Owing to the lack of consistency in the classification across published studies, in this review ethnicity and race are used interchangeably. Ethnicity/race will be categorized as (1) White or Caucasian, (2) Black or African American, (3) Hispanic or Latino, (4) Asian, and (5) others.

Among ethnic minorities, Blacks are disproportionately affected by HIV accounting for 49% of all HIV-infected persons, followed by Hispanics (18%) and other minority groupings (2%) (Fig. 21.1). Furthermore, Blacks are overrepresented among individuals with new HIV infection, perinatal HIV infection, and AIDS-related mortality [1]. A recent retrospective study found a significant ethnic disparity in survival among patients with HIV infection and black race was identified as an independent predictor of poor outcomes [2]. Although this study was not designed to determine the exact reason for the observed ethnic differences in overall survival, the investigators did not find an association with socioeconomic status. Thus, even though Blacks account for only 13% of the US population, they are overrepresented in population-based estimates of HIV incidence, prevalence, and mortality.

In recent years, with the introduction of highly active antiretroviral therapy (HAART) therapy the trends in HIV-related morbidity have shown a shift in chronic disease pattern. Morbidity and mortality from HIV/AIDS has declined, but that due to chronic liver disease and its long-term sequelae of cirrhosis and hepatocellular carcinoma is on the rise. The exact prevalence of liver disease among persons infected with HIV in the US is unknown, but a recent US-based study found that, among those with chronic liver disease, nonalcoholic fatty liver disease (NAFLD) was the most common occurring in 30%, followed by viral hepatitis [hepatitis B virus (HBV) and hepatitis C virus (HCV)] and alcoholic liver disease [3]. Though this study did not evaluate for ethnic-specific differences in liver disease prevalence or etiology, Akhtar and Shaheen [4] – in a retrospective analysis of a large African American and Hispanic population with abnormal liver tests – showed that the subset with AIDS and jaundice had a primary hepatic as opposed to biliary disorder. In this study, the most common etiology was drug-induced hepatotoxicity as defined by elevated liver enzyme tests, followed by infection (nonviral or viral) and alcoholic liver disease. Though the findings of this study are limited by the retrospective nature of the study design and the absence of whites as a comparative ethnic/racial group, it does provide an insight into the possible disease etiologies among ethnic minorities.

Despite the lack of population-based studies addressing ethnic-specific prevalence in chronic liver disease, the reports of an increasing liver-related morbidity and mortality among persons with HIV, and the disproportionate number of HIV-infected ethnic minorities, highlights the importance of understanding the impact and disease burden of chronic liver disease in this population. This review discusses the existing literature on ethnic variations of chronic liver disease in the

N.M. Kemmer (✉)
Department of Internal Medicine, University of Cincinnati,
231 Albert B. Sabin Way MSB6363, Cincinnati, OH 45267, USA
e-mail: nyingi.kemmer@uc.edu

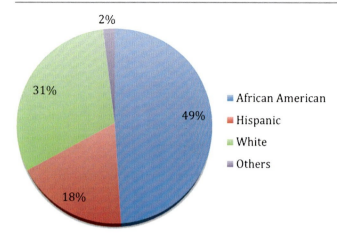

Fig. 21.1 Race/ethnicity of HIV/AIDS diagnosed in 2007 (adapted from http://www.cdc.gov) [1]

HIV population with the purpose of providing a better understanding of ethnic disparities in liver disease and HIV, and to address clinical implications of this disparity, where applicable.

Nonalcoholic Fatty Liver Disease

NAFLD is a clinical spectrum ranging from benign hepatic steatosis to steatohepatitis, with or without fibrosis. In the non-HIV US population, the prevalence of NAFLD is estimated to be between 20 and 30%, and several studies have documented a significant ethnic variation with reports of a higher prevalence among individuals of Hispanic ethnicity [5–7]. In the HIV population, the exact prevalence of NAFLD is unknown and reports from published studies have provided conflicting reports pertaining to the association between ethnicity and hepatic steatosis either by imaging or histopathology. In a study by Crum-Cianflone et al. [8], using imaging (ultrasound) for diagnosis of hepatic steatosis in an HIV population, the investigators reported that African Americans (AA) were less likely to have NAFLD compared to other ethnic groups. This finding is similar to that of Sulkowski et al. [9], in which Caucasians were more likely to have NAFLD compared to AA. In this study, the cohort consisted of an HCV–HIV population and the diagnosis of NAFLD was based on the histologic presence of hepatic steatosis. The finding of a negative association between NAFLD and AA contradicts reports from other published studies. In the study by McGovern et al. [10], the authors reported a higher prevalence of NAFLD in AA compared to non-AA, while Gaslightwala and Bini [11] reported no significant ethnic difference in the presence of NAFLD. In both studies, NAFLD was defined as a histologic presence of hepatic steatosis and the patient population consisted of HCV–HIV coinfected individuals. Therefore, in contrast to the non-HIV population in which reports have consistently shown an ethnic variation in NAFLD, the prevalence of NAFLD in HIV-infected individuals from different ethnic backgrounds is unclear [6, 7]. Furthermore, the published studies evaluating NAFLD in HIV-infected individuals provide very limited information on other ethnic groups since the study population has been predominantly AA and Caucasian. Future studies to better define the prevalence, natural history and burden of NAFLD in the multiethnic HIV population will be invaluable.

Viral Hepatitis: HBV and HCV

Coinfection with HCV or HBV is common in individuals with HIV infection because of the shared route of transmission. The prevalence of HBV–HIV, HCV–HIV, and HBV–HCV–HIV triple infection in the USA is 6–14, 15–30, and 1.6%, respectively [12–14]. Furthermore, in a recent US-based study by Kim et al. [14], the investigators reported Black race to be significantly associated with HBV and HCV coinfection, but not with HBV–HCV–HIV triple infection. Owing to the lower prevalence of triple infection, there is limited population-based data on the natural history and prognosis of these individuals. The following section reviews the available epidemiologic and clinical data available pertaining to HBV and HCV coinfected individuals from different ethnic backgrounds.

Hepatitis C

Although there are no population-based estimates of the prevalence of HCV among HIV individuals of different ethnic backgrounds, the study by Kim et al. [14] report Black race to be associated with the presence of HCV–HIV coinfection. Furthermore, data from an ongoing prospective observational HIV study, found the prevalence of HCV in HIV individuals to be 30.2, 28.6, and 18.9% for AA, Hispanics, and Whites, respectively [15]. This is consistent with reports from several US population studies of a higher prevalence of HCV monoinfection among ethnic minorities [16].

The clinical spectrum of HCV–HIV coinfection, in terms of biochemical and histological parameters, is variable. To date, there are no studies specifically designed to determine if ethnic differences exist in clinical spectrum of individuals with HCV–HIV coinfection. In a study by Shores et al. [17] the investigators found AA were more likely to have a lower alanine transaminase (ALT) in comparison to non-AA, a finding that is consistent with that observed in the monoinfected HCV population. The correlation between ALT and the histologic grade or stage was not provided in this study. However, clinical data from the monoinfected HCV population show a lower histologic grade and stage in AA compared to Whites and Hispanics [18, 19]. A similar finding of a lower hepatic fibrosis score in AA compared to Whites and Hispanics has been observed in patients with HCV–HIV coinfection [20]. This is in contrast to a recent report by Rozenberg et al. [21] showing no significant ethnic difference in the average hepatic fibrosis score as determined by the Ishak scoring scale. In this study, the average Ishak score for AA and CA was 2.3 and 2.1, respectively. The limitation of this study is the small sample size and the lack of Hispanic or Asian representation in the cohort. Therefore, based on the clinical data available from published studies, it is unclear if the clinical presentation of HCV–HIV based on biochemical (i.e., ALT) and histologic parameters differs among ethnic groups, especially in those of Hispanic and Asian heritage.

Although there are no published studies specifically addressing the impact of ethnicity on the natural history and progression of HCV–HIV coinfected individuals, a retrospective analysis of HCV–HIV cohort using data obtained from the Veteran's Administration (VA) Medical center provides useful insights [22]. In this study, the investigators found an ethnic difference in the frequency of biochemical markers of advanced liver disease as demonstrated by thrombocytopenia and hyperbilirubinemia. Whites with HCV–HIV coinfection were more likely to have features of advanced liver disease than Blacks. This may reflect diminished histologic disease, a finding similar to that observed in HCV monoinfected Blacks [18]. In terms of causes of mortality in HCV–HIV coinfected individuals, the authors also found a significant racial disparity in survival, with a higher mortality observed in Whites compared to Blacks; no Hispanics or Asians were included in this study. Therefore, future studies designed to evaluate the clinical spectrum and natural history of HCV–HIV in a multiethnic population is essential because the information derived will represent an indirect measure of the burden of HCV–HIV coinfection among different ethnic groups.

To reduce the liver-related morbidity and mortality of HCV–HIV coinfection, the availability and accessibility of effective antiviral therapies is crucial. Unfortunately, access to antiviral therapy for HCV in this population is not universal. Several studies have implicated health-care access as one of the main reasons for low HCV treatment rates of HCV–HIV coinfected individuals. In a study by Mehta et al. [23] the investigators report low referrals for HCV treatment as a significant factor contributing to poor treatment rates, and AA were less likely to be referred for HCV care. Furthermore, in a multivariate analysis, Cohen et al. [24] found that both AA and Hispanics were negatively associated with referrals for HCV treatment. The reason for the ethnic disparity in referrals for HCV care is uncertain. Ethnic disparity in receipt of antiviral therapy has also been documented in HCV–HIV coinfected individuals. Two large HCV–HIV cohorts [VA and HIV outpatient study (HOPS)] found Black race to be independently associated with nonreceipt of HCV treatment [25, 26]. In addition, the HOPS study found that individuals with elevated ALT had a higher likelihood of receipt of HCV treatment. Similar findings from the Women's Interagency HIV Study (WIHS) found AA and Hispanics were negatively associated with receipt of HCV treatment, but an elevated ALT increased the likelihood of receiving HCV treatment [24]. It is unclear if the lower ALT observed among AA with HCV–HIV coinfection plays a contributory role in treatment decision. Therefore, future studies to elucidate the factors associated with ethnic disparity in receipt of antiviral therapy for HCV is an essential step toward reducing and ultimately eliminating this disparity.

The approved antiviral therapy for HCV in HIV coinfected individuals is a combination of pegylated interferon and ribavirin. For those that receive this combined therapy, the sustained virologic response (SVR) is lower for AA compared to Whites. In a prospective trial of AA and Whites with HCV–HIV coinfection (genotype 1) treated with pegylated interferon (IFN) and Ribavirin, the SVR was 7.6 and 40% for AA and Whites, respectively [21]. In another trial using nonpegylated IFN, Black race was associated with a lower likelihood of early virologic response rate (EVR) at week 12 [20]. The lower response rates in AA with HCV–HIV coinfection is similar to that observed in those with HCV monoinfection [27, 28]. Several studies have attempted to identify the host and viral factors associated with nonresponse in this population. In recent years, much of the research has focused on understanding the possible mechanisms responsible for decreased interferon effectiveness in AA with HCV monoinfection or HCV–HIV coinfection. The studies focusing on viral kinetics have provided useful insights into the host responsiveness to IFN across ethnic groups. Following the subcutaneous administration of IFN, a biphasic pattern of viral reduction is observed. In the first phase, a significant decrease in HCV RNA is observed within 24–48 h followed by a second phase, which is associated with a gradual decrease. The first phase reflects the efficacy of viral inhibition by IFN, while the second phase represents a combination of IFN effectiveness and clearance of infected hepatocytes. In a recent study by Rozenberg et al. [21] the investigators evaluated the viral kinetics and pharmacodynamics of HCV–HIV coinfected individuals receiving IFN therapy. They found a smaller first phase decline in HCV viral load and a much slower second phase decline among AA compared to Whites. Overall, the mean decline in HCV viral load at week 4 and week 12 was significantly lower in AA compared to Whites, and this correlated with an SVR of 7.6 and 40% in AA and Whites, respectively. Despite the small sample size of this study, the findings are similar to that of HCV monoinfected individuals showing a reduced IFN effectiveness among AA [28].

The exact reason for the observed ethnic variation in IFN ineffectiveness is unknown. Several studies have implicated hepatic suppressor of cytokine signaling 3 (SOCS3) as a key factor involved in the cellular mechanisms involving IFN response [29, 30]. IFN mediates its antiviral effect by binding to and activating IFN receptors located on hepatocytes, resulting in a cascade of events that activate IFN stimulated genes via signal transducer and activator of transcription (STAT) pathway. Hepatic SOCS3 are thought to play a role in antagonizing IFN signaling by interfering with STAT pathway. Therefore, a high hepatic SOCS3 expression is presumed to be associated with poor response rate to IFN. The study by Kim et al. [31], investigated the role of hepatic SOCS3 in HCV–HIV coinfected individuals. They found that high hepatic SOCS3 expression correlated with poor response to interferon therapy, and AA had higher hepatic SOCS3 expression than Whites or Hispanics. Though the studies on viral kinetics and IFN signaling provide useful insights into mechanisms involved with IFN ineffectiveness, recent reports implicating genetic variant of IL28B in HCV as a key factor across ethnic groups renders support to a multifactorial mechanism [32, 33]. Therefore, in view of the substantial burden of HCV–HIV coinfection and its sequelae, it is imperative that clinical and translational studies are conducted to better elucidate the underlying pathophysiologic mechanisms responsible for the observed ethnic disparities in this cohort. It is expected that the findings of these studies will pave the way for improved outcomes irrespective of ethnicity.

Hepatitis B

The estimated prevalence of HBV in persons infected with HIV is 6–14% [12]. Among patients with HBV alone, a significantly higher prevalence is found in Asians compared to non-Asians. There are no US-based population studies addressing HBV in HIV-infected individuals of Asian ethnicity. Therefore, the prevalence of HBV–HIV coinfection among Asians Americans is unknown. In a recent HIV outpatient study, the prevalence of HBV based on the presence of HBsAg was 3.5, 8.7, and 9.5% in Hispanics, Whites, and Blacks, respectively [34]. There are no population-based studies addressing ethnic differences in the clinical presentation, natural history and treatment responses of HBV–HIV coinfected individuals. However, in a retrospective analysis using data from the US Military HIV Natural History Study (NHS), the investigators report an ethnic variation in clinical presentation based on three virologic patterns: (1) Chronic HBV classified as the presence of HBsAg, (2) isolated HBcAb, and (3) resolved HBV defined as presence of HBcAb and HBsAb [35]. In this study, the prevalence of chronic HBV was higher in AA compared to Hispanics and Whites, a pattern similar to that of the HIV outpatient study. Additionally, the prevalence of isolated HBcAb was higher in AA (10.9%) compared to Whites (8.1%) and Hispanics (7.2%). The clinical significance or long-term outcome of isolated HBcAb in HIV-positive individuals is uncertain; therefore, the clinical impact of the higher prevalence among AA is unknown. In the WIHS, though the investigators were not able to determine the clinical significance of isolated HBcAb, they found that during a median follow up period of 7.5 years, the majority of the women maintained an isolated HBcAb virologic status, while 20% converted to HBsAb positive and 2% reverted to HBsAg positive [36]. In this study cohort, ethnicity was not a predictor of conversion to HBsAb-positive status.

Future studies focusing on the natural history and treatment outcomes will improve our understanding of the burden of disease among HBV–HIV coinfected individuals from different ethnic backgrounds. In the interim, public health programs focusing on the implementation of strategies to decrease or eliminate HBV transmission in the HIV population should be strongly encouraged. In a study by Kellerman et al. [37] the investigators found low hepatitis B vaccination rates in their HIV cohort. Although the postvaccination response rates in HIV-infected individuals are low, Landrum et al. [38] in their recent hepatitis B vaccination study showed no ethnic differences in vaccine response. Therefore, efforts to increase vaccination rates in HIV-positive individuals irrespective of ethnic background should be encouraged. The application of these preventive strategies in HIV-positive individuals and the conducting of clinical trials and population based studies to better understand the clinical spectrum and natural history of HBV–HIV coinfection across ethnic backgrounds will be invaluable step in confronting ethnic disparity in this population.

Hepatocellular Carcinoma

Hepatocellular carcinoma (HCC) in HIV-infected individuals occurs most frequently in those with HBV or HCV coinfection. In large study using the VA database, the investigators found that in the HCV–HIV coinfection increases the risk of HCC by fivefold [39]. The role of HBV–HIV coinfection on the incidence of HCC was not evaluated. In the non-HIV US population, HCC is more common in Asians and Blacks and most often associated with HBV and HCV, respectively [40]. In the HIV population, reports from a multicenter study revealed that patients with HCC were more likely to be Black in comparison to other racial groups [41]. However, in contrast to the lower survival observed among Blacks with HCC in the non-HIV population, race was not a predictor of survival in HIV cohort. This study did not address the impact of available treatment options including liver transplantation

(LT) on overall survival. Future studies to evaluate the impact of ethnicity on HCC recurrence after regional or systemic treatment in HIV-positive individuals will be provide invaluable information.

Liver Transplantation

The role of LT in end-stage liver disease patients with HIV has evolved from an absolute contraindication to being a viable option in selected patients. Reports from several studies in Europe and North America have consistently shown a reasonable patient and graft survival of LT recipients with HIV infection [42, 43]. In a retrospective analysis of data from the US liver transplant registry, the investigators found that among LT recipients with HIV, the risk of death was significantly higher in Blacks compared to non-Blacks, and the most common indication for LT in this cohort was viral hepatitis [44]. In another study of HCV–HIV coinfected individuals, the authors report that LT recipients of AA ethnicity had a lower survival in contrast to non-AA [45]. The finding of inferior outcomes for AA in HCV–HIV-positive recipients is similar to reports from the HCV LT population [46]. Conversely, reports from a cohort of LT recipients with HBV monoinfection do not show ethnic differences in long-term outcomes [47]. However, it is unknown if the lack of ethnic difference in survival among recipients with HBV monoinfection reflects a similar outcome among HBV–HIV recipients. In a recent study of HBV–HIV cohort, though they report no survival difference between recipients with HBV versus HBV–HIV, no information on race stratification was provided [48]. Therefore, the impact of ethnicity on post-LT survival in HBV–HIV is unknown.

Summary

Ethnic variations exist in the incidence, prevalence, therapeutic and long-term outcomes of chronic liver disease patients with HIV. These ethnic differences present unique challenges to health-care professionals involved in the care of these patients. With the steadily improving life expectancy of individuals living with HIV, the increasing liver-related morbidity highlights the need for a better understanding of liver disease in this population. In view of our ethnically diverse population and the disproportionate rate of HIV among ethnic minorities, a heightened awareness of the existing ethnic variations in liver disease in this population is essential. Furthermore, a better understanding of the impact of ethnicity on liver disease in HIV-positive individuals promises to identify strategies to decrease the prevalence of preventable liver diseases and ultimately improve therapeutic outcomes in this population. Though this review summarizes the complex relationship between ethnicity and liver disease in the HIV population, it also highlights the lack of population-based studies with adequate representation of all ethnic groups. The significance of adequate representation of currently underrepresented ethnic minorities in clinical trials involving HIV and Liver disease outcomes cannot be overemphasized. In order to benefit from clinical research, the active participation of ethnic minorities is essential if the results of these studies are to be applicable to them.

Practicing health-care professionals involved in the care of the HIV patient need to be cognizant of these ethnic differences and be aware of the associated therapeutic and prognostic implications. Future research to clarify and improve the issues addressed in this review will be useful as we strive to understand ethnic disparities in the HIV-positive population.

References

1. CDC: Centers for disease control and prevention. 2010.
2. Oramasionwu CU, Hunter JM, Skinner J, Ryan L, Lawson KA, Brown CM, et al. Black race as a predictor of poor health outcomes among a national cohort of HIV/aids patients admitted to us hospitals: a cohort study. BMC Infect Dis. 2009;9:127.
3. Crum-Cianflone N, Collins G, Medina S, Asher D, Campin R, Bavaro M, et al. Prevalence and factors associated with liver test abnormalities among human immunodeficiency virus-infected persons. Clin Gastroenterol Hepatol. 2010;8:183–91.
4. Akhtar AJ, Shaheen M. Jaundice in African-American and Hispanic patients with aids. J Natl Med Assoc. 2007;99:1381–5.
5. Clark JM, Brancati FL, Diehl AM. The prevalence and etiology of elevated aminotransferase levels in the United States. Am J Gastroenterol. 2003;98:960–7.
6. Browning JD, Szczepaniak LS, Dobbins R, Nuremberg P, Horton JD, Cohen JC, et al. Prevalence of hepatic steatosis in an urban population in the United States: impact of ethnicity. Hepatology. 2004;40:1387–95.
7. Weston SR, Leyden W, Murphy R, Bass NM, Bell BP, Manos MM, et al. Racial and ethnic distribution of nonalcoholic fatty liver in persons with newly diagnosed chronic liver disease. Hepatology. 2005;41:372–9.
8. Crum-Cianflone N, Dilay A, Collins G, Asher D, Campin R, Medina S, et al. Nonalcoholic fatty liver disease among HIV-infected persons. J Acquir Immune Defic Syndr. 2009;50:464–73.
9. Sulkowski MS, Mehta SH, Torbenson MS, Higgins Y, Brinkley SC, de Oca RM, et al. Rapid fibrosis progression among HIV/hepatitis C virus-co-infected adults. AIDS. 2007;21:2209–16.
10. McGovern BH, Ditelberg JS, Taylor LE, Gandhi RT, Christopoulos KA, Chapman S, et al. Hepatic steatosis is associated with fibrosis, nucleoside analogue use, and hepatitis C virus genotype 3 infection in HIV-seropositive patients. Clin Infect Dis. 2006;43:365–72.
11. Gaslightwala I, Bini EJ. Impact of human immunodeficiency virus infection on the prevalence and severity of steatosis in patients with chronic hepatitis C virus infection. J Hepatol. 2006;44:1026–32.
12. Alter MJ. Epidemiology of viral hepatitis and HIV co-infection. J Hepatol. 2006;44:S6–9.
13. Sherman KE, Rouster SD, Chung RT, Rajicic N. Hepatitis C virus prevalence among patients infected with human immunodeficiency virus: a cross-sectional analysis of the US adult aids clinical trials group. Clin Infect Dis. 2002;34:831–7.

14. Kim JH, Psevdos G, Suh J, Sharp VL. Co-infection of hepatitis B and hepatitis C virus in human immunodeficiency virus-infected patients in New York city, United States. World J Gastroenterol. 2008;14:6689–93.
15. Spradling PR, Richardson JT, Buchacz K, Moorman AC, Finelli L, Bell BP, et al. Trends in hepatitis C virus infection among patients in the HIV outpatient study, 1996–2007. J Acquir Immune Defic Syndr. 2010;53:388–96.
16. Armstrong GL, Wasley A, Simard EP, McQuillan GM, Kuhnert WL, Alter MJ. The prevalence of hepatitis C virus infection in the United States, 1999 through 2002. Ann Intern Med. 2006;144:705–14.
17. Shores NJ, Maida I, Perez-Saleme L, Nunez M. Virological rather than host factors are associated with transaminase levels among HIV/HCV-coinfected patients. J Int Assoc Physicians AIDS Care (Chic). 2010;9:15–9.
18. Wiley TE, Brown J, Chan J. Hepatitis C infection in African Americans: its natural history and histological progression. Am J Gastroenterol. 2002;97:700–6.
19. Lepe R, Layden-Almer JE, Layden TJ, Cotler S. Ethnic differences in the presentation of chronic hepatitis C. J Viral Hepat. 2006;13:116–20.
20. Brau N, Rodriguez-Torres M, Prokupek D, Bonacini M, Giffen CA, Smith JJ, et al. Treatment of chronic hepatitis C in HIV/HCV-coinfection with interferon alpha-2b+ full-course vs. 16-week delayed ribavirin. Hepatology. 2004;39:989–98.
21. Rozenberg L, Haagmans BL, Neumann AU, Chen G, McLaughlin M, Levy-Drummer RS, et al. Therapeutic response to peg-ifn-alpha-2b and ribavirin in HIV/HCV co-infected African-American and Caucasian patients as a function of HCV viral kinetics and interferon pharmacodynamics. AIDS. 2009;23:2439–50.
22. Merriman NA, Porter SB, Brensinger CM, Reddy KR, Chang KM. Racial difference in mortality among U.S. Veterans with HCV/HIV coinfection. Am J Gastroenterol. 2006;101:760–7.
23. Mehta SH, Lucas GM, Mirel LB, Torbenson M, Higgins Y, Moore RD, et al. Limited effectiveness of antiviral treatment for hepatitis C in an urban HIV clinic. AIDS. 2006;20:2361–9.
24. Cohen MH, Grey D, Cook JA, Anastos K, Seaberg E, Augenbraun M, et al. Awareness of hepatitis C infection among women with and at risk for HIV. J Gen Intern Med. 2007;22:1689–94.
25. Butt AA, Tsevat J, Leonard AC, Shaikh OS, McMahon D, Khan UA, et al. Effect of race and HIV co-infection upon treatment prescription for hepatitis C virus. Int J Infect Dis. 2009;13:449–55.
26. Vellozzi C, Buchacz K, Baker R, Spradling PR, Richardson J, Moorman A, et al. Treatment of hepatitis C virus (HCV) infection in patients coinfected with HIV in the HIV outpatient study (HOPS), 1999–2007. J Viral Hepat. 2010;18(5):316–24.
27. Muir AJ, Bornstein JD, Killenberg PG. Peginterferon alfa-2b and ribavirin for the treatment of chronic hepatitis C in blacks and non-Hispanic whites. N Engl J Med. 2004;350:2265–71.
28. Conjeevaram HS, Fried MW, Jeffers LJ, Terrault NA, Wiley-Lucas TE, Afdhal N, et al. Peginterferon and ribavirin treatment in African American and Caucasian American patients with hepatitis C genotype 1. Gastroenterology. 2006;131:470–7.
29. Huang Y, Feld JJ, Sapp RK, Nanda S, Lin JH, Blatt LM, et al. Defective hepatic response to interferon and activation of suppressor of cytokine signaling 3 in chronic hepatitis C. Gastroenterology. 2007;132:733–44.
30. Persico M, Capasso M, Russo R, Persico E, Croce L, Tiribelli C, et al. Elevated expression and polymorphisms of SOCS3 influence patient response to antiviral therapy in chronic hepatitis C. Gut. 2008;57:507–15.
31. Kim KA, Lin W, Tai AW, Shao RX, Weinberg E, De Sa Borges CB, et al. Hepatic SOCS3 expression is strongly associated with non-response to therapy and race in HCV and HCV/HIV infection. J Hepatol. 2009;50:705–11.
32. Rauch A, Kutalik Z, Descombes P, Cai T, Di Iulio J, Mueller T, et al. Genetic variation in il28b is associated with chronic hepatitis C and treatment failure: a genome-wide association study. Gastroenterology. 2010;138:1338–45. 1345.e1–17.
33. Thomas DL, Thio CL, Martin MP, Qi Y, Ge D, O'Huigin C, et al. Genetic variation in il28b and spontaneous clearance of hepatitis C virus. Nature. 2009;461:798–801.
34. Spradling PR, Richardson JT, Buchacz K, Moorman AC, Brooks JT. Prevalence of chronic hepatitis B virus infection among patients in the HIV outpatient study, 1996–2007. J Viral Hepat. 2010;17(12):879–86.
35. Landrum ML, Fieberg AM, Chun HM, Crum-Cianflone NF, Marconi VC, Weintrob AC, et al. The effect of human immunodeficiency virus on hepatitis B virus serologic status in co-infected adults. PLoS One. 2010;5:e8687.
36. French AL, Lin MY, Evans CT, Benning L, Glesby MJ, Young MA, et al. Long-term serologic follow-up of isolated hepatitis B core antibody in HIV-infected and HIV-uninfected women. Clin Infect Dis. 2009;49:148–54.
37. Kellerman SE, Hanson DL, McNaghten AD, Fleming PL. Prevalence of chronic hepatitis B and incidence of acute hepatitis B infection in human immunodeficiency virus-infected subjects. J Infect Dis. 2003;188:571–7.
38. Landrum ML, Huppler Hullsiek K, Ganesan A, Weintrob AC, Crum-Cianflone NF, Barthel RV, et al. Hepatitis B vaccine responses in a large U.S. Military cohort of HIV-infected individuals: another benefit of HAART in those with preserved cd4 count. Vaccine. 2009;27:4731–8.
39. Giordano TP, Kramer JR, Souchek J, Richardson P, El-Serag HB. Cirrhosis and hepatocellular carcinoma in HIV-infected veterans with and without the hepatitis C virus: a cohort study, 1992–2001. Arch Intern Med. 2004;164:2349–54.
40. Nguyen MH, Whittemore AS, Garcia RT, Tawfeek SA, Ning J, Lam S, et al. Role of ethnicity in risk for hepatocellular carcinoma in patients with chronic hepatitis C and cirrhosis. Clin Gastroenterol Hepatol. 2004;2:820–4.
41. Brau N, Fox RK, Xiao P, Marks K, Naqvi Z, Taylor LE, et al. Presentation and outcome of hepatocellular carcinoma in HIV-infected patients: a U.S.-Canadian multicenter study. J Hepatol. 2007;47:527–37.
42. Stock PG, Roland ME. Evolving clinical strategies for transplantation in the HIV-positive recipient. Transplantation. 2007;84:563–71.
43. Duclos-Vallee JC, Teicher E, Vittecoq D, Samuel D. Liver transplantation for patients infected with both HIV and HCV or HIV and HBV. Med Sci (Paris). 2007;23:723–8.
44. Mindikoglu AL, Regev A, Magder LS. Impact of human immunodeficiency virus on survival after liver transplantation: analysis of united network for organ sharing database. Transplantation. 2008;85:359–68.
45. de Vera ME, Dvorchik I, Tom K, Eghtesad B, Thai N, Shakil O, et al. Survival of liver transplant patients coinfected with HIV and HCV is adversely impacted by recurrent hepatitis C. Am J Transplant. 2006;6:2983–93.
46. Forman LM, Lewis JD, Berlin JA, Feldman HI, Lucey MR. The association between hepatitis C infection and survival after orthotopic liver transplantation. Gastroenterology. 2002;122:889–96.
47. Bzowej N, Han S, Degertekin B, Keeffe EB, Emre S, Brown R, et al. Liver transplantation outcomes among Caucasians, Asian Americans, and African Americans with hepatitis B. Liver Transpl. 2009;15:1010–20.
48. Coffin CS, Stock PG, Dove LM, Berg CL, Nissen NN, Curry MP, et al. Virologic and clinical outcomes of hepatitis B virus infection in HIV–HBV coinfected transplant recipients. Am J Transplant. 2010;10(5):1268–75.

Quality of Life in Patients with HIV Infection and Liver Disease

Cindy L. Bryce and Joel Tsevat

Introduction

The presence of HIV infection, alone or in combination with other infections and diseases, can have a serious impact on a patient's health and quality of life (QOL). According to the World Health Organization (WHO) Constitution of 1948, "Health is a state of complete physical, mental and social well-being and not merely the absence of disease or infirmity" [1]. Like the definition of health, the definition of QOL is broad and multidimensional, "[An] individual's perception of their position in life in the context of the culture and value systems in which they live and in relation to their goals, expectations, standards and concerns" [2].

While the formal assessment of QOL is a major topic of interest to health services researchers, a general understanding of QOL is crucial for clinicians involved in the care of HIV-infected patients. Issues related to QOL can strongly influence a physician's recommendations for treatment of a particular patient and can even dictate how the patient responds to the recommendations. Although survival and life expectancy are of course major concerns, they are not the only concerns in decision-making about health care. In fact, many medical interventions have no impact on survival or life extension and are performed entirely to improve functional status or other dimensions (domains) of QOL. In cases in which various treatments offer the prospects for equivalent outcomes in terms of survival, life extension, cost, and other objectively quantifiable measures, the choice of treatment is often based on subjective QOL considerations. And, for that matter, even if different types of treatments do not have equivalent life expectancies, patients may place more value on QOL considerations and opt for a therapy that improves their function even as it may hasten their death. As McDowell argues, "Herein lies the central purpose of QOL scales: they provide insight into the perceived discrepancy between actual and ideal states" [3].

Assessing QOL can shed light on attributes of a health state that are unobservable or difficult to measure. Good QOL measures assess, either explicitly or implicitly, how much a patient is bothered, or would be bothered if a particular course of treatment were followed, by perceived deficits in any specific aspect of their physical, emotional, or social well-being [4]. Two people in exactly the same situation might make very different choices about their care. Therefore, it is important for the clinician to determine the individual patient's preferences and develop a plan for what is sometimes called preference-sensitive care.

This chapter is designed to familiarize health-care providers with the concepts related to QOL (Table 22.1) and the types of instruments that can be used to assess QOL, including in patients with HIV and liver disease (Table 22.2).

Characteristics of Quality-of-Life Measures

With the vast number of QOL measures available, choosing an instrument for a particular patient population can be overwhelming. Several characteristics of QOL measures might be helpful to consider when identifying an appropriate measure.

Domains of Quality of Life

Efforts to measure QOL typically involve partitioning the broad, multidimensional concept of QOL into narrow and clearly defined constructs known as domains. Instruments designed to measure health-related QOL generally include

C.L. Bryce (✉)
School of Medicine, University of Pittsburg, 200 Meyran Ave,
Ste 200, Pittsburg, PA 15213, USA
e-mail: brycecl@upmc.edu

Table 22.1 Glossary of terms pertaining to quality-of-life assessment

Term	Definition (reference)
Health	"Health is a state of complete physical, mental and social well-being and not merely the absence of disease or infirmity" [1]
Health state	The health state is the state of being. Examples are life without chronic disease, life with immobility, life with pain, and life without pain, but with impaired cognition
Health status	Health status refers to an individual's health at a particular point in time, in terms of one or more domains (e.g., physical function, mental health, social and role function, general health perceptions) [31, 70]
QOL	"[Quality of life] refers to the adequacy of material circumstances and to [an individual's] feelings about these circumstances," and "Health forms but one of many components in this broad concept." [3] "[An] individual's perception of their position in life in the context of the culture and value systems in which they live and in relation to their goals, expectations, standards and concerns" [2]
Health-related QOL	Health-related QOL includes the aspects of a person's life that are affected strongly by changes in health status and that are important to the individual [70]. Health-related QOL refers to people's subjective evaluations of the influences of their current health status, health care, and health promoting activities on their ability to achieve and maintain a level of overall functioning that allows them to pursue valued life goals and that is reflected in their general well-being [5]. Examples are physical health, mental health, social functioning, role functioning, and general health perceptions
Domains of QOL	In a QOL measure, a domain is a narrow and clearly defined focus of attention [70]. Measures designed to measure health-related QOL generally include physical, psychological/emotional, and social, but they may also include other domains, such as cognition, pain, spirituality, and overall well-being. Each domain may include multiple items
Item	A discrete question within the measure to assess QOL
Measure to assess QOL	
• Health status measure	A health status measure to assess QOL is sometimes called an instrument, questionnaire, scale, or survey to elicit patient-reported outcomes (e.g., information about symptoms or conditions that the patient says are present). Questionnaires or surveys usually consist of multiple items (questions)
• Direct elicitation	An approach that captures patient preferences (e.g., the patient's beliefs about or attitudes toward symptoms or conditions)
• Health state classification system	A questionnaire based on multiattribute utility theory that applies predetermined weights to patient responses and creates a final utility score that represents the value (preference) of the given health state from the perspective of the general public; also known as indirect utility elicitation
• Item response theory	A collection of modeling techniques for analyzing item-level data obtained to measure interindividual variation (e.g., in health status) [71]
Psychometric properties of measures to assess QOL	
• Validity	Validity is the extent to which an instrument measures what it is intended to [3, 4, 72]
• Reliability	Reliability is the consistency with which an instrument measures a domain or construct, [3, 4] the stability of an instrument over repeated measurement [72]
• Sensitivity	Sensitivity (responsiveness) is the ability of the instrument to detect important incremental changes in QOL [3, 4, 72]
Results of measures to assess QOL	
• Profile	In a profile, the results for each item have equal weight in the total score
• Index	In an index, the items for a particular domain are weighted and combined into a final numeric score for that domain
• Utility	A particular metric for valuing the (strength of) preference for a health state. Utilities generally range from 0 to 1, with 0 indicating the worst state and 1 indicating the best state. Utilities are numerical measures that denote the value or strength of preference for a particular state of being (such as a health state, either real or described)
• QALY	A quality-adjusted life-year (QALY) is an example of a QOL metric, using utilities in combination with quantity of life (longevity) to adjust (or weight) the time spent in a particular health state by the desirability of that health state. Only scores expressed as utilities can be used in cost–utility analysis

QOL quality of life

Table 22.2 Characteristics and examples of quality-of-life measures

Type of measure	Characteristics	Examples (reference)
Generic health status questionnaire	*Advantages*: These measures can be used for various populations (i.e., individuals with or without a specific disease and individuals with different types of diseases). Items are generally straightforward and easy to understand. *Disadvantages*: Items may be too broad and may be insensitive to relevant changes in QOL for patients with specific diseases. In many cases, scores for individual domains are kept separate, making it difficult to understand the net impact on QOL. Scores from health status questionnaires may be numeric, but they are not utility-based and cannot be used in cost–utility analysis	• Medical Outcomes Study (MOS) 36-Item Short Form Survey (SF-36) [32] • MOS SF-12 [33]

Disease-specific health status questionnaire	*Advantages*: These measures are sensitive to QOL changes that are important and relevant to a particular patient population. *Disadvantages*: The measures are not intended for other patient groups or for general populations so their results cannot be compared with QOL of people without the condition. However, several measures listed here (LDQOL, HQLQ) are based on the SF-36 plus other items, so these measures can, in fact, generate SF-36 QOL scores for comparison across conditions	• Questionnaires specific for HIV:
		  – MOS-HIV [36, 37]
		  – AIDS Health Assessment Questionnaire (AIDS-HAQ) [40]
		  – HIV/AIDS-Targeted Quality of Life (HAT-QOL) Questionnaire [41]
		• Questionnaires specific for liver disease:
		  – Liver Disease Quality of Life (LDQOL) Questionnaire [44]
		  – Hepatitis Quality of Life Questionnaire (HQLQ) [45]
		  – Chronic Liver Disease Questionnaire (CLDQ) [73]
		  – Chronic Liver Disease-Hepatitis C Virus (CLDQ-HCV) Questionnaire [74, 75]

Direct elicitation (preference-based)	*Advantages*: Standard gamble and time trade-off scores reflect an individual's preferences and do not use a predetermined or prescribed set of weights. Although the results often pertain to specific diseases, the utility values for a given health state (e.g., HIV) can be compared with utility values elicited for other conditions and can be used in cost–utility analysis. *Disadvantages*: Rating scales do not provide utilities and cannot be used to compute quality-adjusted life years. The standard gamble and time trade-off are time-consuming to administer and often difficult for patients to understand because they ask patients to take hypothetical risks or make hypothetical trade-offs vis-à-vis other health conditions	• Rating scale • Standard gamble [14] • Time trade-off [23]
Health state classification system (preference-based)	*Advantages*: These measures can be used for various populations. The items look simple and straightforward, and the results can be used in cost–utility analysis. *Disadvantages*: The domains addressed or items included in the instruments may not capture changes relevant to patients with specific diseases	• EuroQOL (EQ-5D) Questionnaire [18, 19] • MOS SF-6D [20, 21] • Quality of Well-Being Scale [22] • Health Utilities Index [23]

QOL quality of life

physical, psychological/emotional, and social domains, but they may also include other domains, such as role functioning, cognition, pain, fatigue, and overall well-being. Relevant domains for HIV-infected patients include sexual functioning, sexual behaviors, stigma, and spirituality [5, 6].

Health Status Measures

Health status measures are designed to elicit data and descriptive information about the past and current health status of individuals in the population being studied. They are designed to describe functioning in one or more domains of health. The results are generally expressed in terms of a profile (which yields separate scores for each domain) or an index (which combines items from across domains into a summary score of QOL).

The most frequently used instruments in QOL assessment are standardized questionnaires that have been developed and verified in ways that are consistent with principles of survey development or educational testing. The measure development process involves several steps. The first step entails defining the scope and objectives of the instrument (i.e., defining whether the instrument is intended to assess overall QOL or specific domains of QOL) and then compiling, testing, and refining a battery of items or questions to address the objectives. The next step entails evaluating and refining the instrument according to various psychometric standards. These include validity (the extent to which an instrument measures what it is intended to measure), reliability (the consistency with which it measures a domain or construct), and responsiveness or sensitivity (the ability of the instrument to detect important changes in QOL) [3, 4, 7, 8]. The final step involves providing guidelines for scoring a patient's responses and for interpreting the scores.

Generic vs. Disease-Specific Measures

QOL measures may be characterized in terms of whether they are generic or disease-specific. An advantage of generic measures is that they can assess health states for different groups of patients or different populations, allowing the results to be compared. A disadvantage of these measures is that they do not provide detailed information about condition-specific domains and therefore may not be able to detect changes in symptoms that matter most to patients with a particular condition. Disease-specific measures focus more narrowly on symptoms or attributes of a particular condition, such as HIV or liver disease. They are more sensitive to clinically relevant changes that matter to patients who have the particular condition but may not be germane to individuals in the general population or to patients with other conditions.

Preference-Based Measures

Preference-based measures, also known as health utilities or health values, are designed to find out how patients value particular actual or described health states. The results, thus, denote the value or strength of preference for a health state.

By convention, utilities are scaled between 0 and 1, with 0 indicating the worst state (usually, dead) and 1 indicating the best state (usually, full health or perfect health). Every other health state is an intermediate one, with a utility weight that lies somewhere in the [0, 1] interval (except that some measures allow for negative utilities representing states worse than dead). Utility weights can be used to compute quality-adjusted life-years (QALYs). QALYs are useful in that they combine measures of quantity and quality of life into a single metric by adjusting (or weighting) the time spent in a particular health state by the desirability of that health state. For example, spending 10 years in full health (utility = 1.0) would yield 10 QALYs, but spending 10 years in a compromised health state with a utility of 0.7 would yield only 7 QALYs.

There are several approaches for eliciting preferences, but two widely applied methods involve (1) direct assessment via rating scales, the standard gamble method, or the time trade-off method, and (2) indirect assessment via health state classification systems, in which utilities derived from the general public are mapped onto an individual's health state. (Other methods for eliciting preferences, including willingness to pay, conjoint analysis, and person-trade-offs, are described elsewhere [9–12].)

Rating Scale
Rating scales and similar metrics, such as the feeling thermometer and visual analog scale, ask patients to rate a particular health state, e.g., HIV, along a continuum between 0 (worst health state) and 100 (best health state). Although relatively easy to complete, such ratings do not represent true utilities because no trade-offs are involved, and therefore, raw rating scale scores theoretically cannot be used to compute QALYs [13]. When administered in combination with other preference-based measures as an introductory exercise, however, a rating scale may help patients to think in quantitative terms about the quality of health states.

Standard Gamble
The standard gamble is regarded as a true utility elicitation technique that assesses a patient's willingness to risk an immediate bad outcome (usually, death) for a chance to improve the quality of a given health state such as HIV (usually to perfect health). Patients must choose between two options, denoted as the sure thing (HIV) or the gamble. If they choose the "sure thing," then they agree to accept or remain in that current (or described) health state. Alternatively,

they can try to attain the best possible health state by choosing the "gamble," which represents an experimental or risky intervention (e.g., a pill or an operation) that will either successfully restore the patient to full health (with an assigned likelihood of p that can vary between 0 and 1) or cause immediate death (with an assigned probability of $1-p$). Patients are presented with the choice between the sure thing and the gamble over several iterations in which p is varied systematically, until eventually there is a value of p at which the patient cannot decide between the sure thing and the gamble. At this indifference point, the options are considered to be equivalent to the patient, and the magnitude of p is the patient's utility for the given health state.

Time Trade-Off

The time trade-off technique determines the amount of time (if any) by which patients are willing to reduce life expectancy order to improve a given health state [14]. For example, would a patient with HIV prefer a shorter but healthier life to living their remaining life expectancy in their current state of health? [15] Again, patients must choose between two options. One is to remain in the given health state, e.g., HIV, for some specified duration of time (X), usually their life expectancy, followed by death. The other is to live in the best possible health state for some shorter duration of time $(X-t)$, again followed by death. In contrast to the standard gamble, in the time trade-off, there is no risk of immediate death. Instead, death occurs with certainty at the end of the time horizon stated explicitly for both options. But, like the standard gamble, in the time trade-off, the exercise is repeated for different values of t as long as the patient expresses a strict preference between the two options. When the patient reaches the point of indifference, the options are considered to be valued equally and the patient's utility for the given health state is computed as the ratio $(X-t)/X$.

Health State Classification Systems

These indirect utility questionnaires are a hybrid between health status questionnaires and direct utility measures. As with the development of any validated questionnaire, health state classification systems [16] are the end product of substantial data collection efforts, in this case obtaining directly assessed utilities (e.g., standard gamble or time trade-off) for described health states in large groups of participants (community-based samples) and then using these data to estimate and validate quality-of-life weights for those health states [13, 17]. Once completed, health state classification systems can be administered in the same manner as health status questionnaires that ask patients to report their health and level of functioning across various domains. The weights are then mapped to patient responses and combined into a final utility score. The five-item EuroQOL (EQ-5D) questionnaire, [18, 19] Short Form 6D (SF-6D), [20, 21], Quality of Well-Being (QWB) scale [22], and Health Utilities Index systems (HUI2 and HUI3) [16, 23] are all examples of health state classification systems (Table 22.2). Weights for the EQ-5D derived from US samples are available [24, 25].

On the one hand, the health state classification systems questionnaires have several advantages. Their administration is straightforward. They do not require an understanding of probabilities and they do not involve subjecting patients to unfamiliar tasks or unusual experiments, such as trading years of life for perfect health. They can be used as a measure of QOL, even if economic evaluations (e.g., cost-effectiveness analyses) are not intended and utility calculations are not needed. On the contrary, health state classification systems are typically generic rather than disease-specific, so physicians need to consider whether the items included in them are appropriate to use for their targeted patient population. Also, because the questionnaires apply predetermined weights to patients' responses, they treat preferences as homogeneous across individuals. They cannot be used to discern individual differences in preferences or values for health states.

Item Response Theory and Computerized Adaptive Testing

A relatively recent approach to measuring health-related QOL is item response theory (IRT) and computerized adaptive testing (CAT) [26]. IRT draws from a large battery or database of items ("item banks") related to QOL (or domains of QOL). When combined with CAT, IRT provides for more efficient QOL assessment because the full battery of items related to QOL does not need to be administered. Instead, after a respondent completes an item, CAT chooses to administer the next most informative item, based on the individual's previous responses (think of it as "smart skip patterns"). The analogy in educational testing, where IRT originated, is to avoid having test-takers complete either too many easy questions to demonstrate their understanding or too many hard questions to confirm lack of understanding for a given concept; therefore, with each new response, CAT refines its assessment of the test-taker's performance and chooses the next most discriminating item to further refine the assessment. In the case of QOL, IRT is generally sufficiently flexible to administer to many patient groups/populations and also to assess QOL for many different severities of illness within the same diagnosis. In particular, Revicki and Cella [27] described the potential usefulness of IRT for assessing QOL across different stages of illness in patients with HIV. Among the disadvantages of IRT are the upfront costs of developing and validating extensive item banks for QOL domains [27].

Uses of Quality-of-Life Measures

Clinical Decision-Making

Although efforts in developing measures of QOL are largely motivated by research interests, [28] administering QOL measures to patients and assessing change in QOL over time also plays a role in clinical practice. Most commonly, utilities are incorporated into decision analyses comparing two or more diagnostic or therapeutic strategies (e.g., two different threshold CD4 counts for initiating highly active antiretroviral therapy), with the optimal option being the one that maximizes the number of QALYs. The specific questions asked to measure QOL for these purposes may also provide patients with the opportunity to thoughtfully evaluate their own priorities and clarify their preferences. Furthermore, the responses to the questions can help physicians understand their patients' perspectives and serve as "talking points" to improve physician–patient communication. With health status assessment, declines over time in functioning and other QOL domains might indicate a need to manage a patient's condition differently, and changes (whether improvement or deterioration) following an intervention would speak to the success of treatment. On a larger scale, trends in responses to QOL-related questions may help inform developing best practices for specific patient populations.

Economic Evaluation

Health utilities can be incorporated into economic evaluations to help inform decisions about health policy and resource allocation. In cost-effectiveness analysis (CEA), two or more treatments or courses of action are analyzed to assess which course would be the most advantageous and worth pursuing in terms of the resources expended relative to the benefits achieved [13]. For the analysis, direct medical costs and other relevant costs, such as costs of patient's time, are converted into monetary units, but benefits are defined differently from one analysis to the next depending on the most clinically relevant outcomes. For example, in the case of HIV, intervention benefits could be measured in terms of life-years gained, cases of HIV detected, or cases of HIV averted [29, 30]. Once defined and measured, the results are expressed as an incremental cost-effectiveness ratio (ICER). In comparing two treatments, A and B, the ICER is computed as follows:

$$\frac{Cost_A - Cost_B}{Effect_A - Effect_B}$$

where the numerator equals the additional costs of option A over B and the denominator equals the additional benefits.

Lesser ICERs indicate a lower additional cost per unit of benefit and are therefore more desirable than greater ICERs.

Cost–utility analysis (CUA) is a special case of CEA that uses the QALY (defined above) to assess effectiveness in the denominator of the ICER. Because QALYs are a common metric, their use allows analysts to make comparisons of different treatments for a particular condition and also to make comparisons across conditions [13, 31].

In the UK, formal economic evaluation contributes substantially to decision-making about health care. For example, the National Institute for Health and Clinical Excellence applies CUA to assess, recommend, and prioritize best care practices and to influence payment and coverage decisions by the National Health Service. In the USA, economic evaluation has been less influential in shaping health policy. Nevertheless, in the mid-1990s, the US Public Health Service's Panel on Cost-Effectiveness in Health and Medicine issued recommendations for performing economic analyses and recommended CUA as a key component of economic evaluations [31].

Assessment of Quality of Life in Patients with HIV Infection, Liver Disease, or Both

Examples of QOL Measures

Generic Health Status Measures
Several well-known generic health status measures were derived from the Medical Outcomes Study (MOS). These include two of the most common health status questionnaires, the MOS 36-item short form (SF-36) [32] and the 12-item SF-12 [33]. Both instruments address eight domains or subscales – physical function, role limitations due to physical health, role limitations due to emotional health, social functioning, mental health, pain, vitality, and general health – and compute two summary component scores: physical and mental.

Disease-Specific Health Status Measures
Although instruments can be developed de novo for a specific population of patients, generic measures are often modified or supplemented with additional items to assess the needs of specific groups; to wit, Shumaker and colleagues [5] recommend that QOL assessment for a particular patient population (e.g., those with HIV infection) incorporate generic components shared by other patient and community populations.

Several MOS measures have been modified to assess QOL in patients with HIV infection or liver disease. Regarding QOL in HIV, a series of interrelated measures can all be traced back to the SF-36. These include the AIDS Clinical Trials Group (ACTG) questionnaire, [34] the HIV Cost and Service Utilization Study (HCSUS) measures, [35] and the MOS-HIV developed by Wu and colleagues [36–38].

The most widely used instrument, the MOS-HIV, addresses ten domains (physical function, role function, pain, social function, emotional well-being, fatigue, cognitive function, general health, distress, and overall QOL). There are many other health status measures available for assessing QOL in HIV-infected individuals, [39], including the AIDS Health Assessment Questionnaire (AIDS-HAQ) [40] and the HIV/AIDS-Targeted Quality of Life (HAT-QOL) instrument [41]. Additional examples of both HIV-specific measures and generic measures as applied to HIV populations can be found in recent review articles [28, 42, 43].

Regarding liver disease and QOL, some measures have used the SF-36 as a basis and then added several items specifically targeting liver symptoms. Examples are the Liver Disease Quality of Life (LDQOL) measure for chronic liver disease [44] and the Hepatitis Quality of Life Questionnaire (HQLQ) for hepatitis C virus (HCV) infection [45]. Those two measures vary in terms of comprehensiveness/respondent burden: the LDQOL includes 75 additional items to address 12 disease-specific domains (symptoms, activities of daily living, concentration, memory, sexual functioning, sexual problems, sleep, loneliness, hopelessness, social interaction, health distress, and self-perceived stigma), whereas the HQLQ adds only four items related to both generic concerns (sleep and health distress) and condition-specific issues (HCV-related limitations and distress).

Although a large number of individuals are coinfected with HIV and HCV, a targeted QOL instrument has not been developed with this particular population in mind. Instead, QOL in coinfected individuals has been assessed with HIV-specific measures such as the HCSUS measures, [46] the HQLQ, [47] and the MOS-HIV [48]. Only the MOS-HIV has been validated for use in detecting QOL differences between HIV-infected individuals and HIV–HCV-coinfected individuals in terms of both the physical domains and mental domains of QOL [48].

Direct Utility Assessment

Direct assessment methods can be applied to any health state and have been widely used in HIV-related contexts. Direct elicitation methods (e.g., standard gamble and time trade-off) have been used extensively in HIV and HIV–HCV coinfection [49, 50] and in liver disease [51]. Additionally, Mrus and colleagues [52] demonstrated that rating scale scores could be transformed to standard gamble utilities reasonably well.

Health State Classification Systems

There are currently no health state classification measures specific to HIV-infected individuals, but a recent study found that the HUI3 and, to a lesser extent, the EQ-5D were responsive to changes in QOL among patients with advanced HIV and AIDS [53]. The QWB and SF-6D have also been used in patients with HIV [54, 55].

Results of Selected Quality of Life Studies

Quality of Life and HIV Infection

Many studies have assessed QOL in HIV. In one of the largest, as part of the HIV Cost and Services Utilization Study, researchers examined QOL data for a national sample of 2,864 HIV-positive adults at various stages of illness ranging from asymptomatic to AIDS [35]. They computed SF-36 summary measures of physical health and mental health and compared values to the general population and to other patient groups. There was substantial morbidity in the HIV population based primarily on symptoms, but there was also wide variation according to stage of illness. In terms of physical health for example, patients at the least severe stage (asymptomatic) compared favorably with the general population, while those at the most severe stage (AIDS) reported worse physical functioning than all other chronic illnesses considered. Mental health was similar across stage of illness for HIV-positive patients, but substantially worse than other conditions except mental illness.

Mrus and colleagues [56] examined patients from three large HIV studies and compared their self-assessment of overall health using two global rating scales and found QOL was related to measures of illness severity (e.g., CD4 count, salvage therapy) as well as age. They also found that patients enrolled in clinical trials tended to assign higher QOL ratings.

A growing body of research has shown that, perhaps contrary to expectation, self-reported QOL may actually *improve* over time for some HIV-positive patients after their diagnosis. In particular, patients with increased tangible support (e.g., assistance from family, regular medical care), improved emotional support (e.g., family reconciliation, spiritual/faith community), or improved health behaviors (e.g., discontinued drug use) after diagnosis might quite reasonably experience better QOL after diagnosis. Alternatively, patients may rate their QOL as better over time once they adapt to their diagnosis or new health state [15, 57].

Quality of Life and Liver Disease

In testing the Hepatitis Quality of Life Questionnaire (HQLQ), the health burden associated with HCV was substantial. Overall, patients with HCV scored lower than the general population for most domains; they had worse QOL scores than patients with hypertension, were comparable to patients with diabetes, and fared better than patients with depression [45].

More recently, a review of studies examining QOL in HCV patients published from January 2005 to March 2007 has reported that 20 of the 21 studies used the SF-36 [58]. Many studies used multiple measures, but no other measure was used by more than two studies. Groessl and colleagues [58] noted that a negative correlation between HCV infection and QOL in numerous domains is clear but that the cause is not. Questions remain about the roles that physiological mechanisms and psychological mechanisms (e.g., stigma) play in lowering the QOL scores.

Until recently, preference-based estimates of QOL for HCV-related health states have been lacking, except for proxy estimates from physicians. In the past decade, however, several groups of researchers have computed utilities for HCV health states using either direct elicitation methods or health state classification systems. In North America, Sherman and colleagues [59] administered a rating scale, followed by both SG and TTO, while Chong and colleagues [60] used visual analog scale, SG, HUI3, and EQ-5D. Björnsson et al. [61] performed a similar study in Sweden and Norway, administering the EQ-5D (which includes a visual analog scale) to HCV patients. All three of these studies administered some version of the SF-36 in addition to the preference-based measures, and all three studies stratified their utility estimates by severity or stage of illness. Consistently, the studies found that patient-reported values for HCV health states were worse than physician estimates. Still another approach for deriving preference-based estimates of QOL was reported by Thein and colleagues, [62] who conducted a systematic review of studies using the SF-36; in turn, they applied three different methods for "converting" the SF-36 scores into utility scores and compared the results. The comparison highlighted substantial variation in the utility estimates for the same level of illness, depending on the method used. In general, the simplest transformation by Shmueli produced the highest point estimates [63] relative to the other proposed methods based on the QWB and HUI2 [64, 65].

Quality of Life and Comorbid HIV Infection and Liver Disease

Although either HIV infection or liver disease can exacerbate QOL, it is not clear whether the combination of conditions worsens QOL beyond that associated with monoinfection and, if so, whether the effect on QOL is additive or multiplicative. Using the SF-36, Fleming and colleagues [47] studied the QOL of 299 individuals with HIV infection, HCV infection, or HIV–HCV coinfection in the USA and found that each of these three groups had a poorer QOL than did the general US population but that the three groups had similar scores for the eight subscales on the SF-36 and for the summary physical and mental component scores on the SF-36. When Kanwal and colleagues [46] studied the QOL of individuals with HIV infection, HI–HCV coinfection, and HIV–hepatitis B virus (HBV) coinfection by using the HCSUS measure, they found that physical and mental health scores were similar across the three groups at baseline and that, although all three groups experienced declines over a 2-year period, the changes were not statistically significant. And when Henderson and colleagues [48] studied the QOL of individuals with HIV-infection vs. comorbid HIV infection and liver disease by using the MOS-HIV, they found significantly less impairment in the physical functioning of the group with HIV monoinfection.

Mrus and others [66] used multiple approaches, including the SF-12, other health status measures, and direct utility assessment methods to compare QOL values among HIV-infected, HCV-infected, and coinfected groups. The study demonstrated that, as with other health states, the method of QOL assessment matters and is associated with wide variation in the resulting numeric values. In turn, covariates related to QOL values also varied according to the method of assessment, though symptoms and spirituality were consistent across methods. Importantly, coinfected patients appeared similar to those with monoinfection.

In Germany, Tillman and colleagues [67] used the EQ-5D and compared the QOL of individuals with HIV–hepatitis B virus (HBV) coinfection, HIV–HCV coinfection, and HIV–HBV–HCV coinfection. They found that HBV coinfection was not associated with worse QOL among HIV-infected patients; by contrast, HIV-infected patients who were coinfected with HCV exhibited worse QOL and more impairment. This finding was distinct from previously reported data regarding the impact of coinfection on survival outcomes, in which Rockstroh and coworkers [68] found that HBV infection was more harmful than HCV infection.

Summary

QOL is an important, patient-reported measure of wellbeing. Efforts to study and measure QOL are motivated by the realization that clinical outcomes alone (including survival) are often insufficient to differentiate among alternative treatments or to convey the full impact (be it benefit or harm) of a particular course of treatment. As McDowell aptly states in summarizing the relevance of QOL, "… patients want to live, not merely survive" [3].

As an end point in the treatment and management of patients with HIV and HCV infection, QOL is relatively recent and reflects interest in both patient-centered outcomes generally and clinical advances for treating these conditions specifically. Early and appropriate treatment of HIV and HCV infection can now add years to life expectancy, suggesting that attention and resources must also be devoted to improving and maximizing the quality associated with this survival benefit.

With numerous QOL measures in existence, no single QOL measure serves as a gold standard, suggesting that, in general, it is often useful to assess QOL using multiple measures – for example, a generic health status measure, a disease-specific health status measure, and a utility measure. The measures are complementary: direct or indirect utility measures allow for QALYs to be calculated and generic measures in general allow for QOL in HIV/liver disease to be compared in relation to other conditions; meanwhile, disease-specific measures can monitor changes in specific symptoms or concerns as part of the overall management of chronic conditions [69]. In some settings, this multiple-measure approach may not be practical due to patient burden, but advances in IRT and CAT could someday streamline this process.

References

1. World Health Organization. Preamble to the Constitution of the World Health Organization as adopted by the International Health Conference, New York, 19–22 June, 1946; signed on 22 July 1946 by the representatives of 61 States (Official Records of the World Health Organization, no. 2, p. 100) and entered into force on 7 April 1948. http://www.who.int/about/definition/en/print.html. Accessed 12 Apr 2010.
2. The WHOQOL Group. The World Health Organization Quality of Life assessment (WHOQOL): position paper from the World Health Organization. Soc Sci Med. 1995;41:1403–9.
3. McDowell I. Measuring health: a guide to rating scales and questionnaires. 3rd ed. New York: Oxford University Press; 2006.
4. Whalen GF, Ferrans CE. Quality of life as an outcome in clinical trials and cancer care: a primer for surgeons. J Surg Oncol. 2001;77:270–6.
5. Shumaker SA, Ellis S, Naughton M. Assessing health-related quality of life in HIV disease: key measurement issues. Qual Life Res. 1997;6:475–80.
6. Szaflarski M, Ritchey PN, Leonard AC, Mrus JM, Peterman AH, Ellison CG, et al. Modeling the effects of spirituality/religion on patients' perceptions of living with HIV/AIDS. J Gen Intern Med. 2006;21 suppl 5:S28–38.
7. Vetter TR. A primer on health-related quality of life in chronic pain medicine. Anesth Analg. 2007;104(3):703–18.
8. Eisen GM, Locke III GR, Provenzale D. Health-related quality of life: a primer for gastroenterologists. Am J Gastroenterol. 1999;94(8):2017–21.
9. O'Brien B, Gafni A. When do the 'dollars' make sense? Toward a conceptual framework for contingent valuation studies in health care. Med Decis Making. 1996;16:288–99.
10. Ryan M, Farrar M. Using conjoint analysis to elicit preferences for health care. BMJ. 2000;320:1530–3.
11. Beusterien KM, Dziekan K, Flood E, Harding G, Jordan JC. Understanding patient preferences for HIV medications using adaptive conjoint analysis: feasibility assessment. Value Health. 2005;8:453–61.
12. Nord E. The person-trade-off approach to valuing health care programs. Med Decis Making. 1995;15:201–8.
13. Drummond MF, Sculpher MJ, Torrance GW, O'Brien BJ, Stoddart GL. Methods for the economic evaluation of health care programmes. 3rd ed. New York: Oxford University Press; 2005.
14. Torrance GW. Social preference for health states. An empirical evaluation of three measurement techniques. Soc Econ Plan Sci. 1976;10:129–36.
15. Tsevat J, Sherman SN, McElwee JA, Mandell KL, Simbartl LA, Sonnenberg FA, et al. The will to live among HIV-infected patients. Ann Intern Med. 1999;131:194–8.
16. Feeny D, Furlong W, Boyle M, Torrance GW. Multi-attribute health status classification systems: health utilities index. Pharmacoeconomics. 1995;7:490–502.
17. Furlong W, Feeny D, Torrance GW, Goldsmith C, DePauw S, Boyle M, et al. Multiplicative multi-attribute utility function for the Health Utilities Index Mark 3 (HUI3) system: a technical report. 1998. McMaster University Centre for Health Economics and Policy Analysis Working Paper No. 98–11.
18. Group EQ. EuroQOL – a new facility for the measurement of health-related quality of life. Health Policy. 1990;16:199–208.
19. Kind P. The EuroQOL instrument: an index of health-related quality of life. In: Spilker B, editor. Quality of life and pharmacoeconomics in clinical trials. 2nd ed. Philadelphia: Lippincott-Raven; 1996.
20. Brazier J, Usherwood T, Harper R, Thomas K. Deriving a preference-based single index measure from the SF-36 health survey. J Clin Epidemiol. 1998;51:1115–28.
21. Brazier J, Roberts J, Deverill M. The estimation of a preference-based measure of health from the SF-26. J Health Econ. 2002;21:271–92.
22. Kaplan RM, Anderson JP. The general health policy model: an integrated approach. In: Spilker B, editor. Quality of life and pharmacoeconomics in clinical trials. 2nd ed. Philadelphia: Lippincott-Raven; 1996.
23. Torrance GW, Feeny DH, Furlong WJ, Barr RD, Zhang Y, Wang Q. Multiattribute utility function for a comprehensive health status classification system: health utilities index mark 2. Med Care. 1996;34:702–22.
24. Shaw JW, Johnson JA, Coons SJ. US valuation of the EQ-5D health states. Development and testing of the D1 valuation model. Med Care. 2005;43:203–20.
25. Rivero-Arias O, Ouellet M, Gray A, Wolstenholme J, Rothwell PM, Luengo-Fernandez R. Mapping the modified Rankin Scale (mRS) measurement into the generic EuroQol (ED-5D) health outcome. Med Decis Making. 2010;30:341–54.
26. Reeve BB, Hays RD, Bjorner JB, Cook KF, Crane PK, Teresi JA, et al. Psychometric evaluation and calibration of health-related quality of life item banks: plans for the Patient-Reported Outcomes Measurement Information System (PROMIS). Med Care. 2007;45(5 suppl 1):S22–31.
27. Revicki DA, Cella DF. Health status assessment for the twenty-first century: item response theory, item banking and computer adaptive testing. Qual Life Res. 1997;6:595–600.
28. Robinson FP. Measurement of quality of life in HIV disease. J Assoc Nurses AIDS Care. 2004;15(5 suppl):14S–9.
29. Galárraga O, Colchero MA, Wamai RG, Bertozzi SM. HIV prevention cost-effectiveness: a systematic review. BMC Public Health. 2009;18(9 suppl 1):S5.
30. Bayoumi AM, Zaric GS. The cost-effectiveness of Vancouver's supervised injection facility. Can Med Assoc J. 2008;179:1143–51.
31. Gold MR, Siegel JE, Russell LB, Weinstein MC, editors. Cost effectiveness in health and medicine. New York: Oxford University Press; 1996.
32. Ware Jr JE, Sherbourne CD. The MOS 36-item short-form health survey (SF-36). Med Care. 1992;30:473–83.
33. Ware Jr JE, Kosinski M, Keller SD. A 12-item short-form health survey: construction of scales and preliminary tests of reliability and validity. Med Care. 1996;34:220–3.
34. Wu A, The Quality of Life Subcommittee of the AIDS Clinical Trial Group (ACTG) Outcomes Committee. ACTG QOL 601–602 (QOL 601–2) Health Survey Manual, 1999. https://www.fstrf.org/apps/cfmx/apps/actg/html/QOLForms/manualql601-2799.pdf. Accessed 7 Jun 2010.
35. Hays RD, Cunningham WE, Cherbourne CD, Wilson IB, Wu AW, Cleary PD, et al. Health-related quality of life in patients with human immunodeficiency virus infection in the United States: results from the HIV Cost and Services Utilization Study. Am J Med. 2000;108:714–22.
36. Wu AW, Rubin HR, Mathews WC, Ware JE, Brysk LT, Hardy WD, et al. A health status questionnaire using 30 items from the medical outcomes study: preliminary validation in persons with early HIV infection. Med Care. 1991;29(8):786–98.

37. Wu AW, Hays RD, Kelly S, Malitz F, Bozzette SA. Applications of the medical outcomes study health-related quality of life measures in HIV/AIDS. Qual Life Res. 1997;6:531–54.
38. Wu AW, Revicki DA, Jacobson D, Malitz FF. Evidence for reliability, validity and usefulness of the Medical Outcomes Study HIV Health Survey (MOS-HIV). Qual Life Res. 1997;6:481–93.
39. Mapi Research Trust. Patient-Reported Outcome and Quality of Life Instruments Database (ProQolid). http://www.mapi-trust.org/ressources/inhouseandexternaldatabases. Accessed 02 Jul 2010.
40. Lubeck DP, Fries JF. Assessment of quality of life in early stage HIV-infected persons: data from the AIDS Time-oriented Health Outcome Study (ATHOS). Qual Life Res. 1997;6:494–506.
41. Holmes WC, Shea JA. A new HIV/AIDS-targeted quality of life (HAT-QoL) instrument: development, reliability, and validity. Med Care. 1998;36:138–54.
42. Clayson DJ, Wild DJ, Quarterman P, Duprat-Lomon I, Kubin M, Coons SJ. A comparative review of health-related quality-of-life measures for use in HIV/AIDS clinical trials. Pharmacoeconomics. 2006;24:751–65.
43. Garvie PA, Lawford J, Banet MS, West RL. Quality of life measurement in paediatric and adolescent populations with HIV: a review of the literature. Child Care Health Dev. 2009;25:440–53.
44. Gralnek IM, Hays RD, Kilbourne A, Rosen HR, Keeffe EB, Artinian L, et al. Development and evaluation of the liver disease quality of life instrument in persons with advanced, chronic liver disease – the LDQOL 1.0. Am J Gastroenterol. 2000;95:3552–65.
45. Ware Jr JE, Bayliss MS, Mannocchia M, Davis GL, and the International Hepatitis Interventional Therapy Group. Health-related quality of life in chronic hepatitis C: impact of disease and treatment response. Hepatology. 1999;30:550–5.
46. Kanwal F, Gralnek IM, Hays RD, Dulai GS, Brennan MR, Spiegel BMR, et al. Impact of chronic viral hepatitis on health-related quality of life in HIV: results from a nationally representative sample. Am J Gastroenterol. 2005;100:1984–94.
47. Fleming CA, Christiansen D, Nunes D, Heeren T, Thornton D, Horsburgh Jr CR, et al. Health-related quality of life of patients with HIV disease: impact of hepatitis C coinfection. Clin Infect Dis. 2004;38:572–8.
48. Henderson WA, Schlenk EA, Kim KH, Hadigan CM, Martino AC, Sereika SM, et al. Validation of the MOS-HIV as a measure of health-related quality of life in persons living with HIV and liver disease. AIDS Care. 2010;22(4):483–90. doi:10.1080/09540120903207292. http://dx.doi.org/10.1080/09540120903207292.
49. Tengs TO, Lin TH. A meta-analysis of utility estimates for HIV/AIDS. Med Decis Making. 2002;22:475–81.
50. Bult JR, Hunink MGM, Tsevat J, Weinstein MC. Heterogeneity in the relationship between the time tradeoff and Short Form-36 for HIV-infected and primary care patients. Med Care. 1998;36:523–32.
51. Bryce CL, Angus DC, Switala J, Roberts MS, Tsevat J. Health status vs. utilities of patients with end-stage liver disease. Qual Life Res. 2004;13:773–82.
52. Mrus JM, Yi MS, Freedberg KA, Wu AW, Zackin R, Gorski H, et al. Utilities derived from visual analog scale scores in patients with HIV/AIDS. Med Decis Making. 2003;23:414–21.
53. Nosyk B, Sun H, Bansback N, Guh DP, Barnett P, Bayoumi A, et al. The concurrent validity and responsiveness of the health utilities index (HUI 3) among patients with advanced HIV/AIDS. Qual Life Res. 2009;18:815–24.
54. Anderson JP, Kaplan RM, Coons SJ, Schneiderman LJ. Comparison of the Quality of Well-being Scale and the SF-36 results among two samples of ill adults: AIDS and other illnesses. J Clin Epidemiol. 1998;51:755–62.
55. Braithwaite RS, Goulet J, Kudel I, Tsevat J, Justice AC. Quantifying the decrement in utility from perceived side effects of combination antiretroviral therapies in patients with HIV. Value Health. 2008;11:975–9.
56. Mrus JM, Schackman BR, Wu AW, Freedberg KA, Tsevat J, Yi MS, et al. Variations in self-rated health among patients with HIV infection. Qual Life Res. 2006;15:503–14.
57. Tsevat J, Leonard AC, Szaflarski M, Sherman SN, Cotton S, Mrus JM, et al. Change in quality of life after being diagnosed with HIV: a multicenter longitudinal study. AIDS Patient Care STDS. 2009;23:931–7.
58. Groessl EJ, Weingart KR, Kaplan RM, Ho SB. Health-related quality of life in HCV-infected patients. Curr Hepat Rep. 2007;6:169–75.
59. Sherman KE, Sherman SN, Chenier T, Tsevat J. Health values of patients with chronic hepatitis C infection. Arch Intern Med. 2004;164:2377–82.
60. Chong CA, Gulamhussein A, Heathcote EJ, Lilly L, Sherman M, Naglie G, et al. Health-state utilities and quality of life in hepatitis C patients. Am J Gastroenterol. 2003;98:630–8.
61. Björnsson E, Verbaan H, Oksanen A, Frydén A, Johansson J, Friberg S, et al. Health-related quality of life in patients with different stages of liver disease induced by hepatitis C. Scand J Gastroenterol. 2009;44:878–87.
62. Thein HH, Krahn M, Kaldor JM, Dore GJ. Estimation of utilities for chronic hepatitis C from SF-36 scores. Am J Gastroenterol. 2005;100:643–51.
63. Shmueli A. The SF-36 profile and health-related quality of life: an interpretative analysis. Qual Life Res. 1998;7:187–95.
64. Fryback DG, Lawrence WF, Martin PA, Klein R, Klein BE. Predicting quality of well-being scores from the SF-36: results from the beaver Dam health outcomes study. Med Decis Making. 1997;17:1–9.
65. Nichol MB, Sengupta N, Globe DR. Evaluating quality-adjusted life years: estimation of the health utility index (HUI2) from the SF-36. Med Decis Making. 2001;21:105–12.
66. Mrus JM, Sherman KE, Leonard AC, Sherman SN, Mandell KL, Tsevat J. Health values of patients coinfected with HIV/Hepatitis C: are two viruses worse than one? Med Care. 2006;44:158–66.
67. Tillmann HL, Kaiser T, Claes C, Schmidt RE, Manns MP, Stoll M. Differential influence of different hepatitis viruses on quality of life in HIV positive patients. Eur J Med Res. 2006;11:381–5.
68. Rockstroh JK, Mocroft A, Soriano V, Tural C, EuroSIDA Study Group. Hepatitis B and hepatitis C in the EuroSIDA cohort: influence of hepatitis C virus infection on HIV-1 disease progression and response to highly active antiretroviral therapy. J Infect Dis. 2005;192:992–1002.
69. Nader CM, Tsevat J, Justice AC, Mrus JM, Levin F, Kozal MJ, et al. Development of an electronic medical record-based clinical decision support tool to improve HIV symptom management. AIDS Patient Care STDS. 2009;23:521–9.
70. Tully MP, Cantrill JA. Subjective outcome measurement – a primer. Pharm World Sci. 1999;21(3):101–9.
71. Edelen MO, Reeve BB. Applying item response theory (IRT) modeling to questionnaire development, evaluation, and refinement. Qual Life Res. 2007;16:5–18.
72. Hays RD, Anderson R, Revicki D. Psychometric considerations in evaluating health-related quality to life measures. Qual Life Res. 1993;2:441–9.
73. Younossi ZM, Guyatt G, Kiwi M, Boparai N, King D. Development of a disease specific questionnaire to measure health related quality of life in patients with chronic liver disease. Gut. 1999;45:295–300.
74. Two R, Verjee-Lorenz A, Clayson D, Dalal M, Grotzinger K, Younossi ZM. A methodology for successfully producing global translations of patient reported outcome measures for use in multiple countries. Value Health. 2010;13:128–31.
75. The Chronic Liver Disease Questionnaire-HCV (CLDQ-HCV). http://www.ispor.org/publications/value/vihsupplementary/vih13i1_two.asp. Accessed 14 May 2010.

Index

A
a/b T cells, 55
Acute HCV infection
 natural history, 101
 serologies, 153
 treatment, 137–138
Acute hepatitis B virus infection
 clinical features, 116
 incidence of, 158
 natural history of, 107
 serologies, 153
Addiction, alcohol, 182
Addiction Severity Index (ASI), 182
Adefovir dipivoxil, 129, 143
Adenosine monophosphate-dependent protein kinase (AMPK), 48
Adenovirus hepatitis, 25
Adiponectin, 48–49
Alanine aminotransferase (ALT)
 HCV–HIV coinfection, ethnic difference, 190
 hepatotoxicity, 164
Alcoholic liver disease (ALD)
 gut–liver axis, 49–50
 hepatic lipid metabolism
  de novo lipogenesis, 45–46
  fatty acid oxidation, 46
  fatty acid uptake, 46–47
  VLDL secretion, 46
 mechanisms
  adiponectin, 48–49
  AMPK, 48
  oxidative stress, 49
  zinc deficiency, 49
 therapy, 50–51
 transcription factors
  HNF-4a, 47–48
  PPAR-a, 47
  SREBPs, 48
Alcoholic steatosis. See Alcoholic liver disease (ALD)
Alcohol-use disorders
 assessment of patients, 182–184
 definitions, 181–182
 motivated behavior concept, 184–185
 pharmacologic interventions, 187–188
 treatment, 185–187
AMPK. See Adenosine monophosphate-dependent protein kinase (AMPK)

Antiretroviral therapy. See Hepatotoxicity
Apolipoprotein B mRNA-editing enzyme, catalytic polypeptide-like 3G (APOBEC3G), 70
APRI. See AST to platelet ratiop index (APRI)
Aspartate aminotransferase (AST), 164
AST to platelet ratiop index (APRI), 35

B
Bacillary angiomatosis, 26
Bacterial cholangitis. See Cholangitis
B cells
 cell types, liver structure, 57
 in HBV vaccination, 156
Beta-defensin-1 (DEFB1), 71
Bile duct injury
 cholangitis, 28
 liver biopsy, 23
Biliary epithelial cells, 55

C
Candida infections, 26
CC-chemokine receptor 5 (CCR5) gene, 68
CCR5. See CC-chemokine receptor 5 (CCR5) gene
CDC. See Centers for Disease Control (CDC)
Centers for Disease Control (CDC), 1, 2
Child–Turcotte–Pugh (CTP) score, 39
Cholangitis, 28
Chronic HCV infection
 Amsterdam Cohort study, 102
 APRI, 35
 cytokine response, 86
 DAD study, 102
 end-stage liver disease (ESLD), 101
 FDA-approved therapy, 18
 genome wide association studies (GWAS), 61
 hepatic fibrosis, 33
 HIV/HCV coinfection, 102, 103
 IL28B, 72
 parenteral transmission, 152
 serologies, 153
 TNF-a, 73
 treatment of, 133

Chronic hepatitis B virus infection
    ART, 110
    ethnic differences, 192
    HDV infection, 115
    HIV-positive men, 24
    isolated anti-HBc pattern, 109
    laboratory testing, 152
    lamivudine, 129
    natural history of, 108
    prevalence of, 10
Chronic viral hepatitis, in HIV-infected patients, 23
Clinical decision-making, 200
Coccidioides infections, 27
Combination antiretroviral therapy (CART)
    HIV/AIDS, 15
    limitation, 17
    liver disease, 9–10
Combination therapy, HBV infection, 144–145
Computerized adaptive testing (CAT), 199
Cost–utility analysis (CUA), 200
Cryptococcus infections, 26–27
CTLA4, 74
Cytomegalovirus infection, 25

D
DAD study. *See* Data Collection on adverse events of anti-HIV drugs (DAD) study
DARC. *See* Duffy antigen receptor for chemokines (DARC)
Data collection on adverse events of anti-HIV drugs (DAD) study, 102
DC-SIGN (CD209), 71
DEFB1. *See* Beta-defensin-1 (DEFB1)
De novo lipogenesis, 45–46
Department of health and human services (DHHS) guidelines, 15
Direct-acting antiviral agents (DAAs), 18
Direct hepatotoxicity, 164
Drug Abuse Screening Tool (DAST), 182, 183
Drug hypersensitivity, 71
Drug-induced liver injury (DILI)
    FDA evaluation guidance, 163
    incidence rates comparison, 19
Duffy antigen receptor for chemokines (DARC), 68–69

E
Early HIV-1 gene, 92–93
Early virologic response rate (EVR), 191
Economic evaluations, 200
Emtricitabine, 142–143
End-stage liver disease (ESLD)
    coinfected patients, mortality rate, 33
    liver transplantation, management
        HAART, 177
        HBV and HCV coinfection, 177
        immunosuppression, 175–177
        malignancy screening, 177–178
    management
        ascites, 173
        cirrhosis, 171
        decompensated cirrhosis, 171–173
        esophagogastric varices, 173–174
        Hepatic encephalopathy, 174–175
        HRS, 174
        SBP, 173
    mortality, 17
Entecavir, 129, 143–144
env gene, 91

Epidemiology
    alcohol use, 10
    combination antiretroviral therapy, 9–10
    HAV, 113–114
    HCV coinfection, 10
    HDV, 115–116
    HEV, 119–120
    noninfectious complications, 10–11
Epstein–Barr virus (EBV) infection, 25
Ethnic categories, 189

F
Fas induced apoptosis, 60
Fatty acid oxidation, 46
Fatty acid uptake, 46–47
FIB-4 index, 36
Fibrosing cholestatic hepatitis, 108
Forns index, 35–36

G
g/d T cells, 57
gp120, 82
Granulomas, 23
Granulomatous hepatitis, 23

H
HAART. *See* Highly active antiretroviral therapy (HAART)
HAV. *See* Hepatitis A virus (HAV)
HBV. *See* Hepatitis B Virus (HBV)
HBV–HIV coinfection, ethnic disparity, 192
HBV X protein (HBx), 128
HCV. *See* Hepatitis C virus (HCV)
HCV genotype 1, 74
HCV–HIV coinfection
    ethnic disparity, 190–192
    prevalence of, 10
HDV. *See* Hepatitis D virus (HDV)
Health, definition of, 195
Hepatic dendritic cells, 57
Hepatic fibrosis assessment, coinfected populations
    biomarkers role, 35
    liver biopsy, 33
    noninvasive assessment models
        biochemical tests, 34–37
        comparative studies, 38
        imaging methods, 37–38
Hepatic steatosis, 11
Hepatic stellate cells (HSCs)
    Fas receptors, 60
    HIV effects, 84
    liver immunopathogenesis, 55
Hepatitis A virus (HAV)
    clinical manifestations, 114
    epidemiology, 113–114
    prevention, 114–115, 151
    virology, 113
Hepatitis B e antigen (HBeAg), 141
Hepatitis B surface antigen (HBsAg), 141
Hepatitis B virus (HBV)
    evolution
        genotypic variability, 130
        mechanisms, 130
        Occult HBV infection, 131
        phenotypic variability, 131

infection
  acute, 107
  ART, 110
  chronic, 108
  HCC, 109–110
  HIV-coinfected patients, 24, 145–147
  isolated anti-HBc serological pattern, 109
  prevention, 151–152
  seroreversion, 108–109
  treatment, 141–145
mutation
  drug resistance, 129
  multidrug resistance, 129–130
  vs. retroviral genes, 128–129
prevention, 151
replication cycle
  (−)DNA strand synthesis, 127
  (+)DNA synthesis, 127–128
  overlapping reading frames, genome, 125–126
  protein X, 128
  release of virions, 127
  reverse transcription, 126–127
  step-wise process of, 125
  transcription, 126
  virion entry, 126
Hepatitis C virus (HCV) infection
  acute, 101
  chronic
    Amsterdam Cohort study, 102
    DAD study, 102
    end-stage liver disease (ESLD), 101
    risk ratios, HIV/HCV coinfection, 102, 103
  clearance, frequency of, 101
  frequency of, 102
  HIV-coinfected patients, 24–25
  HIV effects, 104
  prevention, 152
  treatment
    acute HCV, 137
    adverse effects, 135–136
    direct acting antiviral agents (DAAs), 136
    drug interactions, 136
    initiation, treatment, 133
    non-responders/relapsers, 137
    pegylated-interferon-alpha (IFN), 134
    PNALT, 133
    response predictors, 136
    treatment, 134–135
    viral kinetics, 135
Hepatitis D virus (HDV)
  clinical manifestations, 116
  diagnosis, 116–117
  epidemiology, 115–116
  treatment, 117–118
  virology, 115
Hepatitis E virus (HEV)
  clinical manifestations, 120
  diagnosis, 120
  epidemiology, 119–120
  treatment, 121
  virology, 119
Hepatitis infection prevention
  behavioural interventions, 153
  HAV, 151
  HBV, 151–152
  HCV, 152
  issues, HBV core positivity, 156–157
  laboratory testing, 152–153
  needle exchange programs (NEP), 154
  opioid replacement therapy, 154
  substance abuse treatment, 153–154
  vaccination
    HAV, 155
    HBV, 155–156
    perceptions, 157–158
Hepatitis Quality of Life Questionnaire (HQLQ), 201
Hepatocellular carcinoma (HCC)
  epidemiology of, 11
  ethnic disparity, 192–193
  HBV infection, natural history, 109–110
  liver tumors, 27
Hepatocytes
  cell types, liver structure, 55
  HIV effects, 82–84
Hepatomegaly, 23
Hepatorenal syndrome (HRS), 174
Hepatotoxicity
  ALT/AST elevations, 164
  definition, 163–164
  incidence, 166
  mechanisms
    direct hepatotoxicity, 164
    hyperbilirubinemia, 166
    hypersensitivity reactions, 164–165
    immune reconstitution, 165
    mitochondrial toxicity, 164
    steatohepatitis, 165
  predictors and risk factors, 167
Herpes simplex virus infection, 25
HEV. See Hepatitis E virus (HEV)
Highly active antiretroviral therapy (HAART)
  morbidity and mortality, 4–5
  opportunistic infections, 23
Histoplasma infections, 27
HIV-associated biliary disease. See Cholangitis
HIV-associated liver disease
  bacterial infections, 25–26
  cholangitis, 28
  drug toxicity, 28
  fungal infections, 26–27
  general features of, 23
  HAART, 23
  hepatocellular carcinomas, 27
  Kaposi's sarcoma, 27
  lymphoma, 27–28
  protozoal infections, 27
  viral hepatitis, 24–25
HIV-associated sclerosing cholangitis. See Cholangitis
HIV care providers, challenges for, 151
HIV Cost and Services Utilization Study, 201
HIV-1 dependency factors (TSG101 and PPIA), 69
HIV epidemics, USA
  active combination antiretroviral therapy, 2–3
  AIDS diagnosis, 2–3
  CDC estimation, 1
  incidence rate, 2
  late diagnoses, 3–4
  morbidity and mortality
    HAART, 4–5
    non-AIDS defining illnesses, 5
  non morbidity and mortality, 5–6
  prevalence rates, 1
  race/gender differences, 1–2
  routine testing, 4

HIV–1 integrase (IN), 96
HIV Medicine Association (HIVMA), 152
HIV replication
  assembly, 97
  encoded genes, 91–93
  integration, 96
  maturation, 97–98
  process steps, 91
  reverse transcription, 94–96
  transcription, 96–97
  viral fusion, 94
HIV treatment guidelines, 15–19
HLA. See Human leukocyte antigen (HLA) system
Hospital Gregorio Marañón (HGM) indices, 36
Host gene polymorphisms
  HCV–HIV coinfection
    CTLA4 and KIR, 74
    HLA system, 73–74
    IFN-g, 73
    interferon-inducible MxA protein, 74
    interleukin, 72–73
    TGF-b and TNF-a, 73
  HIV–1 disease
    DARC, 68–69
    DC-SIGN (CD209), 71
    DEFB1, 71
    HIV–1 dependency factors, 69
    HLA and drug hypersensitivity, 70–71
    intrinsic antiretroviral factors, 69–70
  HIV–HBV coinfection, 74
HRS. See Hepatorenal syndrome (HRS)
Human leukocyte antigen (HLA) system, 73–74
Hyperbilirubinemia, 166
Hypersensitivity reactions, 164–165

I
IFN-a, 141–142
IFN-g, 73
IL–6, 72
IL–10, 73
IL–12, 73
IL–28B, 72
Immune reconstitution, 165
Immunopathogenesis, liver injury
  apoptosis
    Fas receptors, 60
    TNF, 60–61
    TNF-a, 60
  cell types, 55
  HCV infection, 61
  HIV infection, 62
  immune responses
    Ag-specific responses, 58
    innate responses, 57
  tolerance, 58
Incremental cost-effectiveness ratio (ICER), 200
Inflammatory syndrome. See Immune reconstitution
Interferon-inducible MxA protein, 74
Interferon therapy
  HBV infection, 141–142
  HCV–HIV coinfection, racial disparity, 191
Intrinsic antiretroviral factors, 69–70
Isolated anti-HBc serological pattern, 109
Item response theory (IRT), 199
36-Item Short Form Survey (SF-36), 197, 200

K
Kaposi's sarcoma, 27
Killer cell immunoglobulin-like receptors (KIR)
  HCV–HIV coinfection, 74
  HIV–1 disease, 71
Kupffer cells
  HIV effects, 85–86
  liver immunopathogenesis, 57

L
Lamivudine, 129, 142
Late HIV–1 gene, 93
Leishmaniasis, 27
Liver cell populations, HIV effects
  blood supply, 81
  cytokine dysregulation, 86–87
  HBV infection, 87–88
  HCV infection, 87–88
  hepatic stellate cells, 84
  hepatocytes, 82–84
  Kupffer cells, 85–86
  liver sinusoidal endothelial cells, 85
  microbial translocation, 87
  viral antigens, 81
Liver cirrhosis, 9
Liver Disease Quality of Life (LDQOL) measure, 201
Liver sinusoidal endothelial cells
  HIV effects, 85
  liver immunopathogenesis, 57
Liver transplantation
  candidacy for, 175, 176
  ethnic disparity, 193
  HCV, 152
Lymphocytes, 55
Lymphoma, 27–28

M
Macrovesicular steatosis, 23
Magnetic resonance elastography (MRE), 37
Major Histocompatibility Complex (MHC), 70–71
Mannose-binding lectin (MBL), 72
MBL. See Mannose-binding lectin (MBL)
Medical Outcomes Study (MOS), 200
MHC. See Major Histocompatibility Complex (MHC)
Mitochondrial toxicity, 164
Model for End-Stage Liver Disease (MELD) score, 39
Motivated behavior model, 185
MRE. See Magnetic resonance elastography (MRE)
Mycobacterium avium complex infection, 26
Mycobacterium tuberculosis infection, 25–26

N
Natural killer cells, 57
Needle exchange programs (NEP), 154
Negative factor (*Nef*) gene, 92
NEP. See Needle exchange programs (NEP)
NKT cells, 57
Nodular regenerative hyperplasia, 11
Nonalcoholic fatty liver disease (NAFLD)
  epidemiology, 10–11
  ethnic disparity, 190
  hepatic steatosis, 165

Noninvasive fibrosis assessment
  algorithm for, 42
  biochemical tests
    nonroutine tests, 36–37
    routine laboratory tests, 34–36
  comparative studies, 38
  imaging methods
    SPECT, 37–38
    TE and MRE, 37
  liver stiffness measurements (LSM), 39
Nonnucleoside reverse transcriptase inhibitor (NNRTI), 15
Nuclear factor kappa B (NF-kB), 96
Nucleoside analog inhibitors, 142–144
Nucleoside reverse transcriptase inhibitor (NRTI), 15

O
OAT. *See* Opioid agonist therapy (OAT)
Opioid agonist therapy (OAT), 154
Opioid replacement therapy, 154
Opportunistic infections, 10
Oxidative stress, 49

P
Pegylated-interferon alpha (PegIFN), 134. *See also* IFN-a
Persistently normal alanine aminotransferase (PNALT), 133
Pneumocystis pneumonia, 27
pol gene, 91
Portal granuloma, 24
Preference-sensitive care, 195

Q
Q fever, 26
Quality-adjusted life-years (QALYs), 198
Quality-of-life (QOL) measures
  assessment, 200–201
  characteristics, 195, 197–199
  coinfection, 202
  concepts, 196
  considerations, 195
  definition of, 195
  domains, 195, 198
  generic *vs.* disease-specific measures, 198
  HCV-related health states, 201–202
  health state classification systems, 199
  health status measures, 198
  HIV Cost and Services Utilization Study, 201
  preference-based measures, 198
  rating scales, 198
  time trade-off technique, 199
  uses
    clinical decision-making, 200
    economic evaluations, 200

R
Racial categories, 189
Ribavirin (RBV), 134

S
SBP. *See* Spontaneous bacterial peritonitis (SBP)
Seroreversion, 108–109
SHASTA index, 36
Single photon emission computed tomography (SPECT), 37–38
SPECT. *See* Single photon emission computed tomography (SPECT)
Spontaneous bacterial peritonitis (SBP), 173
Standard gamble technique, 198–199
Steatohepatitis, 165. *See also* Alcoholic liver disease (ALD)
Stellate cells, 55
Strategic timing of ART (START), 16
Substance abuse, 182
Substance dependence, 182
Substance misuse, 181
Substance-use disorders. *See* Alcohol-use disorders
Suppressor of cytokine signaling 3 (SOCS3), 192
Sustained virologic response (SVR), 133

T
Tat gene, 91, 93
TE. *See* Transient elastography (TE)
Telbivudine, 129, 144
Tenofavir disoproxil fumarate, 143
Tenofovir, 129
TGF-b. *See* Transforming growth factor (TGF-b)
Time trade-off technique, 199
TLR. *See* Toll-like receptor (TLR)
TNF-a. *See* Tumor necrosis factor (TNF-a)
TNF related apoptosis, 60–61
Toll-like receptor (TLR), 72
Toxoplasmosis, 27
Transforming growth factor (TGF-b), 73
Transient elastography (TE), 37
Treatment
  Hepatitis B virus (HBV) infection
    combination therapy, 144–145
    interferon therapy, 141–142
    nucleoside analog inhibitors, 142–144
  Hepatitis D virus (HDV), 117–118
  Hepatitis E virus (HEV), 121
TRIM5a. *See* Tripartite interaction motif 5a (TRIM5a)
Tripartite interaction motif 5a (TRIM5a), 70
Tumor necrosis factor (TNF-a)
  apoptosis, 60
  HCV–HIV coinfection, 73

V
Varicella zoster virus infection, 25
Very low density lipoproteins (VLDL) Secretion, 46
Viral infectivity factor (*Vif*) gene, 92
Viral protein R (*Vpr*) gene, 92
Viral protein U (*Vpu*) gene, 92
VLDL. *See* Very low density lipoproteins (VLDL) secretion

Z
Zinc deficiency, 49